MEDICAL RADIOLOGY

Diagnostic Imaging

Editors:
A. L. Baert, Leuven
M. Knauth, Göttingen
K. Sartor, Heidelberg

S. Grampp (Ed.)

Radiology of Osteoporosis

2nd Revised Edition

With Contributions by

J. E. Adams · R. Barkmann · P. M. Bernecker · D. Diacinti · K. Engelke · H. K. Genant
S. Grampp · R. Gruber · G. Guglielmi · G. Holzer · H. Imhof · M. Jergas · C. Krestan
T. M. Link · M. Peterlik · P. Pietschmann · S. Prevrhal · H. Resch · C. van Kuijk
R. R. van Rijn

Foreword by

A. L. Baert

With 169 Figures in 225 Separate Illustrations, 15 in Color and 17 Tables

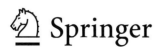 Springer

STEPHAN GRAMPP, MD
Univ. Dozent
Dr. Grampp & Dr. Henk OEG
Röntgenordination
Lenaustrasse 23
2000 Stockerau
Austria

MEDICAL RADIOLOGY · Diagnostic Imaging and Radiation Oncology
Series Editors:
A. L. Baert · L. W. Brady · H.-P. Heilmann · M. Knauth · M. Molls · C. Nieder · K. Sartor

Continuation of Handbuch der medizinischen Radiologie
            Encyclopedia of Medical Radiology

ISBN 978-3-540-25888-9   e-ISBN 978-3-540-68604-0

DOI 10.007/b 136255

Medical Radiology · Diagnostic Imaging and Radiation Oncology ISSN 0942-5373

Library of Congress Control Number: 2005934451

© 2008 Springer-Verlag Berlin Heidelberg

Cover design and Typesetting: Verlagsservice Teichmann, Mauer

Printed on acid-free paper

9 8 7 6 5 4 3 2 1

springer.com

Foreword

It is a great pleasure to introduce this second fully revised and updated edition of *Radiology of Osteoporosis*.

The need for the publication of this second edition, only 4 years following the first edition, indicates the great interest among radiologists, and several other medical disciplines, in the diagnosis and management of this very common condition and its possible complications.

One of the great merits of this book is that it deals with all aspects of osteoporosis, including morphology and function.

The outstanding qualifications and high level of expertise of the editor, Prof. S. Grampp, and of the contributing authors are a guarantee for the up-to-date and comprehensive contents of this outstanding volume.

I am confident that this volume will again meet with great interest among radiologists and all other clinicians involved in the care of patients with osteoporosis and that it will enjoy the same success as the first edition.

Leuven   ALBERT L. BAERT

Preface

There is almost universal agreement among the clinical community that the measurement of bone mineral density in potentially healthy individuals is the only means of assessing fracture risk and skeletal status. In patients with risk factors, measurement of BMD adds substantially to the assessment of fracture risk. For each of the methods and related skeletal sites, there is a wealth of scientific data emphasising the relationship between decreasing bone density and mass on the one hand and increasing fracture risk on the other.

Indeed, all measurement techniques presented here are able to provide valuable information in most clinical circumstances, as well as information that cannot be obtained by other means.

Selection of any of the available methods for clinical practice can be governed by practical considerations such as availability, cost and reimbursement, time and effort involved, as well as patient acceptance.

We wrote this book to guide the clinical practitioner through this minefield of scientific knowledge and it is our sincere hope that it will assist in daily practice.

Due to the success of the first edition, we decided to update and upgrade this volume to the very latest clinical and scientific knowledge. (Since the first edition sold so rapidly, we are confident of continued success. We do not expect the same sort of popular movement to the bookstores as historically seen in the Nika insurrection of 532 [Byzantium], the Harry Potter craze [Europe, beginning of the millennium], or the Cavalli Fashion Massacre [Central Europe 2007 – if you do not know about this and are not female, ask someone who is]. But still an editor can hope.)

I am especially grateful to the authors who are amongst the most prominent and knowledgeable in this particular scientific field for their effort and dedication.

Stockerau   STEPHAN GRAMPP

Contents

Introduction to Bone Development, Remodelling and Repair

REINHARD GRUBER, PETER PIETSCHMANN, and MEINRAD PETERLIK

CONTENTS

1.1 Introduction

Bone is a specialized form of mineralized connective tissue that is build by various types of metabolically active cells during embryonic and postnatal development. In the adult, the same cells contribute to the maintenance of structural and functional integrity, and accomplish the healing process following injury. Bone not only shows a marked rigidity and mechanical stability while still maintaining some degree of elasticity, but also constitutes the most important storage site for calcium and inorganic phosphate (BARON 1993). Osteoporosis is a systemic disease where rigidity and mechanical stability of bone declines, until bone loses the ability to withstand functional loading or weak traumata. A transient but disproportional bone loss of 20%–30% trabecular and 5%–10% cortical bone is most apparent in women during the first postmenopausal decade. The following slow phase accounts for 20%–30% of trabecular and cortical bone loss in both sexes. Epidemiologic data show that the lifetime risk to acquire hip fractures is 17% for white women and 6% for white men (CUMMINGS and MELTON 2002; MELTON 1995). Progress in medical care and education has contributed to an increased average life span, which

R. GRUBER, PhD
Associate Professor, Department of Oral Surgery, Vienna University Clinic of Dentistry, Medical University of Vienna, Waehringer Strasse 25a, 1090 Vienna, Austria
P. PIETSCHMANN, MD
Associate Professor of Pathophysiology and Internal Medicine, Department of Pathophysiology, Medical University of Vienna, Waehringer Guertel 18–20, 1090 Vienna, Austria
and
Ludwig Boltzmann-Institute of Aging Research, Langobardenstrasse 122, 1220 Vienna, Austria
M. PETERLIK, MD, PhD
Professor and Head of the Department of Pathophysiology, Medical University of Vienna, Waehringer Guertel 18–20, 1090 Vienna, Austria

is, however, associated with a higher risk of acquiring age-related diseases such as osteoporosis. On the other hand, progress has been made on diagnosing osteoporosis and monitoring disease progression. Potent drugs are available that help reduce the risk of fracture and new pharmacologic substances are already in the pipeline (DELMAS 2002; RODAN and MARTIN 2000). Improvement in patient care is possible because of a substantial increase in the functional understanding of the genetic and molecular mechanism on bone development, remodelling and repair, and as a result, the pathophysiology of osteoporosis. The aim of this chapter is to give an update on the fundamental aspects of bone biology with regard to the coordinated action of bone cells during development, remodelling and repair. We briefly review the structural and cellular composition of the bone matrix and focus on genetic and molecular mechanisms that control cell differentiation and activity. This information is considered a scientific basis for the following chapters on the pathophysiology of age-related bone loss (see Chap. 2), bone loss associated with chronic inflammation (see Chap. 3), as well as the chapter dealing with the current approaches in osteoporosis therapy (see Chap. 4).

1.2
Structure, Cells and Matrix

1.2.1
Structural Organization and Parameters of Bone Strength

At the structural level, two different forms of bone can be distinguished: cortical or compact bone, which, for example, forms the diaphysis of long bones, thus providing protection for the medullary cavity. Trabecular, cancellous, or spongy bone, which in long bones is found at their ends, at the epiphyses, makes up the greater part of vertebral bodies. The total skeleton comprises around 20% trabecular bone. Trabecular bone has a porosity of 50%–90%, cortical bone of approximately 10% (SIKAVITSAS et al. 2001). The high surface-to-volume ratio of trabecular bone involves its metabolic function, whereas cortical bone has mainly a structural and protective role.

The outer bone surface is in contact with the surrounding soft tissue via the periosteum. The inner bone surface faces the medullary cavity and is covered by the endosteum. Both periosteum and endosteum are connective tissues organized in layers. The cambium layer is in intimate contact with the mineralized structure and provides a pool of mesenchymal cells with the potential to differentiate into the chondrogenic and the osteogenic lineage.

Trabecular bone and cortical bone are composed of the same microstructural elements: cells, organic matrix, crystalline inorganic matrix and soluble factors. The calcified matrix of adult bone is built up in multiple layers of oriented collagen fibers, giving rise to the typical structure of lamellar bone. The lamellae are arranged parallel to each other, as on the surface of flat bones and trabecular structures, or in concentric layers around blood vessels and nerves, forming the haversian system synonymic for osteons in the corticalis. The haversian canals are connected to the periosteum and the endosteum by Volkmann's canals. Blood flow in bone totals 200–400 ml/min in adult humans, indicating that bone is a highly vascularized tissue.

Under conditions in which rapid formation of new bone is required, e.g. during skeletal growth in early childhood and in periods of bone regeneration, or in particular metabolic bone disorders, instead of lamellar bone, immature "woven" bone is formed, in which the collagen fibers are randomly oriented and the degree of mineralization is relatively low. Woven bone is later remodelled into lamellar bone, which has better mechanical properties. Formation, remodelling, and repair of the structural elements require the coordinated action of the bone cells: osteoblasts, osteocytes, lining cells, and osteoclasts (BARON 1993; MARKS 2002; SCHENK and HUNZIKER 1994).

Bone strength is defined by the parameters mass, geometry, material properties, and microstructure. The bone mass accounts for about half of the decrease in bone strength in the elderly. The diameter of the corticalis is a parameter of bone geometry. Material properties are modulated by the mineral crystals and the correct synthesis of the single components of the bone matrix. The diameter of the trabeculae as well their horizontal and vertical interconnectivity are further determinants that together define bone strength (PARIS et al. 2000; RIGGS and PARFITT 2005).

1.2.2
The Bone Cells

Osteocytes are cells that are embedded in the mineralized matrix of both woven and lamellar bone. They emerge at the end stage of osteoblast differentiation and become trapped within the mineralized matrix. Osteocytes reside singly in small lacunae but are connected to neighbouring cells through cytoplasmic protrusions, which form a dense network of canaliculi. This syncytium permits direct communication between neighbouring osteocytes, as well as with lining cells and osteoblasts on the bone surface. Nutritional and oxygen transport within this network is limited to the diffusion distance, which is approximately 100 µm, equivalent to the wall thickness of trabecular structures and the outer diameter of an osteon. Osteocytes probably act as mechanosensors that signal the need for bone modelling to adapt the bone to functional loading according to Wolff's law (FROST 2004) and remodelling to repair microstructural changes within the bone matrix. Osteocytes can detect changes in the levels of hormones, such as oestrogen and glucocorticoids that influence their survival rate. Since osteocytes form a network spanning the skeletal system, they may well, through their residual metabolic activity, play a role in bone turnover (KNOTHE TATE et al. 2004; MANOLAGAS 2000; MARKS 2002; NIJWEIDE 2002).

Osteoblasts are mesenchymal cells located on the surface of the mineralized matrix and are responsible for formation of new bone; that is, they synthesize and regulate the deposition and mineralization of the extracellular matrix (Fig 1.1). Osteoblasts form a dense monolayer of approximately 100–400 cells clustering at each bone-forming site. They exhibit a prominent Golgi apparatus and a well-developed rough endoplasmic reticulum. Osteoblasts secrete mainly type I collagen as well as a large number of noncollagenous proteins. The layer of unmineralized bone matrix, termed osteoid, serves as a template for the initiation and propagation of mineralization. During development and the early stages of bone regeneration, woven bone is produced by pinching of matrix vesicles from osteoblasts similar to mineralized hypertrophic cartilage (ANDERSON et al. 2005). Osteoblasts lay down lamellar bone onto the previously formed woven bone, at about 1–2 µm per day. Mean thickness of osteoid is 10 µm, indicating that the mineralization time of lamellar bone is approximately 10 days (SCHENK 1994). After ceasing matrix-forming activity, osteoblasts can undergo apoptosis, terminal differentia-

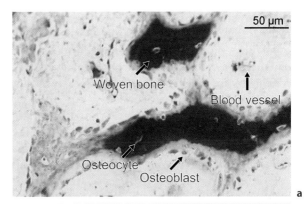

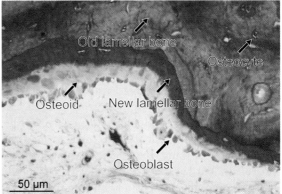

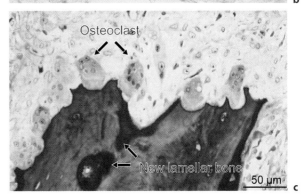

Fig. 1.1. a Woven bone forms struts and ridges within a blood vessel-rich granulation tissue. The origin of osteoblasts has not been clearly demonstrated. Likely sources are the vascular pericytes and the blood. Woven bone appears dark blue. **b** Osteoblasts originate in the mesenchyma and lay down osteoid onto the pre-existing bone surface, which mineralizes at a distance of approximately 10 µm. Osteoblast is forming a seam. Osteocytes form a network within the mineralized matrix and can signal the need for bone remodelling. Less mineralized newly formed bone showed more intense purple staining than old bone. **c** Osteoclasts are multinucleated cells of the haematopoietic lineage that have the unique potential to resorb bone. They attach to the mineralized bone matrix and form a sealing zone. Resorption of the bone matrix is a consequence of the low pH and the proteases cathepsin K and matrix metalloproteinase-9. The protons for the H^+ ATPase are provided by carboanhydrase II, which catalyses the hydration of CO_2 to the unstable H_2CO_3

tion into osteocytes, or remain in inactive form as so-called lining cells on the bone surface (MARKS 2002). In addition, endosteal osteoblasts provide the micro-environment, or niches, for haematopoietic stem cells, which give rise to cells of the myeloid lineage, including osteoclasts (TAICHMAN 2005).

Osteoclasts are large polykaryons containing between 3 and 30 nuclei, and are considered to be the exclusive bone-resorbing cell. This cell type contains large numbers of lysosomes, mitochondria, and an extensive Golgi complex. Osteoclasts are located at bone surfaces within Howship's lacunae, also called resorption lacunae. Under normal conditions, osteoclasts are rarely found in bone, i.e. only 2–3/μm^3, but they appear in increased numbers at sites of high bone turnover, such as in the metaphysis of growing bone or in trabecular bone in postmenopausal osteoporosis. A characteristic feature of active osteoclasts, which distinguishes them from polynuclear macrophages, is the development of a ruffled border surrounded by an organelle-free area, termed the sealing zone. Through the finger-like structures of the ruffled border, osteoclasts secrete proteolytic enzymes, such as cathepsin K and matrix metalloproteinase 9, as well as hydrogen ion. The acidic pH of approximately 4.5 provides the environment for the mobilization of hydroxyapatite and optimal conditions for the proteolytic enzymes to degrade the bone matrix. The degraded matrix components are released in the periosteoclastic environment by transcytosis (MARKS 2002; ROODMAN 1996; SALO et al. 1997; TEITELBAUM 2000)

1.2.3
The Organic Matrix

The organic matrix contains approximately 90% type I collagen; the remaining 10% consist of noncollagenous components. Type I collagen serves as the main structural element which has the ability to bind a large number of noncollagenous proteins. Type I collagen is composed of two α_1 chains and one α_2 chain, which share a common amino acid sequence consisting of Gly-X-Y repeats. X represents a proline residue, Y is in most cases modified by a post-translational reaction into hydroxyproline. The latter is essential for stabilization of the triple-helical structure. Before the procollagen molecules assemble to form a triple-helical structure, the N- and C-terminal propeptides are removed by proteolytic cleavage and serve as metabolic markers of bone formation. The

single triple-helical structures are interconnected by the formation of covalent cross-links. The corresponding cleavage products, pyridinoline and deoxypyridinoline, as well as the not completely digested N- and C-terminal telopeptides, are metabolic markers of bone resorption (ROSSERT and DE CROMBRUGGHE 2002; SWAMINATHAN 2001).

Proteoglycans and glycoproteins are the noncollagenous components of the organic bone matrix. Proteoglycans are large macromolecules composed of glycosaminoglycans (GAGs) covalently linked to a core protein from which the molecule derives its name, e.g. decorin, biglycan, versican and fibromodulin. Each GAG, such as chondroitin sulfate or heparan sulfate, is made up of repeating disaccharide units that contain a sulfated amino sugar. Proteoglycans not only serve as anchoring sites for collagen fibers, but also contain binding sites for growth factors (ROBEY 2002). Gene deletion of biglycan in mice causes a phenotype characterized by a reduced growth rate and decreased bone mass (XU et al. 1998).

Glycoproteins, which are produced at different stages of osteoblast maturation, are post-translationally modified proteins with N- or O-linked oligosaccharides. Thrombospondin, fibronectin, osteopontin, and bone sialoprotein are glycoproteins that exhibit a RGD sequence (Arg-Gly-Asp), which constitute binding domains for cell membrane receptors of the integrin class. Osteocalcin and matrix Gla protein are characterized by their content of multiple γ-carboxy glutamic acid residues, which exhibit high affinity for mineral ions such as Ca^{2+}. Mice deficient in osteocalcin show a higher bone mass when compared to wild type animals (DUCY et al. 1996). Mice deficient in matrix Gla protein are normal at birth, but develop severe calcification of their arteries (LUO et al. 1997). It seems likely that both glycoproteins are involved in the regulation of matrix mineralization. Alkaline phosphatase and osteonectin are also extracellular proteins, which contain neither an RGD sequence nor a γ-carboxy glutamic acid group. Gene deletion of tissue nonspecific alkaline phosphatase in the mouse indicates that the enzyme plays a role in bone mineral deposition during bone remodelling (NARISAWA et al. 1997; WAYMIRE et al. 1995).

The expression of the genes coding for matrix molecules is linked to different stages of osteogenic differentiation (STEIN and LIAN 1993). The extracellular matrix is also an important storage pool of growth factors that are believed to play a role during bone remodelling (ROBEY 2002).

1.3
Bone Development, Remodelling and Regeneration

1.3.1
Bone Development

The skeleton comprises more than 200 elements with different locations and shapes. Skeletal development requires two main events that have to be coordinated in their special and temporal sequence: patterning and differentiation. Patterning is the process defining the shape, size, and location of the skeletal elements. Differentiation involves the multistep process where uncommitted mesenchymal progenitor cells receive signals that activate the transcription of genes that control proliferation and differentiation of osteoblasts, chondrocytes, and osteoclasts.

Skeletal development requires intramembranous and endochondral ossification. Intramembranous ossification starts with mesenchymal progenitor cells differentiating into bone-forming osteoblasts, a process that generates the flat bones of the cranial vault, some facial bones, and parts of the mandible and clavicle. In addition, concentric bone growth is achieved by intramembranous ossification. Osteoblasts originating from periosteum deposit new bone on the outer surface, while at the same time old bone is resorbed by osteoclasts at endosteal sites. Also the bony collar, as exemplified below, develops by the intramembranous route.

Bones that are part of joints and thus have to bear weight are formed by endochondral ossification. In this process, mesenchymal progenitor cells condense in a special and temporal sequence during development, thereby forming the anlagen, which prefigures the future skeletal structures. Mesenchymal cells differentiate into the chondrogenic lineage, characteristically expressing collagen type II and aggrecan. Chondrocytes undergo a program of proliferation, followed by the differentiation into the prehypertrophic and the hypertrophic state. Hypertrophic chondrocytes express collagen type X and produce a calcified matrix before they die by apoptosis. Endochondral and intramembranous ossification are functionally linked, as a mineralized bone collar directly develops from mesenchymal cells that surround the cartilage anlagen. Hypertrophic chondrocytes in turn release angiogenic molecules that induce invasion of blood capillaries originating from the bone collar. Along with the blood capillaries come progenitor cells of osteoblasts and chondroclasts. Mature osteoblasts deposit new bone on the calcified matrix previously produced by the hypertrophic chondrocytes, and chondroclasts excavate the marrow cavity. Chondroclasts resemble osteoclasts specialized to resorb the mineralized matrix produced by the hypertrophic chondrocytes. The sequence of endochondral bone formation continues in the formation of the growth plates, which are responsible for longitudinal bone growth at the epiphyses. During the process of endochondral bone formation, all remaining mineralized cartilaginous structures are replaced by new bone. Structural adaptation of bone to functional loading is termed bone modelling and causes changes in shape. The coordination action of osteoblast and osteoclast to maintain bone integrity is termed bone remodelling.

During development, mesenchymal progenitor cells of the craniofacial skeleton originate from the cranial neural crest. The axial skeleton and the limbs derive from the somites and the lateral plate mesoderm, respectively. Independent of their origin, dysostoses are disorders caused by mutations in patterning genes, osteochondrodysplasia occurs when genes responsible for growth and differentiation are affected (KARSENTY and WAGNER 2002; KRONENBERG 2003; ZELZER and OLSEN 2003).

1.3.2
Bone Remodelling

After cessation of growth, the skeleton is completely renewed about every 10 years, thereby maintaining its structural and functional integrity. Bone remodelling is the result of the coordinated action of bone-resorbing osteoclasts and bone-forming osteoblasts. Osteoblasts and osteoclasts interact within a spatial structure known as the basic multicellular unit (BMU) in cortical bone and in analogy, bone structural units in trabecular bone. In the following text, the term "BMU" will be used for remodelling units in cortical and trabecular bone. BMUs are functional in the developing and growing skeleton during the process of modelling and during remodelling of mature bone. Histological examinations of BMUs demonstrate that osteoclasts excavate a resorption canal in the corticalis and a cavity in the trabecular structures. The resorption phase requires about 2–4 weeks. It is hypothesized that growth factors released from the bone matrix and the osteoclasts can attract mesenchymal progenitor cells provided by the blood capillaries and stimulate their differentiation into functional osteoblasts (MARTIN and SIMS 2005). Osteoblasts deposit osteoid onto the previously resorbed channel or cavity that is later mineralized, a process that takes about 4–6 months. In cortical bone, the resorption canal is continuously filled with layers of lamellar bone with a blood vessel remaining in the middle. The end-stage product is the secondary osteon. BMUs are approximately 2–3 mm long and 200–250 μm in diameter, with 50–80 μm for the vascular channel. The mean depth of trabecular cavities is around 50 μm. An estimated one million BMUs exist at any time in the adult skeleton. The life span of a BMU is 6–9 months, much longer than the life span of osteoblasts and osteoclasts. Hence, to replace old cells, their respective progenitors have to be recruited and caused to differentiate into their mature phenotypes. Potential sources of progenitor cells are the blood capillaries, centrally located within each BMU. Osteoblast progenitors can originate from pericytes, covering the outer basal membrane of the capillaries, and from a subpopulation of circulating mononucleated cells (DOHERTY et al. 1998; EGHBALI-FATOURECHI et al. 2005). Osteoclasts arise from circulating cells of the monocytic lineage, which possibly receive a specific "area code" of adhesion molecules expressed by the endothelial cells (MANOLAGAS 2000; PARFITT 1998, 2000, 2002).

The birth, life, and death of osteoblasts and osteoclasts within the BMU is fundamental to understand the pathophysiology of skeletal diseases such as osteoporosis (MANOLAGAS 2000). Osteoblasts, osteoclasts, and their respective progenitors are exposed to a variety of systemic hormones and local factors that regulate the tight balance of bone remodelling. Systemic hormones are brought into the BMU by means of blood capillaries and cells release local factors in an autocrine/paracrine mode of action. Local and systemic factors can influence the activation frequency, which defines the number of BMUs at a given time point, in addition to the remodelling balance of the cells within each BMU. Therapeutic agents that can cause bone loss such as glucocorticoids and osteoporosis regimes act through modulating the balance of bone remodelling. Bisphosphonate treatment, for example, lowers high bone remodelling in postmenopausal osteoporosis by decreasing the

activation frequency of BMUs and the average life span and activity of osteoclasts. Under the bisphosphonate alendronate, activation frequency was reduced by 87%, and osteoblasts have more time to rebuild the excavated resorption site, leading to a positive remodelling balance (CHAVASSIEUX et al. 1997). Lower bone remodelling is reflected by the decrease in resorption parameters by about 40%–60% (DELMAS et al. 2000). Under bisphosphonate therapy, osteoblasts produce a higher mineralized structure and lower the porosity of cortical bone that together increase the strength of osteoporotic bone (ROSCHGER et al. 2001). A decreased number of BMUs can add to the mechanical properties of osteoporotic bone.

Another strategy of osteoporosis treatment is based on the intermediate injections of parathyroid hormone (PTH), which leads to a temporal increase in formation over resorption markers for 6 months. Bone mass continues to increase thereafter. PTH treatment increases the activation frequency of BMUs and causes positively balanced bone remodelling. Positive remodelling is related to an increased osteoblast activity, indicated by the heterogenous mineralization of cortical and trabecular bone (MISOF et al. 2003) and a decrease in osteoblast apoptosis (JILKA et al. 1999). In contrast, glucocorticoid treatment is associated with a high apoptosis rate in osteocytes, and osteoblasts culminate in pathologic bone loss (MANOLAGAS 2000). Sodium fluoride can increase bone mass by affecting bone cristal structure; the fracture risk, however, was not decreased in osteoporotic patients, suggesting that not only bone remodelling, also the nanostructure defines bone strength (MEUNIER et al. 1998). Bone remodelling not only effects bone mass, but also the geometry, material properties and microstructure, all of which are parameters of bone that help withstand fractures. Osteoporosis therapies modulate bone remodelling and consequently bone quality (RIGGS and PARFITT 2005).

The current theory of the coupling phenomenon between resorption and formation is based on the following mechanism: growth factors, which were originally produced by the osteoblasts, are released from the bone matrix during the course of bone resorption. Osteogenic cells respond to these factors and to paracrine factors expressed by osteoclasts, thereby receiving signals that stimulate bone formation (MARTIN and SIMS 2005). Osteoclast formation requires close contact with stromal cells and osteoblasts. This interrelationship between bone formation and resorption makes it obvious why both cell types are restricted to a BMU.

What are the triggers that signal the need for bone remodelling and culminate in the initiation of a new BMU? Osteocytes are considered to act as sensors that can recognize changes in the interstitial flow rate within the canaliculi system that occur upon functional loading of bone. Osteocytes are connected to osteoblasts and lining cells, so that the demand to establish a new BMU is transmitted to the bone surface. Once the canaliculi network is interrupted due to microfractures, surgical interventions, or circulating molecules such as glucocorticoids, osteocytes die. Osteocytes might release signals to lining cells that suppress osteoclastogenesis, which disappears once the osteocyte network is interrupted. Lining cells in turn express collagenase, which digest the extracellular matrix and free the mineralized structures to allow osteoclastogenesis to take place. Lining cells also contract to make space for the development of the new BMUs, and likely also express factors that attract osteoclast progenitors and stimulate their differentiation (KNOTHE TATE et al. 2004; MANOLAGAS 2000; NIJWEIDE 2002).

1.3.3
Bone Regeneration

Bone holds the intrinsic capacity to regenerate without the formation of a scar. The basic mechanisms of bone regeneration are very similar to those during bone development, except that early stages are linked with an inflammatory response. Immediately following bone injury, e.g. fractures, reconstruction surgery, placement of dental or orthopedic implants and tooth extraction, blood vessel disruption leads to the development of a blood clot that fills the defect site with a provisional fibrin-rich extracellular matrix. Accumulating platelets and the immigrating neutrophils and macrophages provide a source of growth factors such as platelet-derived growth factor (PDGF), vascular endothelial growth factor (VEGF), basic fibroblast growth factor (bFGF) and a broad spectrum of other bioactive molecules that target mesenchymal progenitor cells with their osteochondrogenic potential. Blood capillaries sprout into the blood clot by a process termed angiogenesis (CARMELIET 2000; RISAU 1997). In parallel, endothelial progenitor cells that originate from the bone marrow are

transported via the blood stream to the site of blood vessel formation where they contribute to capillary sprouting. This process is termed vasculogenesis (ASAHARA and KAWAMOTO 2004). Once the blood clot is replaced by the blood vessel-rich granulation tissue, differentiation of mesenchymal progenitor cells into functional osteoblasts is initiated, e.g. as observed in tooth extraction sites (CARDAROPOLI et al. 2003) and during osseointegration of dental implants (BERGLUNDH et al. 2003). Low oxygen tension and the instability of a fracture, however, favor the differentiation of mesenchymal progenitor cells into the chondrogenic lineage. Cartilaginous tissue, which stabilizes the defect site, is then replaced by bone via endochondral ossification. Lamellar bone is laid appositionally onto immature woven- and pre-existing bone, as well as onto osteoconductive surfaces of implants and grafting materials (BARNES et al. 1999; GERSTENFELD et al. 2003; SCHENK and HUNZIKER 1994).

Bone regeneration also involves the process of adaptive modelling and remodelling. This mechanism is based on the sensing of mechanical extension and mechanotransduction. Conversion of mechanical forces into cellular response involves activation of intercellular signals, which are induced by stretched cytoskeletal molecules and piezoelectric potentials. Stress and strains should not overwhelm the microdamage threshold of approximately 3,000 microstrains, which stands for shortened bone by 0.3% of original length. Bone modelling occurs best around 1,000 microstrains (FROST 1994, 2004). Biophysical stimulations such as pulsed electromagnetic fields and low-intensity pulsed ultrasounds are considered to have positive effects on bone regeneration (EISMAN 2001; FINI et al. 2004). Other therapeutic concepts are based on the application of growth factors, cells, and matrices that play a role during bone regeneration. Growth and differentiation factors for mesenchymal cells can be of either natural sources such as autologous preparations of platelet-rich plasma (MARX et al. 1998) or from biotechnology such as recombinant BMP-2 or BMP-7, which are approved for the treatment of nonhealing fractures and for spinal fusion (MONT et al. 2004). In addition, metabolites that activate prostaglandin receptors 2 and 4 can stimulate bone regeneration (PARALKAR et al. 2003; TANAKA et al. 2004). Angiogenic factors are investigated based on the understanding that blood capillaries are essential for bone regeneration (ITO et al. 2005; MURPHY et al. 2004). Another strategy to enhance bone regeneration is supplementation of the defect site with additional osteogenic cells that can be isolated from autologous sources, e.g. bone marrow aspirates and the periosteum (CANCEDDA et al. 2003; CAPLAN and BRUDER 2001; SCHMELZEISEN et al. 2003). Gene therapeutic approaches follow the concept that the transfected cells serve as a bioreactor for therapeutic growth factors over a prolonged time, but this method has not reached the level of routine clinical use (DAI et al. 2004; JADLOWIEC et al. 2003; LEACH and MOONEY 2004).

Bone development, remodelling and regeneration basically depend on the same elements: mesenchymal progenitor cells that differentiate into osteoblasts or chondrocytes, haematopoietic progenitors that give rise to osteoclasts, local clues that attract the cells and control their proliferation and differentiation into the mature phenotypes, and a provisional matrix, which defines the area for these dynamic processes (Fig. 1.2). In the next section, the genetic and molecular mechanisms that control bone cell differentiation will be exemplified.

1.4
Regulatory Mechanisms of Development and Function

Bone marrow contains a population of mesenchymal cells that can differentiate into various cell types such as osteoblasts, chondrocytes, adipocytes and myotubes. The commitment of pluripotent mesenchymal cells into each of these lineages is genetically controlled by series of master genes encoding various lineage-specific transcription factors. Among these, C/EBPα,β,γ (CCAAT-enhancer-binding protein) and peroxisome proliferator-activated receptor-γ control adipogenesis. Myogenic regulatory factors (including MyoD, myogenin, myogenic factor 5 and myogenic regulatory factor 4) and myocyte-enhancer factor 2 have been identified to control myoblast differentiation (HARADA and RODAN 2003; MANOLAGAS 2000). In this chapter, we focus on mechanisms that regulate the differen-

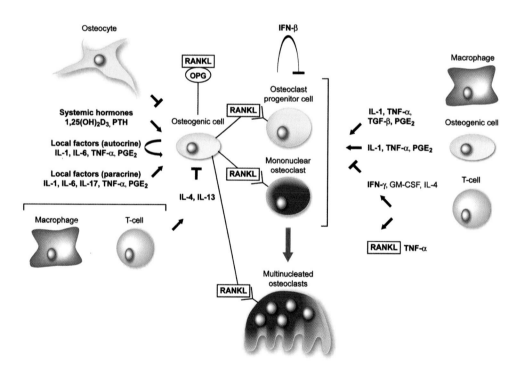

Fig. 1.2. Differentiation of haematopoietic progenitor cells into highly specialized bone-resorbing osteoclasts, which is controlled by indirect and direct mechanisms. Indirect mechanisms require the presence of cells of the osteogenic lineage that express the key factor of osteoclastogenesis RANKL under the control of systemic hormones and autocrine/paracrine mechanisms. OPG can bind a neutralized RANKL acting as a negative regulator of osteoclast formation and activity. Direct mechanisms involve the stimulation of osteoclastogenesis under permissive levels of RANKL. Again, systemic, autocrine and paracrine mediators are involved in the control of this process. Overall, osteoclastogenesis is considered a highly controlled multistep process of formation, activation and survival of osteoclasts. Pathologic conditions such as chronic inflammation can boost the process, causing increased local and systemic bone loss

tiation of mesenchymal cells into the chondrogenic and osteogenic lineage, a process that is likely to be conserved throughout bone development, remodelling and repair.

1.4.1
Regulatory Mechanisms in Chondrocytes

The transcription factor Sox-9, which has a high-mobility-group (HMG)-box DNA-binding domain, is required for the transition of mesenchymal progenitors into chondrocytes and their condensation within the skeletal anlagen, as concluded from mouse models and genetic studies in humans. In addition, chondrocytes in Sox-5 and Sox-6 double knock-out mice failed to undergo hypertrophy, and consequently columnar organization of the growth plate is affected (KARSENTY and WAGNER 2002; KRONENBERG 2003; PROVOT and SCHIPANI 2005).

Genetic studies further suggest the involvement of the functional axis fibroblast growth factor (FGF)-18/FGF receptor 3 (FGFR-3) in chondrocyte proliferation. Constitutive activation of the FGFR-3 tyrosine kinase receptor causes the virtual absence of prehypertrophic chondrocytes, whereas gene deletion models show larger zones of proliferating chondrocytes. FGF-18 produced by the perichondrium binds to FGFR-3 on proliferating chondrocytes. FGF-18 gene ablation similarly results in larger zones of proliferating chondrocytes, suggesting that FGF-18 is the predicted ligand for FGFR-3, which inhibits chondrocyte proliferation (KARSENTY and WAGNER 2002; KRONENBERG 2003; PROVOT and SCHIPANI 2005).

Chondrocyte proliferation is positively regulated by the PTHrP/Indian Hedgehog (Ihh) feedback loop. PTHrP is produced by cells of the periarticular perichondrium and by early stages of proliferating chondrocytes and acts as a mitogen for late proliferating and prehypertrophic chondrocytes. With increasing distance from the PTHrP source, the mitogenic activity fades and prehypertrophic chondrocytes can develop. Prehypertrophic chondrocytes are the main source of the soluble factor Ihh, which stimulates the production of PTHrP by an unknown mechanism. Ihh is also a mitogen for proliferating chondrocytes directly and through BMP signalling. Thus, PTHrP expression regulated by Ihh can control the length of the zone of proliferating chondrocytes and their transition into the prehypertrophic phenotype. Moreover, mice without a functional Ihh gene lack the bony collar because Ihh regulates the master gene of osteogenic differentiation, the transcription factors Runx-2 (ST-JACQUES et al. 1999) (see below). Ihh is not required for osteoblastogenesis in bones formed through intramembranous ossification. Runx-2 is further expressed by chondrocyte condensations, prehypertrophic and hypertrophic chondrocytes. The transcription factor drives differentiation into hypertrophic chondrocytes. Even though in some growth plates hypertrophic chondrocytes can be detected in the absence of functional Runx-2, they fail to mineralize (KARSENTY and WAGNER 2002; KRONENBERG 2003; PROVOT and SCHIPANI 2005).

Bone morphogenetic proteins (BMPs) belong to the TGF superfamily. The function of BMPs was originally recognized by the ability of decalcified bone matrix to induce endochondral bone formation at ectopic sites (URIST 1965). At least 15 different BMPs have been characterized at the molecular level. During development, BMPs are expressed within mesenchymal condensations (BMP-5), in the perichondrium (BMP-2, BMP-4, BMP-5, BMP-7), and in the future zones of joint formation growth and differentiation factor-5 (GDF-5). BMP-7 is expressed in proliferating chondrocytes and BMP-2 and BMP-6 are found in hypertrophic chondrocytes. Overall, BMPs are mitogenic for chondrocytes and negatively regulate their terminal differentiation. The importance of BMPs for growth and development is further underscored by results from studies on knock-out mice, which die in utero (BMP-2, BMP-4), or shortly after birth (BMP-7). Severe skeletal defects involving joint formation caused by GDF-5 mutations of the gene were reported (FRANCIS-WEST et al. 1999; THOMAS et al. 1996, 1997). BMPs bind to serine–threonine receptors termed BMP-receptor type IA or IB, each of which forms a heterodimer with a type II receptor. BMPRIA controls the pace of chondrocyte proliferation, whereas BMPRIB is involved in cartilage formation and apoptosis (ZOU et al. 1997). At the extracellular level, the biologic activity of BMPs is modulated by a number of antagonists known as noggin, chordin, gremlin, and follistatin. Of these, noggin and chordin have been shown to bind to BMP-2 and BMP-4 with high affinity, and noggin-null mutations indicate the involvement of this molecule in patterning of the neural tube, somites, and cartilage. Overexpression of noggin in the osteoblastic lineage causes a decreased trabecular bone volume and impaired osteoblastic function (DEVLIN et al. 2003; WU et al. 2003). Mouse models where the expression of BMPs and their receptors is controlled by cartilage-specific genes are awaited (Yu et al. 2005). During the postnatal phase, BMPs and their corresponding receptors are expressed during fracture repair (Onishi et al. 1998). For review see: (Canalis et al. 2003; Karsenty and Wagner 2002; Kronenberg 2003; Provot and Schipani 2005; Reddi 1998).

Once the chondrocytes have undergone hypertrophy, they express the key angiogenic molecule VEGF in response to transcriptional activation by hypoxia-inducible factor-1. Conditional knock out of VEGF in chondrocytes results in delayed blood vessel invasion. Matrix metalloproteinase-9 (MMP-9), highly expressed in chondroclasts and osteoclasts, is involved in the release of VEGF from the mineralized extracellular matrix. Interestingly, Runx-2 is required for vascular invasion, via regulation of VEGF expression. VEGF also plays a key role in fracture healing (Carano and Filvaroff 2003; Karsenty and Wagner 2002; Kronenberg 2003; Provot and Schipani 2005).

For information on further mechanisms that regulate endochondral bone formation involving the growth hormone–insulin-like growth factor (IGF) axis, the reader is referred to recent reviews (Olney 2003; van der Eerden et al. 2003; Veldhuis et al. 2005).

1.4.2
Regulatory Mechanisms in Osteoblasts

Runx-2, also termed CBFA1/PEBP2αA/AML2, encodes a member of the runt family of transcription factors whose expression precedes the appearance of osteoblasts. Null mutation causes the formation of a cartilaginous skeleton without any evidence of bone (Komori et al. 1997; Otto et al. 1997). Heterozygote mutations of Runx-2 have been detected in mice and humans, correlating with the phenotype of cleidocranial dysplasia: hypoplastic clavicles and nasal bones and retarded ossification of parietal, interparietal, and supraoccipital bones (Lee et al. 1997; Mundlos et al. 1997; Otto et al. 1997). Runx-2 is also important for the continuing activity of osteoblasts in adults. In addition, the transcription factor plays a role in the transition of proliferating chondrocytes into pre- and hypertrophic chondrocytes (Kronenberg 2003; Zelzer and Olsen 2003). Runx-2 activity is transiently inhibited at the posttranscriptional levels by Twist proteins, basic helix-loop-helix transcription factors, which

are expressed in Runx2-positive cells throughout the skeleton early in development. The interaction between a C-terminal region of Twist and the Runt domain of Runx-2 prevents DNA binding and gene activation (Bialek et al. 2004). Runx-2 activity is further modulated by co-activator core binding factor β (CBFβ), and other transcription factors such as the Smads, Rb, and MAP kinases and corepressors (Kronenberg 2004; Kundu et al. 2002; Yoshida et al. 2002). Among the factors that control Runx-2 transcription are BMPs and Ihh (Ducy et al. 1997; St-Jacques et al. 1999). Moreover, BMPs and Runx-2 are also involved in the transition of mesenchymal cells into a phenotype with the potential to support osteoclastogenesis (Abe et al. 2000; Geoffroy et al. 2002; Hoshi et al. 1999).

Another transcription factor that controls osteoblast fate is called osterix (Nakashima et al. 2002). Osterix knockout animals express Runx-2 but not vice-versa, suggesting that osterix acts downstream in the signalling cascade. Osterix-deficient mice show all stages of cartilage development up to mineralized hypertrophic chondrocytes. The catabolic effects of immunosuppression on bone metabolism may involve the decreased nuclear factor of activated T (NFAT) that is required to form a complex with osterix to activate target genes (Koga et al. 2005). Distal-less homeobox 5 (Dlx5), msh homeobox homologue 2 (Msx2) and members of the Fos family are additional transcription factors that regulate bone development (Harada and Rodan 2003; Karsenty and Wagner 2002).

Signalling via the Wnt pathway is also involved in the regulation of bone remodelling. Wnt ligands bind to a receptor complex composed of low-density lipoprotein receptor protein (LRP) 5 and LRP6, and a member of the frizzled family of seven transmembrane-spanning proteins. Activation of the frizzled receptor complex causes stabilization of intracellular β-catenin by inhibition of its phosphorylation. Unphosphorylated β-catenin accumulates in the cytoplasm and translocates to the nucleus, where it associates with LEF/TCF transcription factors and controls gene transcription. Phosphorylated β-catenin is rapidly degraded. Heterozygous gain-of-function mutations in the gene coding for LRP5 are associated with a high bone mass (Boyden et al. 2002; Little et al. 2002). The mutation reduced the affinity of LRB5 for the inhibitor Dickkopf-1 (Ai et al. 2005). Loss of function mutation causes the osteoporosis pseudoglioma syndrome, which is characterized by low bone density (Gong et al. 2001). Both phenotypes could be confirmed in mouse models (GONG et al. 2001). Genetic mouse models further indicate that β-catenin is essential in determining that mesenchymal progenitors become osteoblasts and not chondrocytes, regardless of regional locations or ossification mechanisms (DAY et al. 2005; HILL et al. 2005). Animal models based on stabilization and destabilization of β-catenin in osteoblasts showed that these mutations primarily affect bone resorption rather than bone formation (GLASS et al. 2005). Whether modulation of Wnt signalling, for example by blocking binding of Dkk-1 to LRP-5, will be a therapeutic opportunity in osteoporosis remains to be determined (For review see HARADA and RODAN 2003; HE et al. 2004; LOGAN and NUSSE 2004).

Sclerostin is an inhibitor of osteoblast function, and inactivating mutations cause generalized progressive bone overgrowth termed osteosclerosis. Sclerostin binds LRP5 and 6 and inhibits canonical Wnt signalling, suggesting that increased Wnt signalling is linked with osteosclerosis (LI et al. 2005; WINKLER et al. 2003). PTH can inhibit sclerostin transcription (BELLIDO et al. 2005; KELLER and KNEISSEL 2005). Its unique expression by osteocytes and action on osteoblasts suggest that sclerostin may be an osteocyte-derived factor that is transported to osteoblasts at the bone surface and modulates bone formation (VAN BEZOOIJEN et al. 2004).

1.4.3
Regulatory Mechanisms in Osteoclast Development and Function

Osteotropic hormones such as 1,25-dihydroxyvitamin D_3 [$1,25(OH)_2D_3$] and PTH, and local factors such as prostaglandins or cytokines [interleukin (IL)-1, IL-6, IL-11, tumour necrosis factor (TNF)] can induce the expression of a membrane-associated osteoclast differentiation factor in osteoblasts/stromal cells. Osteoclast precursors recognize this factor through cell–cell interaction, thereby receive the signal necessary for differentiation into mature osteoclasts (SUDA et al. 1992). Factors that are instrumental in osteoclast differentiation are members of the TNF/TNF receptor superfamily, viz. the receptor activator of nuclear factor-κB (RANK), the RANK ligand (RANKL), and osteoprotegerin (OPG) (BOYLE et al. 2003; SUDA et al. 1999). RANK is expressed on mononuclear osteoclast precursors of the monocyte/macrophage lineage, while RANKL, which is identical with the aforementioned osteoclast differ-entiation factor, is expressed on stromal/osteoblast cells (Fig. 1.3) as well as on activated T lymphocytes. RANK/RANKL interaction and the presence of macrophage colony-stimulating factor (M-CSF) are sufficient to induce the formation of osteoclasts, and are also important for their activation and survival. OPG, a soluble member of the TNF-receptor superfamily, acts as a decoy receptor that competes with RANK for RANKL (Fig. 1.3). This explains why overexpression of OPG in mice leads to osteopetrosis, whereas OPG knockout mice develop severe osteoporosis. This illustrates the importance of the balance between RANKL and OPG in control of bone remodelling. Other synonyms used in the literature for RANKL are osteoclast differentiation factor (ODF), osteoprotegerin ligand (OPG-L) and TNF-related activation-induced cytokine (TRANCE). The decoy receptor OPG is also known as osteoclastogenesis inhibitory factor (OCIF) and TNF receptor-like molecule 1 (TR1) (For review see BOYLE et al. 2003; SUDA et al. 1999; TEITELBAUM 2000).

RANKL, RANK and OPG, although considered the bottleneck of osteoclastogenesis, represent approximately one-tenth of genes and loci that can control osteoclastogenesis and activation (BOYLE et al. 2003). On the basis of knockout models, it is possible to delineate a genetic cascade that controls osteoclast differentiation. The *PU.1* gene apparently acts at the earliest stages in this cascade, since mice with a loss of function mutation lack both osteoclasts and macrophages. *PU.1* is suggested to regulate the expression of the M-CSF receptor on cells of the monocyte/macrophage lineage (TONDRAVI et al. 1997). Mice with a severe defect in their *M-CSF* gene (*op/op* mice) generate only immature macrophages and are deficient in osteoclasts (CECCHINI et al. 1997). The next steps of osteoclast differentiation are impaired by the absence of cytoplasmic tumour necrosis factor receptor-associated factor (TRAF)-2, -5, and -6, which interact with the intercellular domain of RANK. Among the six major downstream signalling pathways are NFATc1, NF-κB, Akt/PKB, and the three mitogen-activated protein kinases (MAPK): extracellular signal-regulated kinase (ERK), p38, and c-Jun NH (2)-terminal kinase (JNK), which play distinct roles in osteoclast differentiation, function and survival. Intracellular signalling pathways can be modulated by interferon (IFN)-γ, which promotes degradation of TRAF-6, and IFN-β, which down-regulates one of the master genes of osteoclastogenesis c-fos. Activation of the co-stimulatory receptors Fc receptor common gamma chain

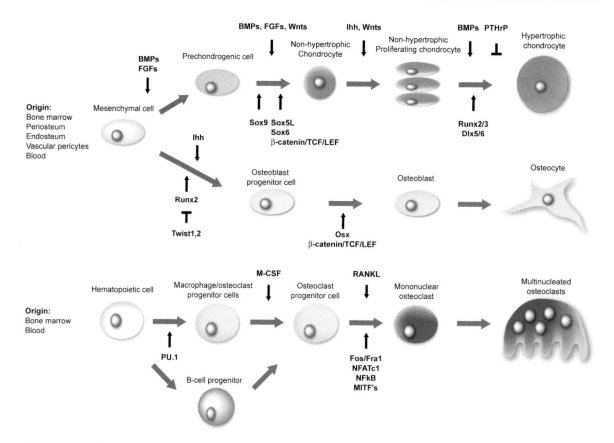

Fig. 1.3. Bone formation during development, remodelling and repair requires the continuous supply of mesenchymal progenitor cells that can differentiate into the chondrogenic and the osteogenic lineage. The phenotypic changes associated with the specialization of the cells is a multistep process, which is controlled by growth and differentiation factors that bind to their respective receptor on the cell surface and initiate a signalling cascade within the cells. These signals can regulate the expression of transcription factors, some of which are master genes that control the transition from one stem cell to the next in the differentiation cascade and the activity of the mature phenotype. Osteoclasts originate from haematopoietic lineage cells. Among the signalling molecules required for obtaining functional osteoclasts are M-CSF and RANKL. M-CSF controls the early transition of progenitor cells into the macrophage/osteoclastogenesis lineage and the proliferation and survival of more mature phenotypes. RANKL is the key regulator of osteoclast formation, activation and survival, and controls downstream transcription factors that can also be considered master genes. Inactivation of these particular genes arrests the process of osteoclastogenesis at a transition step or the resorptive activity. (KOBAYASHI and KRONENBERG)

(FcRγ) and DNAX-activating protein 12 (DAP12), both of which harbour the immunoreceptor tyrosine-based activation motif (ITAM), can activate calcium signalling, thereby mediating activation of NFATc1 (TAKAYANAGI 2005). Mice in which the genes for either αvβ3 integrin or the tyrosine kinase c-Src were knocked out generate differentiated but functionally impaired osteoclasts. Finally, failure to produce functional proteins such as H⁺-ATPase, carboanhydrase II, or cathepsin K renders osteoclasts incapable of bone resorption. Human phenotypes caused by mutation show the same characteristics; for example juvenile Paget's disease is associated with a mutation in the gene coding for OPG (WHYTE

et al. 2002), and mutation of carboanhydrase II produces osteopetrosis (SLY et al. 1983).

Inflammatory cytokines provide co-stimulatory signals that directly modulate osteoclastogenesis, besides their indirect activity via increasing the expression of RANKL by stromal cells/osteoblasts. Hence, IL-1 and TNF-α, which are highly abundant at sites of chronic inflammation, can amplify the process of osteoclastogenesis under permissive levels of RANKL (LAM et al. 2000; WEI et al. 2005). Both cytokines are pathologic factors in the progression of bone resorption in rheumatoid arthritis, and neutralization of their bioactivity by intravenous infusion of antagonists or antibodies is an approved therapy

(FLEISCHMANN et al. 2004; MIHARA et al. 2005). However, neither cytokine appears to be required for bone development, since disruption of either of the cytokine receptors in mice results in a minimal bone phenotype (LORENZO et al. 1998; PESCHON et al. 1998).

Bisphosphonates, which are considered first-line therapies for osteoporosis, also target osteoclasts. Bisphosphonates are incorporated into the bone matrix, and once released and endocytosed by the osteoclast, they inhibit farnesyl diphosphate synthase, which is required for the synthesis of GTB-binding proteins such as Rho, Rab and Cdc42. As these proteins are essential for osteoclast activity and survival, the overall resorption rate of osteoclasts is diminished and bone remodelling slows down. Other targets for inhibition of osteoclast function involve the RANKL–RANK–OPG axis, H^+-ATPase, carboanhydrase II, or cathepsin K, the $\alpha v \beta 3$ integrin receptor, the c-src kinase, and p38 (RODAN and MARTIN 2000). One should take into account that the osteoclasts provide a paracrine microenvironment with osteoblasts and their progenitor cells are potential target cells. New concepts of antiresorptive therapy should therefore not trigger osteoclast apoptosis, but only block the resorptive activity (MARTIN and SIMS 2005).

1.5
Local and Systemic Regulation of Bone Remodelling

The control of bone remodelling is complex and orchestrated by numerous local and systemic factors, and their expression and release is controlled by regulatory loops. Furthermore, the number and the responsiveness of the bone cells have an impact on bone remodelling. Local and systemic factors can affect bone remodelling by directly or indirectly targeting mature cells and their respective progenitor cells. The following is a brief report on some of the main actions of local factors and a summary of the physiologic function of systemic factors that regulate bone mass. Fig. 1.4, Fig. 1.5

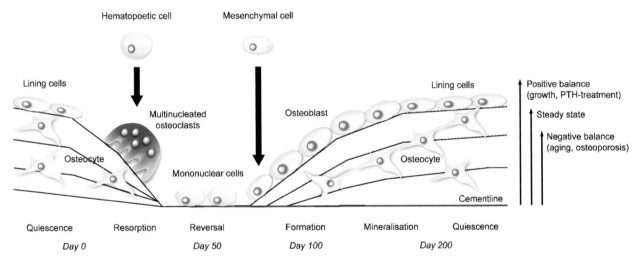

Fig. 1.4. Bone remodelling is a highly coordinated process where the space resorbed by osteoclasts is rebuilt by a team of osteoblasts. The need for bone to remodel is likely to be sensed by the osteocytes, which signal to the bone lining cells. Lining cells contract and digest the underlying nonmineralized matrix. Osteoclast progenitors are attracted and differentiated into bone-resorbing phenotypes. In trabecular bone, the Howship lacunas are approximately 50 µm deep when osteoclast sundergo apoptosis. Mononuclear cells appear, which are suggested to smooth the bone surface and stimulate the formation of the cementlines. The cementlines represent the transition of bone resorption and bone formation. Hence, osteoblast progenitor cells invade the remodelling site and differentiate into mature osteoblasts. Bone is rebuilt up to the original level before osteoblasts are thought to differentiate into lining cells. The other osteoblasts are buried in the bone matrix as osteocytes or die by apoptosis. Bone resorption requires less time than the formation phase. A negative balance of this remodelling unit causes bone loss and can culminate in the pathologic picture of osteoporosis. Osteoporosis therapies try to bring the remodelling unit back into balance. Bisphosphonates mainly decrease bone resorption, which causes the decrease in the formation rate, as both processes are combined. Intermediated PTH can reactivate bone lining cells and increase the lifespan of the osteoclasts and can thereby cause a positive net balance of bone formation over resorption

Stimulation of bone formation: Stimulation of bone resorption:

BMP   **Oestrogen Deficiencey**
LRP5/Wnt   **Immobilisation**
(β-blockers)   **Low Ca (PTH)**
Intermittent PTH
Mechanical Load   Multinucleated
Androgens   osteoclasts

Osteoblast

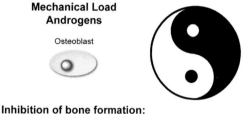

Inhibition of bone formation: Inhibition of bone resorption:

SOST   **Oestrogen**
Leptin/β-adrenergic   **SERMs**
Immobilisation   **Bisphosphonates**
Ageing   **Calcitonin**
                                         Calcium, Vitamin D

Fig. 1.5. The steady state levels of bone remodelling can be controlled on the side of bone resorption and bone formation. On both sides, local cues and systemic factors including pharmacologic substances for osteoporosis therapy can act as inhibitors and activators of either of the two sides of bone remodelling. A constant skeletal haemostasis and bone mass is achieved by feedback regulatory mechanisms that combines bone formation and bone resorption

1.5.1
Local Regulation of Bone Mass by Growth Factors, Cytokines and Prostaglandins

Members of the BMP family, Wnt family, hedgehog family and growth factors such as transforming growth factor-β, platelet-derived growth factor, fibroblast growth factor, and insulin-like growth factor can modulate the various steps of osteoblastogenesis, e.g. commit pluripotent mesenchymal cells to the osteoblastic lineage, stimulate migration and proliferation and promote their further differentiation into mature cells (Govoni et al. 2005; Marie 2003; Roelen and Dijke 2003).

Moreover, local growth factors can also enhance or inhibit osteoclast formation and function. Interleukin-1 (IL-1), IL-3, IL-6, IL-11, leukaemia inhibitory factor (LIF), ciliary neutrophilic factor (CNTF), tumour necrosis factor (TNF), granulocyte macrophage-colony stimulating factor (GM-CSF), M-CSF, and c-kit ligand are among those growth factors that enhance osteoclast activity, whereas cytokines such as IL-4, IL-10, IL-18, and interferon-γ inhibit the development of osteoclasts. Prostaglandins are also centrally involved in bone remodelling and repair and target osteogenic cells as well as osteoclasts (Okada et al. 2000; Zhang et al. 2002). Deviations from the coordinated expression of these cytokines and growth factors in various cell types such as

osteoblasts/stromal cells, monocytes/macrophages, lymphocytes, and malignant cells have been implicated in several pathologic conditions associated with increased bone loss such as osteoporosis, Paget's disease, and tumour hypercalcaemia. Moreover, it should be clearly stated that most of the local factors influence both the osteoblastic and the osteoclastic lineage (Manolagas 2000; Roodman 1996; Takayanagi 2005).

1.5.2
Systemic Factors that Regulate Bone Mass

1.5.2.1
Parathyroid Hormone

Parathyroid hormone (PTH) is an 84-amino acid peptide and the main factor responsible for the short-term regulation of calcium homeostasis. Extracellular calcium levels provide the signals for PTH secretion, a process controlled by the calcium-sensing receptor on the parathyroid cell. PTH increases renal tubular absorption of calcium, whereas it inhibits the tubular reabsorption of phosphate. PTH also stimulates the renal synthesis of $1,25(OH)_2D_3$, thereby increasing calcium and phosphate absorption through the intestinal tract. Moreover, PTH enhances bone resorption.

The biologic activity of PTH resides in the N-terminus, with most clinical studies using the first 34-amino acids, now termed teriparatide (NEER et al. 2001). After 1 year of anabolic therapy with teriparatide, bisphosphonates can further increase bone mineral density (BLACK et al. 2005). In the serum, however, C-terminal fragments are the major PTH species, which do not bind to the classical PTH receptor and the existence of a separate receptor for the C-terminus is postulated (MURRAY et al. 2005). Intermittently administered PTH and N-terminal PTH peptide fragments or analogues also augment bone mass and currently are being introduced into clinical practice as therapies for osteoporosis. The mechanism of action can be based on an increase of the bone-remodelling rate by activating previously quiescent lining cells and increased motility of osteogenic cells in their BMUs (DOBNIG and TURNER 1997). PTH can also prevent osteoblast apoptosis (JILKA et al. 1999). Together, a larger osteoid-covered surface, an increase in trabecular connectivity and a greater radial outer dimension of the cortex characterize teriparatide treatment. The clinical aspects of the anabolic therapy will be covered in the chapter by P.M. Bernecker (HODSMAN et al. 2005; SHRADER and RAGUCCI 2005).

1.5.2.2
1,25-Dihydroxyvitamin D_3

Sources of vitamin D are either dietary or endogenously produced in the skin from 7-dehydrocholesterol under the influence of ultraviolet light in the epidermis. Bound to a specific vitamin D-binding protein in the blood, it is transported to the liver where it is hydroxylated at the C-25 position, thus being converted to $25(OH)_2D_3$. A second hydroxylation at the C-1 position takes place in the kidney, resulting in the formation of the most potent metabolite, $1,25(OH)_2D_3$. In addition, the local production of $1,25(OH)_2D_3$ by the extrarenal 1-hydroxylase has been described. When serum calcium levels are high, the kidney increases the 24-hydroxylase activity, which ensures the synthesis of the relatively inactive metabolites $24,25(OH)_2D_3$ and $1,24,25(OH)_2D_3$. A complex of $1,25(OH)_2D_3$ together with the vitamin D receptor (VDR) binds to a vitamin D-responsive element on the DNA, which has been identified in, for example, the promoter region of osteocalcin, 24-hydroxylase and calbindin D_{28k}. Vitamin D metabolites are also considered to have rapid actions mediated via membrane receptors

(NORMAN et al. 2004). Since $1,25(OH)_2D_3$ has potent effects on calcium homeostasis, its production has to be strictly regulated. High levels of PTH as a result of hypocalcaemia stimulate 1-hydroxylase activities in the kidney, whereas high levels of calcium and $1,25(OH)_2D_3$ have inhibitory effects. The enzymatic activity of the 24-hydroxylase is reciprocally regulated. The classical target tissues of $1,25(OH)_2D_3$ are bone, intestine, and the kidney. In bone, the active vitamin D metabolite stimulates the activity of the osteoclasts and also has effects on the osteoblasts, where it increases the production of extracellular matrix proteins such as osteocalcin and osteopontin. The effects of $1,25(OH)_2D_3$ on intestinal calcium absorption involve stimulation of the synthesis of calbindins. This group of proteins is known to bind calcium and transports it against a concentration gradient. Calbindins have also been found in the kidney and may be involved in $1,25(OH)_2D_3$-dependent reabsorption of calcium. In addition, $1,25(OH)_2D_3$ inhibits the synthesis and secretion of PTH in the parathyroid gland. Therapeutic application of $1,25(OH)_2D_3$ and calcium can lower the probability of hip and all nonvertebral fractures in elderly women who lived in care homes by 29% and 24%, respectively (CHAPUY et al. 1992, 1994) (For review see BOUILLON et al. 1995; CHRISTAKOS et al. 2003; DELUCA 1988; DUSSO et al. 2005).

1.5.2.3
Calcitonin

Calcitonin is a 32-amino-acid peptide hormone produced by the C cells of the thyroid gland. In contrast to PTH and $1,25(OH)_2D_3$, both of which increase calcium release from the mineralized matrix, calcitonin is an inhibitor of osteoclast activity. Calcitonin is not secreted until plasma calcium levels reached approximately 9.5 mg/dl. In addition, β-adrenergic agonists, dopamine, and oestradiol stimulate calcitonin secretion. Calcitonin is approved as a treatment for osteoporosis, but is not considered first-line therapy (DELMAS 2002). Nevertheless, the physiologic role of calcitonin in humans is largely unclear (INZERILLO et al. 2004).

1.5.2.4
Oestradiol

Oestrogens can regulate calcium homeostasis, which is an essential requirement during fetal development and postnatal lactation. Oestrogen deficiency, after menopause or following ovariectomy is associated with a progressive loss of trabecular bone structure, also increasing the perforation of cortical bone. Oestrogen loss causes high bone remodelling rates, where bone formation cannot compensate for the increased resorption. To study the mechanisms of oestradiol function on bone turnover, mouse models with impaired oestradiol receptor (ER) isoforms were developed. ERα-deficient mice showed decreased bone remodelling, a higher trabecular bone volume and a thinner cortex, in both sexes. In the ERβ-deficient models, female mice show a similar picture to ERα-deficient mice, whereas the male counterparts have no aberrant bone phenotype. It was concluded that ERα is relevant in male mice, but in female both receptors are of critical importance for bone remodelling (SIMS et al. 2002). Also nongenotropic effects of sex steroids by synthetic ligand can prevent bone loss induced in ovariectomized and orchidectomized mice, without affecting reproductive organs (KOUSTENI et al. 2002).

Androgen receptor (AR)-deficient mouse models also have increased bone turnover, which is associated with low testosterone levels. Interestingly, substitution of testosterone but not dihydrotestosterone, which cannot be converted to oestradiol by the aromatase, can compensate for orchiedectomy-induced bone loss. These findings further suggest that the ERs are of critical importance for bone preservation in male mice (KAWANO et al. 2003). In humans, testosterone is more potently converted into oestradiol by the aromatase expressed in bone and adipose tissue, leading to oestradiol levels of about 30 pg/ml in men (KHOSLA et al. 2001).

The effects of oestrogen on bone cells is complex and occurs at multiple sites: Oestrogen deficiency is associated with increasing medullary numbers of mesenchymal progenitor cells and progenitors of osteoclasts, in mice (JILKA et al. 1995, 1998). Monocytes, T cells and B cells from individuals with postmenopausal osteoporosis have a higher density of RANKL on their cell membrane (EGHBALI-FATOURECHI et al. 2003), and oestrogen can positively regulate OPG expression (HOFBAUER et al. 1999). Oestrogen levels can also regulate the expression of cytokines of blood and marrow-derived cells, e.g. IL-1 and TNF-α, which in turn can influence the formation, activation and survival of osteoclasts (BISMAR et al. 1995; LAM et al. 2000; WEI et al. 2005; ZHENG et al. 1997). Cytokines and other bioactive molecules, which are regulated by oestradiol presumably, act in cooperation, control each other's

expression and may have synergistic effects on their target cells (JILKA 1998). Blocking of each single cytokine, IL-1, IL-6 and TNF-α, can counteract bone loss in the ovariectomy mouse model (JILKA et al. 1992; KITAZAWA et al. 1994). T-cell-derived TNF-α is suggested to be a key factor of bone loss in this model, involving the TGF-β-mediated mechanism (GAO et al. 2004; ROGGIA et al. 2001). Also B cells, which provide a subset of osteoclast progenitors and the cytokine IL-7, are considered to be players in the process of ovariectomy-induced bone loss (MIYAURA et al. 1997; TORALDO et al. 2003).

Oestrogen and androgen are also a proapoptotic factor for osteoclasts, implying that steroid deficiency extends the lifetime of the bone-resorbing cell (HUGHES et al. 1996; KAMEDA et al. 1997). Oestradiol deficiency can lower the lifespan of osteoblasts and osteocytes, thereby signalling the need for increased bone remodelling. Oestradiol can trigger the differentiation of progenitor cells into the osteogenic vs the adipogenic lineage (VERMA et al. 2002) and can stimulate the expression of RUNX-2, which parallels the increased osteogenic differentiation of in vitro cell cultures. However, growing concern about the efficacy and safety of existing hormone replacement therapies makes them no longer first-line therapy for osteoporosis. Future clinical trials that fully integrate the complex pleiotropic actions of oestrogens and progesterone and their analogues will provide answers to questions on postmenopausal roles for HT (TURGEON et al. 2004) (For review see SYED and KHOSLA 2005).

1.5.3
Sympathic Nervous System

The central nervous system can contribute to the control of bone remodelling. Leptin is a hormone produced by adipocytes that, besides its function in regulating body weight and gonadal function, can also act as an inhibitor of bone formation, as confirmed by leptin-deficient (*ob/ob*), leptin receptor-deficient and lipodystrophic mouse models (DUCY et al. 2000a). In the absence of leptin signalling, the bone mass increases. Interestingly, leptin deficiency is the only known condition resulting in the coexistence of high bone mass and hypogonadism, a condition that otherwise favours bone loss. Blocking of β-adrenergic receptors with propranolol in wild type and ovariectomized mice can simulate the bone-protective effects of leptin deficiency, whereas activation of the receptor with isoproterenol led to a decrease in the bone mass in leptin-deficient and wild type mice (TAKEDA et al. 2002). Propranolol was also reported to stimulate fracture healing in a rat model (MINKOWITZ et al. 1991). In agreement with these findings, mice lacking the β2-adrenergic receptor or those that lack the dopamine hydroxylase necessary to synthesize the neurotransmitter released by sympathetic neurons have increased bone mass in wild type and ovariectomized mice. β2-adrenergic receptor-deficient mice further showed that the sympathetic nervous system decreases bone formation parameters but enhances bone resorption by increasing expression of RANKL (ELEFTERIOU et al. 2005). Together these findings led to the speculation that the postmenopausal decrease in oestradiol levels may be linked to sympathetic nervous activity, e.g. ovariectomy in mice causes a dramatic loss of the nerves that usually penetrate bone (BURT-PICHAT et al. 2005). Moreover, treatment of hypertension with β-blockers is associated with a reduced risk of fractures, taken alone as well as in combination with thiazide diuretics (PASCO et al. 2004; SCHLIENGER et al. 2004), although in other studies, β-blocker use and bone mineral density are unrelated, and associations with fracture risk inconsistent (REID et al. 2005). Besides leptin, signalling via one receptor for neuropeptide Y in neurons (BALDOCK et al. 2002) and thyroid-stimulating hormone (TSH) can regulate bone mass (ABE et al. 2003) (For review see DUCY et al. 2000b; HARADA and RODAN 2003; TAKEDA 2005).

1.6 Discussion of Current Status and Perspectives

Within the last decade, much knowledge has been gained on the local and systemic regulation of bone development. Animal models on gain- or loss-of-function mutations as well as genetic studies of disease that affect the skeletal development provided insights into the orchestration of this multistep process. Systemic hormones and local growth and differentiation factors regulate the expression of transcription factors, the interface and master regulators that control the commitment and differentiation of mesenchymal and haematopoietic

progenitor cells into the mature phenotypes, osteoblasts, osteocytes and osteoclasts, respectively. This book presents the diagnostic and imaging of osteoporotic bone rather than treating growing bone. The control of bone remodelling is central to this work because increased bone remodelling associated with an over-proportional bone resorption causes postmenopausal osteoporosis. This first chapter has extensively covered the control of bone development because there is increasing evidence that the same mechanisms are also functional in the adult organism during remodelling. Intensive research is required to understand the common pathways of bone development and remodelling and how alteration of these mechanisms can add to the development of osteoporosis.

Changes in the bone remodelling rate can be monitored by biochemical parameters. Bone mineral density imaging with dual X-ray absorptiometry (DXA) provides the current definition of osteoporosis by the WHO. However, biochemical parameters and DXA's usefulness for making predictions on the fracture risk is limited. High-resolution imaging techniques such as computed tomography (CT) and magnet resonance imaging (MRI) that take the three-dimensional bone architecture into account are evaluated to assess the fracture risk in large studies. Moreover, finite element analysis comprises mathematical models where the 3D structural information provides the basis for calculating how much load bone can bear. Understanding the process of bone remodelling allows interpretation of bone histology, and hopefully in the near future high-resolution pictures made by noninvasive radiologic imaging techniques (STOKSTAD 2005).

Potent drugs help to reduce the fracture risk, but fractures still occur. Fracture repair in the compromised osteoporotic patient has not gained that much attention and the treatment options are currently rather conventional. Based on the knowledge of the local mechanisms of bone regeneration that basically recapitulate the program of bone development, new therapies have been developed that support the naturally occurring progress and support the healing cascade in fractures that sometimes refuse to heal.

Bone remodelling is the key to understanding the pathophysiology of systemic bone loss: postmenopausal and senile osteoporosis, glucocorticoid-induced osteoporosis, osteoporosis associated with chronic inflammation and osteoporosis following organ transplantation are to be distinguished. Other causes of osteoporosis are tumour burden, low mechanical loading due to bed rest or space flight and malnutrition. Each type of osteoporosis has its particular causes that influence the parameters of bone remodelling. Moreover, therapeutic options to decrease the fracture risk in osteoporotic patients such as bisphosphonates, selective oestrogen-receptor modulators (SERMs), PTH, strontium renelate, hormone replacement therapy, calcitonin, and vitamin D and calcium supplements all affect bone remodelling through different means. The BMU is the door to osteoporosis diagnosis and therapy and for the new recommended nomenclature of drugs used to treat osteoporosis: the new term "anticatabolic" it is consistent not only with a decrease in resorption but also with a decrease in the total number of BMUs, hence a reduction of bone remodelling. Anabolic drugs increase formation more than resorption. The terms "anabolic" and "anticatabolic" not only describe the therapeutic effects more clearly but are semantically more appropriate because the literal definition of "anabolic" is to build up and that of "catabolic" is to break down (RIGGS and PARFITT 2005).

References

Abe E, Yamamoto M, Taguchi Y, Lecka-Czernik B, O'Brien CA, Economides AN, Stahl N, Jilka RL, Manolagas SC (2000) Essential requirement of BMPs-2/4 for both osteoblast and osteoclast formation in murine bone marrow cultures from adult mice: antagonism by noggin. J Bone Miner Res 15:663–673

Abe E, Marians RC, Yu W, Wu XB, Ando T, Li Y, Iqbal J, Eldeiry L, Rajendren G, Blair HC, Davies TF, Zaidi M (2003) TSH is a negative regulator of skeletal remodeling. Cell 115:151–162

Ai M, Holmen SL, Van Hul W, Williams BO, Warman ML (2005) Reduced affinity to and inhibition by DKK1 form a common mechanism by which high bone mass-associated missense mutations in LRP5 affect canonical Wnt signaling. Mol Cell Biol 25:4946–4955

Anderson HC, Garimella R, Tague SE (2005) The role of matrix vesicles in growth plate development and biomineralization. Front Biosci 10:822–837

Asahara T, Kawamoto A (2004) Endothelial progenitor cells for postnatal vasculogenesis. Am J Physiol Cell Physiol 287:C572–C579

Baldock PA, Sainsbury A, Couzens M, Enriquez RF, Thomas GP, Gardiner EM, Herzog H (2002) Hypothalamic Y2 receptors regulate bone formation. J Clin Invest 109:915–921

Barnes GL, Kostenuik PJ, Gerstenfeld LC, Einhorn TA (1999) Growth factor regulation of fracture repair. J Bone Miner Res 14:1805–1815

Baron R (1993) Anatomy and ultrastructure of bone. In: Favus MJ (ed) Primer on the metabolic bone diseases and disorders of mineral metabolism. Raven, New York, pp 3–9

Bellido T, Ali AA, Gubrij I, Plotkin LI, Fu Q, O'Brien C A, Manolagas SC, Jilka RL (2005) Chronic elevation of PTH in mice reduces expression of sclerostin by osteocytes: a novel mechanism for hormonal control of osteoblastogenesis. Endocrinology 146:4577–4583

Berglundh T, Abrahamsson I, Lang NP, Lindhe J (2003) De novo alveolar bone formation adjacent to endosseous implants. Clin Oral Implants Res 14:251–262

Bialek P, Kern B, Yang X, Schrock M, Sosic D, Hong N, Wu H, Yu K, Ornitz DM, Olson EN, Justice MJ, Karsenty G (2004) A twist code determines the onset of osteoblast differentiation. Dev Cell 6:423–35

Bismar H, Diel I, Ziegler R, Pfeilschifter J (1995) Increased cytokine secretion by human bone marrow cells after menopause or discontinuation of estrogen replacement. J Clin Endocrinol Metab 80:3351–3355

Black DM, Bilezikian JP, Ensrud KE, Greenspan SL, Palermo L, Hue T, Lang TF, McGowan JA, Rosen CJ (2005) One year of alendronate after one year of parathyroid hormone (1–84) for osteoporosis. N Engl J Med 353:555–565

Bouillon R, Okamura WH, Norman AW (1995) Structure-function relationships in the vitamin D endocrine system. Endocr Rev 16:200–257

Boyden LM, Mao J, Belsky J, Mitzner L, Farhi A, Mitnick MA, Wu D, Insogna K, Lifton RP (2002) High bone density due to a mutation in LDL-receptor-related protein 5. N Engl J Med 346:1513–1521

Boyle WJ, Simonet WS, Lacey DL (2003) Osteoclast differentiation and activation. Nature 423:337–342

Burt-Pichat B, Lafage-Proust MH, Duboeuf F, Laroche N, Itzstein C, Vico L, Delmas PD, Chenu C (2005) Dramatic decrease of innervation density in bone after ovariectomy. Endocrinology 146:503–510

Canalis E, Economides AN, Gazzerro E (2003) Bone morphogenetic proteins, their antagonists, and the skeleton. Endocr Rev 24:218–235

Cancedda R, Dozin B, Giannoni P, Quarto R (2003) Tissue engineering and cell therapy of cartilage and bone. Matrix Biol 22:81–91

Caplan AI, Bruder SP (2001) Mesenchymal stem cells: building blocks for molecular medicine in the 21st century. Trends Mol Med 7:259–264

Carano RA, Filvaroff EH (2003) Angiogenesis and bone repair. Drug Discov Today 8:980–989

Cardaropoli G, Araujo M, Lindhe J (2003) Dynamics of bone tissue formation in tooth extraction sites. An experimental study in dogs. J Clin Periodontol 30:809–818

Carmeliet P (2000) Mechanisms of angiogenesis and arteriogenesis. Nat Med 6:389–395

Cecchini MG, Hofstetter W, Halasy J, Wetterwald A, Felix R (1997) Role of CSF-1 in bone and bone marrow development. Mol Reprod Dev 46:75–83; discussion 83 84

Chapuy MC, Arlot ME, Duboeuf F, Brun J, Crouzet B, Arnaud S, Delmas PD, Meunier PJ (1992) Vitamin D3 and calcium to prevent hip fractures in the elderly women. N Engl J Med 327:1637–1642

Chapuy MC, Arlot ME, Delmas PD, Meunier PJ (1994) Effect of calcium and cholecalciferol treatment for three years on hip fractures in elderly women. BMJ 308:1081–1082

Chavassieux PM, Arlot ME, Reda C, Wei L, Yates AJ, Meunier PJ (1997) Histomorphometric assessment of the long-term effects of alendronate on bone quality and remodeling in patients with osteoporosis. J Clin Invest 100:1475–1480

Christakos S, Dhawan P, Liu Y, Peng X, Porta A (2003) New insights into the mechanisms of vitamin D action. J Cell Biochem 88:695–705

Cummings SR, Melton LJ (2002) Epidemiology and outcomes of osteoporotic fractures. Lancet 359:1761–1767

Dai J, Rabie AB, Hagg U, Xu R (2004) Alternative gene therapy strategies for the repair of craniofacial bone defects. Curr Gene Ther 4:469–485

Day TF, Guo X, Garrett-Beal L, Yang Y (2005) Wnt/beta-catenin signaling in mesenchymal progenitors controls osteoblast and chondrocyte differentiation during vertebrate skeletogenesis. Dev Cell 8:739–750

Delmas PD (2002) Treatment of postmenopausal osteoporosis. Lancet 359:2018–2026

Delmas PD, Hardy P, Garnero P, Dain M (2000) Monitoring individual response to hormone replacement therapy with bone markers. Bone 26:553–560

DeLuca HF (1988) The vitamin D story: a collaborative effort of basic science and clinical medicine. FASEB J 2:224–36

Devlin RD, Du Z, Pereira RC, Kimble RB, Economides AN, Jorgetti V, Canalis E (2003) Skeletal overexpression of noggin results in osteopenia and reduced bone formation. Endocrinology 144:1972–1978

Dobnig H, Turner RT (1997) The effects of programmed administration of human parathyroid hormone fragment (1–34) on bone histomorphometry and serum chemistry in rats. Endocrinology 138:4607–4612

Doherty MJ, Ashton BA, Walsh S, Beresford JN, Grant ME, Canfield AE (1998) Vascular pericytes express osteogenic potential in vitro and in vivo. J Bone Miner Res 13:828–838

Ducy P, Desbois C, Boyce B, Pinero G, Story B, Dunstan C, Smith E, Bonadio J, Goldstein S, Gundberg C, Bradley A, Karsenty G (1996) Increased bone formation in osteocalcin-deficient mice. Nature 382:448–452

Ducy P, Zhang R, Geoffroy V, Ridall AL, Karsenty G (1997) Osf2/Cbfa1: a transcriptional activator of osteoblast differentiation. Cell 89:747–754

Ducy P, Amling M, Takeda S, Priemel M, Schilling AF, Beil FT, Shen J, Vinson C, Rueger JM, Karsenty G (2000a) Leptin inhibits bone formation through a hypothalamic relay: a central control of bone mass. Cell 100:197–207

Ducy P, Schinke T, Karsenty G (2000b) The osteoblast: a sophisticated fibroblast under central surveillance. Science 289:1501–1504

Dusso AS, Brown AJ, Slatopolsky E (2005) Vitamin D. Am J Physiol Renal Physiol 289:F8–F28

Eghbali-Fatourechi G, Khosla S, Sanyal A, Boyle WJ, Lacey DL, Riggs BL (2003) Role of RANK ligand in mediating increased bone resorption in early postmenopausal women. J Clin Invest 111:1221–1230

Eghbali-Fatourechi GZ, Lamsam J, Fraser D, Nagel D, Riggs BL, Khosla S (2005) Circulating osteoblast-lineage cells in humans. N Engl J Med 352:1959–1966

Eisman JA (2001) Good, good, good... good vibrations: the best option for better bones? Lancet 358:1924–1925

Elefteriou F, Ahn JD, Takeda S, Starbuck M, Yang X, Liu X, Kondo H, Richards WG, Bannon TW, Noda M, Clement K, Vaisse C, Karsenty G (2005) Leptin regulation of bone resorption by the sympathetic nervous system and CART. Nature 434:514–520

Fini M, Giavaresi G, Setti S, Martini L, Torricelli P, Giardino R (2004) Current trends in the enhancement of biomaterial osteointegration: biophysical stimulation. Int J Artif Organs 27:681–690

Fleischmann RM, Iqbal I, Stern RL (2004) Considerations with the use of biological therapy in the treatment of rheumatoid arthritis. Expert Opin Drug Saf 3:391–403

Francis-West PH, Parish J, Lee K, Archer CW (1999) BMP/GDF-signalling interactions during synovial joint development. Cell Tissue Res 296:111–119

Frost HM (1994) Wolff's Law and bone's structural adaptations to mechanical usage: an overview for clinicians. Angle Orthod 64:175–188

Frost HM (2004) A 2003 update of bone physiology and Wolff's Law for clinicians. Angle Orthod 74:3–15

Gao Y, Qian WP, Dark K, Toraldo G, Lin AS, Guldberg RE, Flavell RA, Weitzmann MN, Pacifici R (2004) Estrogen prevents bone loss through transforming growth factor beta signaling in T cells. Proc Natl Acad Sci U S A 101:16618–16623

Geoffroy V, Kneissel M, Fournier B, Boyde A, Matthias P (2002) High bone resorption in adult aging transgenic mice overexpressing cbfa1/runx2 in cells of the osteoblastic lineage. Mol Cell Biol 22:6222–6233

Gerstenfeld LC, Cullinane DM, Barnes GL, Graves DT, Einhorn TA (2003) Fracture healing as a post-natal developmental process: molecular, spatial, and temporal aspects of its regulation. J Cell Biochem 88:873–884

Glass DA 2nd, Bialek P, Ahn JD, Starbuck M, Patel MS, Clevers H, Taketo MM, Long F, McMahon AP, Lang RA, Karsenty G (2005) Canonical Wnt signaling in differentiated osteoblasts controls osteoclast differentiation. Dev Cell 8:751–764

Gong Y, Slee RB, Fukai N, Rawadi G, Roman-Roman S, Reginato AM, Wang H, Cundy T, Glorieux FH, Lev D, Zacharin M, Oexle K, Marcelino J, Suwairi W, Heeger S, Sabatakos G, Apte S, Adkins WN, Allgrove J, Arslan-Kirchner M, Batch JA, Beighton P, Black GC, Boles RG, Boon LM, Borrone C, Brunner HG, Carle GF, Dallapiccola B, De Paepe A, Floege B, Halfhide ML, Hall B, Hennekam RC, Hirose T, Jans A, Juppner H, Kim CA, Keppler-Noreuil K, Kohlschuetter A, LaCombe D, Lambert M, Lemyre E, Letteboer T, Peltonen L, Ramesar RS, Romanengo M, Somer H, Steichen-Gersdorf E, Steinmann B, Sullivan B, Superti-Furga A, Swoboda W, van den Boogaard MJ, Van Hul W, Vikkula M, Votruba M, Zabel B, Garcia T, Baron R, Olsen BR, Warman ML (2001) LDL receptor-related protein 5 (LRP5) affects bone accrual and eye development. Cell 107:513–523

Govoni KE, Baylink DJ, Mohan S (2005) The multi-functional role of insulin-like growth factor binding proteins in bone. Pediatr Nephrol 20:261–268

Harada S, Rodan GA (2003) Control of osteoblast function and regulation of bone mass. Nature 423:349–355

He X, Semenov M, Tamai K, Zeng X (2004) LDL receptor-related proteins 5 and 6 in Wnt/beta-catenin signaling: arrows point the way. Development 131:1663–1677

Hill TP, Spater D, Taketo MM, Birchmeier W, Hartmann C (2005) Canonical Wnt/beta-catenin signaling prevents osteoblasts from differentiating into chondrocytes. Dev Cell 8:727–738

Hodsman AB, Bauer DC, Dempster DW, Dian L, Hanley DA, Harris ST, Kendler DL, McClung MR, Miller PD, Olszynski WP, Orwoll E, Yuen CK (2005) Parathyroid Hormone and Teriparatide for the Treatment of Osteoporosis: A Review of the Evidence and Suggested Guidelines for Its Use. Endocr Rev 26:688–703

Hofbauer LC, Khosla S, Dunstan CR, Lacey DL, Spelsberg TC, Riggs BL (1999) Estrogen stimulates gene expression and protein production of osteoprotegerin in human osteoblastic cells. Endocrinology 140:4367–4370

Hoshi K, Komori T, Ozawa H (1999) Morphological characterization of skeletal cells in Cbfa1-deficient mice. Bone 25:639–651

Hughes DE, Dai A, Tiffee JC, Li HH, Mundy GR, Boyce BF (1996) Estrogen promotes apoptosis of murine osteoclasts mediated by TGF-beta. Nat Med 2:1132–1136

Inzerillo AM, Zaidi M, Huang CL (2004) Calcitonin: physiological actions and clinical applications. J Pediatr Endocrinol Metab 17:931–940

Ito H, Koefoed M, Tiyapatanaputi P, Gromov K, Goater JJ, Carmouche J, Zhang X, Rubery PT, Rabinowitz J, Samulski RJ, Nakamura T, Soballe K, O'Keefe RJ, Boyce BF, Schwarz EM (2005) Remodeling of cortical bone allografts mediated by adherent rAAV-RANKL and VEGF gene therapy. Nat Med 11:291–297

Jadlowiec JA, Celil AB, Hollinger JO (2003) Bone tissue engineering: recent advances and promising therapeutic agents. Expert Opin Biol Ther 3:409–423

Jilka RL (1998) Cytokines, bone remodeling, and estrogen deficiency: a 1998 update. Bone 23:75–81

Jilka RL, Hangoc G, Girasole G, Passeri G, Williams DC, Abrams JS, Boyce B, Broxmeyer H, Manolagas SC (1992) Increased osteoclast development after estrogen loss: mediation by interleukin-6. Science 257:88–91

Jilka RL, Passeri G, Girasole G, Cooper S, Abrams J, Broxmeyer H, Manolagas SC (1995) Estrogen loss upregulates hematopoiesis in the mouse: a mediating role of IL-6. Exp Hematol 23:500–506

Jilka RL, Takahashi K, Munshi M, Williams DC, Roberson PK, Manolagas SC (1998) Loss of estrogen upregulates osteoblastogenesis in the murine bone marrow. Evidence for autonomy from factors released during bone resorption. J Clin Invest 101:1942–1950

Jilka RL, Weinstein RS, Bellido T, Roberson P, Parfitt AM, Manolagas SC (1999) Increased bone formation by prevention of osteoblast apoptosis with parathyroid hormone. J Clin Invest 104:439–446

Kameda T, Mano H, Yuasa T, Mori Y, Miyazawa K, Shiokawa M, Nakamaru Y, Hiroi E, Hiura K, Kameda A, Yang NN, Hakeda Y, Kumegawa M (1997) Estrogen inhibits bone resorption by directly inducing apoptosis of the bone-resorbing osteoclasts. J Exp Med 186:489–495

Karsenty G, Wagner EF (2002) Reaching a genetic and molecular understanding of skeletal development. Dev Cell 2:389–406

Kawano H, Sato T, Yamada T, Matsumoto T, Sekine K, Watanabe T, Nakamura T, Fukuda T, Yoshimura K, Yoshizawa T, Aihara K, Yamamoto Y, Nakamichi Y, Metzger D, Chambon P, Nakamura K, Kawaguchi H, Kato S (2003) Suppressive function of androgen receptor in bone resorption. Proc Natl Acad Sci U S A 100:9416–9421

Keller H, Kneissel M (2005) SOST is a target gene for PTH in bone. Bone 37:148–158

Khosla S, Melton LJ 3rd, Atkinson EJ, O'Fallon WM (2001) Relationship of serum sex steroid levels to longitudinal changes in bone density in young versus elderly men. J Clin Endocrinol Metab 86:3555–3561

Kitazawa R, Kimble RB, Vannice JL, Kung VT, Pacifici R (1994) Interleukin-1 receptor antagonist and tumor necrosis factor binding protein decrease osteoclast formation and bone resorption in ovariectomized mice. J Clin Invest 94:2397–2406

Knothe Tate ML, Adamson JR, Tami AE, Bauer TW (2004) The osteocyte. Int J Biochem Cell Biol 36:1–8

Kobayashi T, Kronenberg H. Minireview: transcriptional regulation in development of bone. Endocrinology (2005) 146(3):1012–7

Koga T, Matsui Y, Asagiri M, Kodama T, de Crombrugghe B, Nakashima K, Takayanagi H (2005) NFAT and Osterix cooperatively regulate bone formation. Nat Med 11:880–885

Komori T, Yagi H, Nomura S, Yamaguchi A, Sasaki K, Deguchi K, Shimizu Y, Bronson RT, Gao YH, Inada M, Sato M, Okamoto R, Kitamura Y, Yoshiki S, Kishimoto T (1997) Targeted disruption of Cbfa1 results in a complete lack of bone formation owing to maturational arrest of osteoblasts. Cell 89:755–764

Kousteni S, Chen JR, Bellido T, Han L, Ali AA, O'Brien CA, Plotkin L, Fu Q, Mancino AT, Wen Y, Vertino AM, Powers CC, Stewart SA, Ebert R, Parfitt AM, Weinstein RS, Jilka RL, Manolagas SC (2002) Reversal of bone loss in mice by nongenotropic signaling of sex steroids. Science 298:843–846

Kronenberg HM (2003) Developmental regulation of the growth plate. Nature 423:332–336

Kronenberg HM (2004) Twist genes regulate Runx2 and bone formation. Dev Cell 6:317–318

Kundu M, Javed A, Jeon JP, Horner A, Shum L, Eckhaus M, Muenke M, Lian JB, Yang Y, Nuckolls GH, Stein GS, Liu PP (2002) Cbfbeta interacts with Runx2 and has a critical role in bone development. Nat Genet 32:639–644

Lam J, Takeshita S, Barker JE, Kanagawa O, Ross FP, Teitelbaum SL (2000) TNF-alpha induces osteoclastogenesis by direct stimulation of macrophages exposed to permissive levels of RANK ligand. J Clin Invest 106:1481–1488

Leach JK, Mooney DJ (2004) Bone engineering by controlled delivery of osteoinductive molecules and cells. Expert Opin Biol Ther 4:1015–1027

Lee B, Thirunavukkarasu K, Zhou L, Pastore L, Baldini A, Hecht J, Geoffroy V, Ducy P, Karsenty G (1997) Missense mutations abolishing DNA binding of the osteoblast-specific transcription factor OSF2/CBFA1 in cleidocranial dysplasia. Nat Genet 16:307–310

Li X, Zhang Y, Kang H, Liu W, Liu P, Zhang J, Harris SE, Wu D (2005) Sclerostin binds to LRP5/6 and antagonizes canonical Wnt signaling. J Biol Chem 280:19883–19887

Little RD, Carulli JP, Del Mastro RG, Dupuis J, Osborne M, Folz C, Manning SP, Swain PM, Zhao SC, Eustace B, Lappe MM, Spitzer L, Zweier S, Braunschweiger K, Benchekroun Y, Hu X, Adair R, Chee L, FitzGerald MG, Tulig C, Caruso A, Tzellas N, Bawa A, Franklin B, McGuire S, Nogues X, Gong G, Allen KM, Anisowicz A, Morales AJ, Lomedico PT, Recker SM, Van Eerdewegh P, Recker RR, Johnson ML (2002) A mutation in the LDL receptor-related protein 5 gene results in the autosomal dominant high-bone-mass trait. Am J Hum Genet 70:11–19

Logan CY, Nusse R (2004) The Wnt signaling pathway in development and disease. Annu Rev Cell Dev Biol 20:781–810

Lorenzo JA, Naprta A, Rao Y, Alander C, Glaccum M, Widmer M, Gronowicz G, Kalinowski J, Pilbeam CC (1998) Mice lacking the type I interleukin-1 receptor do not lose bone mass after ovariectomy. Endocrinology 139:3022–3025

Luo G, Ducy P, McKee MD, Pinero GJ, Loyer E, Behringer RR, Karsenty G (1997) Spontaneous calcification of arteries and cartilage in mice lacking matrix GLA protein. Nature 386:78–81

Manolagas SC (2000) Birth and death of bone cells: basic regulatory mechanisms and implications for the pathogenesis and treatment of osteoporosis. Endocr Rev 21:115–137

Marie PJ (2003) Fibroblast growth factor signaling controlling osteoblast differentiation. Gene 316:23–32

Marks S, Odgren PR (2002) The structure and development of bone. In: Bilezikian JB, Raize LG, Rodan GA (eds). Principles of bone biology II. Academic, San Diego, pp 3–15

Martin TJ, Sims NA (2005) Osteoclast-derived activity in the coupling of bone formation to resorption. Trends Mol Med 11:76–81

Marx RE, Carlson ER, Eichstaedt RM, Schimmele SR, Strauss JE, Georgeff KR (1998) Platelet-rich plasma: Growth factor enhancement for bone grafts. Oral Surg Oral Med Oral Pathol Oral Radiol Endod 85:638–646

Melton LJ 3rd (1995) How many women have osteoporosis now? J Bone Miner Res 10:175–177

Meunier PJ, Sebert JL, Reginster JY, Briancon D, Appelboom T, Netter P, Loeb G, Rouillon A, Barry S, Evreux JC, Avouac B, Marchandise X (1998) Fluoride salts are no better at preventing new vertebral fractures than calcium-vitamin D in postmenopausal osteoporosis: the FAVOStudy. Osteoporos Int 8:4–12

Mihara M, Nishimoto N, Ohsugi Y (2005) The therapy of autoimmune diseases by anti-interleukin-6 receptor antibody. Expert Opin Biol Ther 5:683–690

Minkowitz B, Boskey AL, Lane JM, Pearlman HS, Vigorita VJ (1991) Effects of propranolol on bone metabolism in the rat. J Orthop Res 9:869–875

Misof BM, Roschger P, Cosman F, Kurland ES, Tesch W, Messmer P, Dempster DW, Nieves J, Shane E, Fratzl P, Klaushofer K, Bilezikian J, Lindsay R (2003) Effects of intermittent parathyroid hormone administration on bone mineralization density in iliac crest biopsies from patients with osteoporosis: a paired study before and after treatment. J Clin Endocrinol Metab 88:1150–1156

Miyaura C, Onoe Y, Inada M, Maki K, Ikuta K, Ito M, Suda T (1997) Increased B-lymphopoiesis by interleukin 7 induces bone loss in mice with intact ovarian function: similarity to estrogen deficiency. Proc Natl Acad Sci U S A 94:9360–9365

Mont MA, Ragland PS, Biggins B, Friedlaender G, Patel T, Cook S, Etienne G, Shimmin A, Kildey R, Rueger DC, Einhorn TA (2004) Use of bone morphogenetic proteins for musculoskeletal applications. An overview. J Bone Joint Surg Am 86-A Suppl 2:41–55

Mundlos S, Otto F, Mundlos C, Mulliken JB, Aylsworth AS, Albright S, Lindhout D, Cole WG, Henn W, Knoll JH, Owen MJ, Mertelsmann R, Zabel BU, Olsen BR (1997) Mutations involving the transcription factor CBFA1 cause cleidocranial dysplasia. Cell 89:773–779

Murphy WL, Simmons CA, Kaigler D, Mooney DJ (2004) Bone regeneration via a mineral substrate and induced angiogenesis. J Dent Res 83:204–210

Murray TM, Rao LG, Divieti P, Bringhurst FR (2005) Parathyroid hormone secretion and action: evidence for discrete receptors for the carboxyl-terminal region and related biological actions of carboxyl-terminal ligands. Endocr Rev 26:78–113

Nakashima K, Zhou X, Kunkel G, Zhang Z, Deng JM, Behringer RR, de Crombrugghe B (2002) The novel zinc finger-containing transcription factor osterix is required for osteoblast differentiation and bone formation. Cell 108:17–29

Narisawa S, Frohlander N, Millan JL (1997) Inactivation of two mouse alkaline phosphatase genes and establishment of a model of infantile hypophosphatasia. Dev Dyn 208:432–446

Neer RM, Arnaud CD, Zanchetta JR, Prince R, Gaich GA, Reginster JY, Hodsman AB, Eriksen EF, Ish-Shalom S, Genant HK, Wang O, Mitlak BH (2001) Effect of parathyroid hormone (1–34) on fractures and bone mineral density in postmenopausal women with osteoporosis. N Engl J Med 344:1434–1441

Nijweide PBE, Klein-Nulend J (2002) The osteocyte. In: Bilezikian JP, Raisz CG, Rodan GA (eds) Principles in bone biology. Academic, San Diego, pp 93–107

Norman AW, Mizwicki MT, Norman DP (2004) Steroid-hormone rapid actions, membrane receptors and a conformational ensemble model. Nat Rev Drug Discov 3:27–41

Okada Y, Lorenzo JA, Freeman AM, Tomita M, Morham SG, Raisz LG, Pilbeam CC (2000) Prostaglandin G/H synthase-2 is required for maximal formation of osteoclast-like cells in culture. J Clin Invest 105:823–832

Olney RC (2003) Regulation of bone mass by growth hormone. Med Pediatr Oncol 41:228–234

Onishi T, Ishidou Y, Nagamine T, Yone K, Imamura T, Kato M, Sampath TK, ten Dijke P, Sakou T (1998) Distinct and overlapping patterns of localization of bone morphogenetic protein (BMP) family members and a BMP type II receptor during fracture healing in rats. Bone 22:605–612

Otto F, Thornell AP, Crompton T, Denzel A, Gilmour KC, Rosewell IR, Stamp GW, Beddington RS, Mundlos S, Olsen BR, Selby PB, Owen MJ (1997) Cbfa1, a candidate gene for cleidocranial dysplasia syndrome, is essential for osteoblast differentiation and bone development. Cell 89:765–771

Paralkar VM, Borovecki F, Ke HZ, Cameron KO, Lefker B, Grasser WA, Owen TA, Li M, DaSilva-Jardine P, Zhou M, Dunn RL, Dumont F, Korsmeyer R, Krasney P, Brown TA, Plowchalk D, Vukicevic S, Thompson DD (2003) An EP2 receptor-selective prostaglandin E2 agonist induces bone healing. Proc Natl Acad Sci U S A 100:6736–6740

Parfitt AM (1998) Osteoclast precursors as leukocytes: importance of the area code. Bone 23:491–494

Parfitt AM (2000) The mechanism of coupling: a role for the vasculature. Bone 26:319–323

Parfitt AM (2002) Targeted and nontargeted bone remodeling: relationship to basic multicellular unit origination and progression. Bone 30:5–7

Paris O, Zizak I, Lichtenegger H, Roschger P, Klaushofer K, Fratzl P (2000) Analysis of the hierarchical structure of biological tissues by scanning X-ray scattering using a micro-beam. Cell Mol Biol (Noisy-le-Grand) 46:993–1004

Pasco JA, Henry MJ, Sanders KM, Kotowicz MA, Seeman E, Nicholson GC (2004) Beta-adrenergic blockers reduce the risk of fracture partly by increasing bone mineral density: Geelong Osteoporosis Study. J Bone Miner Res 19:19–24

Peschon JJ, Torrance DS, Stocking KL, Glaccum MB, Otten C, Willis CR, Charrier K, Morrissey PJ, Ware CB, Mohler KM (1998) TNF receptor-deficient mice reveal divergent roles for p55 and p75 in several models of inflammation. J Immunol 160:943–952

Provot S, Schipani E (2005) Molecular mechanisms of endochondral bone development. Biochem Biophys Res Commun 328:658–665

Reddi AH (1998) Role of morphogenetic proteins in skeletal tissue engineering and regeneration. Nat Biotechnol 16:247–252

Reid IR, Gamble GD, Grey AB, Black DM, Ensrud KE, Browner WS, Bauer DC (2005) Beta-blocker use, BMD, and fractures in the study of osteoporotic fractures. J Bone Miner Res 20:613–618

Riggs BL, Parfitt AM (2005) Drugs used to treat osteoporosis: the critical need for a uniform nomenclature based on their action on bone remodeling. J Bone Miner Res 20:177–184

Risau W (1997) Mechanisms of angiogenesis. Nature 386:671–674

Robey PG (2002) Bone matrix proteoglycans and glycoproteins. In: Bilezikian JB, Raize LG, Rodan GA (eds) Principles of bone biology. Academic, San Diego, Connect Tissue Res 35:225–237

Rodan GA, Martin TJ (2000) Therapeutic approaches to bone diseases. Science 289:1508–1514

Roelen BA, Dijke P (2003) Controlling mesenchymal stem cell differentiation by TGFBeta family members. J Orthop Sci 8:740–748

Roggia C, Gao Y, Cenci S, Weitzmann MN, Toraldo G, Isaia G, Pacifici R (2001) Up-regulation of TNF-producing T cells in the bone marrow: a key mechanism by which estrogen deficiency induces bone loss in vivo. Proc Natl Acad Sci USA 98:13960–13965

Roodman GD (1996) Advances in bone biology: the osteoclast. Endocr Rev 17:308–332

Roschger P, Rinnerthaler S, Yates J, Rodan GA, Fratzl P, Klaushofer K (2001) Alendronate increases degree and uniformity of mineralization in cancellous bone and decreases the porosity in cortical bone of osteoporotic women. Bone 29:185–191

Rossert J, de Crombrugghe B (2002) In: Bilezikian JP, Raisz CG, Rodan GA (eds) Type I collagen: structure, synthesis and regulation. Principles in bone biology. Academic, San Diego, pp 189–210

Salo J, Lehenkari P, Mulari M, Metsikko K, Vaananen HK (1997) Removal of osteoclast bone resorption products by transcytosis. Science 276:270 273

Schenk RK (1994) Bone regeneration. In Buser D, Dahlin C, Schenk RK (eds) Guided bone regeneration in implant dentistr. Quintessence Publishing, pp 49–100

Schenk RK, Hunziker EB (1994) Histologic and ultrastructural features of fracture healing. In: Brighton CT, Fried-

laender G, Lane JM, eds. Bone Formation and Repair. American Academy of Orthopaedic Surgeons, Rosemont, IL, pp 117–145

Schlienger RG, Kraenzlin ME, Jick SS, Meier CR (2004) Use of beta-blockers and risk of fractures. JAMA 292:1326–1332

Schmelzeisen R, Schimming R, Sittinger M (2003) Making bone: implant insertion into tissue-engineered bone for maxillary sinus floor augmentation-a preliminary report. J Craniomaxillofac Surg 31:34–39

Shrader SP, Ragucci KR (2005) Parathyroid hormone (1–84) and treatment of osteoporosis. Ann Pharmacother 39:1511–1516

Sikavitsas VI, Temenoff JS, Mikos AG (2001) Biomaterials and bone mechanotransduction. Biomaterials 22:2581–2593

Sims NA, Dupont S, Krust A, Clement-Lacroix P, Minet D, Resche-Rigon M, Gaillard-Kelly M, Baron R (2002) Deletion of estrogen receptors reveals a regulatory role for estrogen receptors-beta in bone remodeling in females but not in males. Bone 30:18–25

Sly WS, Hewett-Emmett D, Whyte MP, Yu YS, Tashian RE (1983) Carbonic anhydrase II deficiency identified as the primary defect in the autosomal recessive syndrome of osteopetrosis with renal tubular acidosis and cerebral calcification. Proc Natl Acad Sci U S A 80:2752–2756

Stein GS, Lian JB (1993) Molecular mechanisms mediating proliferation/differentiation interrelationships during progressive development of the osteoblast phenotype. Endocr Rev 14:424–442

St-Jacques B, Hammerschmidt M, McMahon AP (1999) Indian hedgehog signaling regulates proliferation and differentiation of chondrocytes and is essential for bone formation. Genes Dev 13:2072–2086

Stokstad E (2005) Bone quality fills holes in fracture risk. Science 308:1580

Suda T, Takahashi N, Martin TJ (1992) Modulation of osteoclast differentiation. Endocr Rev 13:66–80

Suda T, Takahashi N, Udagawa N, Jimi E, Gillespie MT, Martin TJ (1999) Modulation of osteoclast differentiation and function by the new members of the tumor necrosis factor receptor and ligand families. Endocr Rev 20:345–357

Swaminathan R (2001) Biochemical markers of bone turnover. Clin Chim Acta 313:95–105

Syed F, Khosla S (2005) Mechanisms of sex steroid effects on bone. Biochem Biophys Res Commun 328:688–96

Taichman RS (2005) Blood and bone: two tissues whose fates are intertwined to create the hematopoietic stem-cell niche. Blood 105:2631–2639

Takayanagi H (2005) Mechanistic insight into osteoclast differentiation in osteoimmunology. J Mol Med 83:170–179

Takeda S (2005) Central control of bone remodeling. Biochem Biophys Res Commun 328:697–699

Takeda S, Elefteriou F, Levasseur R, Liu X, Zhao L, Parker KL, Armstrong D, Ducy P, Karsenty G (2002) Leptin regulates bone formation via the sympathetic nervous system. Cell 111:305–317

Tanaka M, Sakai A, Uchida S, Tanaka S, Nagashima M, Katayama T, Yamaguchi K, Nakamura T (2004) Prostaglandin E2 receptor (EP4) selective agonist (ONO-4819.CD) accelerates bone repair of femoral cortex after drill-hole injury associated with local upregulation of bone turnover in mature rats. Bone 34:940–948

Teitelbaum SL (2000) Bone resorption by osteoclasts. Science 289:1504–1508

Thomas JT, Lin K, Nandedkar M, Camargo M, Cervenka J, Luyten FP (1996) A human chondrodysplasia due to a mutation in a TGF-beta superfamily member. Nat Genet 12:315–317

Thomas JT, Kilpatrick MW, Lin K, Erlacher L, Lembessis P, Costa T, Tsipouras P, Luyten FP (1997) Disruption of human limb morphogenesis by a dominant negative mutation in CDMP1. Nat Genet 17:58–64

Tondravi MM, McKercher SR, Anderson K, Erdmann JM, Quiroz M, Maki R, Teitelbaum SL (1997) Osteopetrosis in mice lacking haematopoietic transcription factor PU.1. Nature 386:81–84

Toraldo G, Roggia C, Qian WP, Pacifici R, Weitzmann MN (2003) IL-7 induces bone loss in vivo by induction of receptor activator of nuclear factor kappa B ligand and tumor necrosis factor alpha from T cells. Proc Natl Acad Sci USA 100:125–130

Turgeon JL, McDonnell DP, Martin KA, Wise PM (2004) Hormone therapy: physiological complexity belies therapeutic simplicity. Science 304:1269–1273

Urist MR (1965) Bone: formation by autoinduction. Science 150:893–899

van Bezooijen RL, Roelen BA, Visser A, van der Wee-Pals L, de Wilt E, Karperien M, Hamersma H, Papapoulos SE, ten Dijke P, Lowik CW (2004) Sclerostin is an osteocyte-expressed negative regulator of bone formation, but not a classical BMP antagonist. J Exp Med 199:805–814

van der Eerden BC, Karperien M, Wit JM (2003) Systemic and local regulation of the growth plate. Endocr Rev 24:782–801

Veldhuis JD, Roemmich JN, Richmond EJ, Rogol AD, Lovejoy JC, Sheffield-Moore M, Mauras N, Bowers CY (2005) Endocrine control of body composition in infancy, childhood, and puberty. Endocr Rev 26:114–146

Verma S, Rajaratnam JH, Denton J, Hoyland JA, Byers RJ (2002) Adipocytic proportion of bone marrow is inversely related to bone formation in osteoporosis. J Clin Pathol 55:693–698

Waymire KG, Mahuren JD, Jaje JM, Guilarte TR, Coburn SP, MacGregor GR (1995) Mice lacking tissue non-specific alkaline phosphatase die from seizures due to defective metabolism of vitamin B-6. Nat Genet 11:45–51

Wei S, Kitaura H, Zhou P, Ross FP, Teitelbaum SL (2005) IL-1 mediates TNF-induced osteoclastogenesis. J Clin Invest 115:282–290

Whyte MP, Obrecht SE, Finnegan PM, Jones JL, Podgornik MN, McAlister WH, Mumm S (2002) Osteoprotegerin deficiency and juvenile Paget's disease. N Engl J Med 347:175–184

Winkler DG, Sutherland MK, Geoghegan JC, Yu C, Hayes T, Skonier JE, Shpektor D, Jonas M, Kovacevich BR, Staehling-Hampton K, Appleby M, Brunkow ME, Latham JA (2003) Osteocyte control of bone formation via sclerostin, a novel BMP antagonist. EMBO J 22:6267–6276

Wu XB, Li Y, Schneider A, Yu W, Rajendren G, Iqbal J, Yamamoto M, Alam M, Brunet LJ, Blair HC, Zaidi M, Abe E (2003) Impaired osteoblastic differentiation, reduced bone formation, and severe osteoporosis in noggin-over-expressing mice. J Clin Invest 112:924–934

Xu T, Bianco P, Fisher LW, Longenecker G, Smith E, Goldstein S, Bonadio J, Boskey A, Heegaard AM, Sommer B, Satomura K, Dominguez P, Zhao C, Kulkarni AB, Robey PG, Young MF (1998) Targeted disruption of the biglycan gene leads to an osteoporosis-like phenotype in mice. Nat Genet 20:78–82

Yoshida CA, Furuichi T, Fujita T, Fukuyama R, Kanatani N, Kobayashi S, Satake M, Takada K, Komori T (2002) Core-binding factor beta interacts with Runx2 and is required for skeletal development. Nat Genet 32:633–638

Yu PB, Beppu H, Kawai N, Li E, Bloch KD (2005) Bone morphogenetic protein (BMP) type II receptor deletion reveals BMP ligand-specific gain of signaling in pulmonary artery smooth muscle cells. J Biol Chem 280:24443–24450

Zelzer E, Olsen BR (2003) The genetic basis for skeletal diseases. Nature 423:343–348

Zhang X, Schwarz EM, Young DA, Puzas JE, Rosier RN, O'Keefe RJ (2002) Cyclooxygenase-2 regulates mesenchymal cell differentiation into the osteoblast lineage and is critically involved in bone repair. J Clin Invest 109:1405–1415

Zheng SX, Vrindts Y, Lopez M, De Groote D, Zangerle PF, Collette J, Franchimont N, Geenen V, Albert A, Reginster JY (1997) Increase in cytokine production (IL-1 beta, IL-6, TNF-alpha but not IFN-gamma, GM-CSF or LIF) by stimulated whole blood cells in postmenopausal osteoporosis. Maturitas 26:63–71

Zou H, Wieser R, Massague J, Niswander L (1997) Distinct roles of type I bone morphogenetic protein receptors in the formation and differentiation of cartilage. Genes Dev 11:2191–2203

Pathophysiology and Aging of Bone

PETER PIETSCHMANN, REINHARD GRUBER, and MEINRAD PETERLIK

CONTENTS

P. PIETSCHMANN, MD
Associate Professor of Pathophysiology and Internal Medicine,
Department of Pathophysiology, Medical University of Vienna,
Waehringer Guertel 18–20, 1090 Vienna, Austria
and
Ludwig Boltzmann Institute of Aging Research, Langobarden-
strasse 122, 1220 Vienna, Austria
R. GRUBER, PhD
Associate Professor, Department of Oral Surgery, Vienna
University Clinic of Dentistry, Medical University of Vienna,
Waehringer Strasse 25a, 1090 Vienna, Austria
M. PETERLIK, PhD, MD
Professor and Head of the Department of Pathophysiology,
Medical University of Vienna, Waehringer Guertel 18–20, 1090
Vienna, Austria

2.1
Aging of Bone

2.1.1
Cellular Mechanisms

Human aging is a complex process which, as a result of multiple genetically programmed mechanisms as well as stochastic events, leads to accumulation of damaging alterations in vital cellular functions. A variety of in vitro studies indicate that aging is associated with an overall decline in protein synthesis and protein turnover as well as with an accumulation of damaged molecules (GLOWACKI 1999). With respect to bone turnover, several authors investigated the effects of age on generation, maturation, and function of osteoblasts in experimental animals as well as in humans. In rats, for example, a defect in maturation of preosteoblasts into osteoblasts was demonstrated, which led to a more than ten-fold decrease in the number of osteoblasts with age (ROHOLL et al. 1994). QUARTO et al. (1995) determined the number of osteoprogenitor cells in bone marrow from adult and aged rats as well as their ability to differentiate and form bone. The number of adherent colony forming cells was significantly lower in marrow cells from aged rats than in those from adult rats. BERGMAN and colleagues (1996) found that primary marrow stromal mesenchymal stem cell cultures from older BALB/c mice yielded markedly fewer osteogenic progenitor cell colonies than those from younger animals. PFEILSCHIFTER and coworkers (1993) studied the outgrowth of osteoblast-like cells from human bone explants; they observed that cells from 61- to 70-year-old donors required substantially higher concentrations of growth factors and hormones to yield comparable increases in DNA synthesis than did cells from 51- to 60-year-old donors. In particular, a significant negative correlation between age and mitogenic responsiveness to platelet-derived growth factor and growth hormone was observed. BATTMANN and coworkers (1997) demonstrated impaired growth of human endosteal bone cells from men aged over 50 years. In addition, the production of osteocalcin after stimulation with 1,25-$(OH)_2D_3$ was lower, regardless of gender, in older donors than in younger ones. In summary, cumulative results obtained in different models consistently demonstrate an age-related deficit in osteoblast maturation and function.

The senescence-accelerated mouse P6 (SAMP6) is an interesting model of involutional osteopenia with spontaneous fractures at old age (MATSUSHITA 1986). SAMP6 mice exhibit decreased osteoblastogenesis in the bone marrow that is associated with a low rate of bone formation and reduced bone mineral density (JILKA et al. 1996). Secondary to impaired osteoblast formation, osteoclastogenesis is also decreased in these mice. In contrast to their impaired osteoblastogenesis, SAMP6 mice exhibit increased adipogenesis and myelopoiesis (KAJKENOVA et al. 1997). Recent data indicate that despite reduced endocortical bone formation, periosteal bone formation is unimpaired in SAMP6 mice (SILVA et al. 2005).

PERKINS et al. (1994) studied the composition of mouse bone marrow to assess whether increased numbers of monocyte/macrophage/osteoclast precursor cells were present in marrow from aged mice compared to young animals. The authors found a significant increase in the pool size of hematopoietic osteoclast precursor cells in marrow from long bones of aged mice. In addition, co-culture of bone marrow cells from aged mice with a stromal cell line gave rise to twice as many osteoclast-like cells as did marrow from young animals. Similar data were reported by KAHN and coworkers (1995), who also found a considerable increase in the number of marrow cells capable of forming osteoclasts in 24-month-old mice compared to 4- to 6-month-old mice. MAKLUF et al. (2000) reported that osteoprotegerin mRNA expression in human bone marrow cells declines with age. Consequently, this may increase the ability of stromal cells/osteoblasts to support osteoclastogenesis. CAO et al. (2003) studied the effect of age on RANKL and osteoprotegerin mRNA levels in male C57BL/6 mice. RANKL levels in whole bone were higher in old than in young mice whereas osteoprotegerin levels decreased with age. Also in cultivated osteoblast-like cells from older animals expression of RANKL was higher and osteoprotegerin lower than in young animals.

In conclusion, age-related osteopenia may result from inversely related changes in the pool size of hematopoietic osteoclast precursor cells and osteogenic stromal cells; reduced production of osteoprotegerin and enhanced RANKL expression would additionally promote the formation of osteoclasts.

2.1.2
Effect of Age on Bone Histology

In humans (and animals), static and dynamic markers of bone structure and remodeling can be established by histomorphometric analysis of microscopic sections of bone biopsies. Many studies have demonstrated an age-related decline in trabecular bone volume in both men and women (e.g., VEDI et al. 1982; BALLANTI et al. 1990; CLARKE et al. 1996). In both sexes a negative effect of aging on cortical bone mass has also been demonstrated (BROCKSTEDT et al. 1993). Some authors described an age-related increase of osteoid volume (KAJKENOVA et al. 1997), which was not confirmed by others (KAHN et al. 1995). Variations in the prevalence of vitamin D deficiency in the subjects studied may, at least in part, explain these differences.

One clearly established age-related alteration in trabecular bone is a reduction in wall width (JILKA et al. 1996; KAJKENOVA et al. 1997), which reflects a decrease in bone formation rate. Thus, age-related bone loss traditionally has been regarded as a consequence of decreased osteoblast activity. This notion, however, has been contested by the findings of EASTELL et al. (1988), who used histomorphometry of iliac biopsies and determination of bone turnover markers to provide evidence of a higher bone formation rate in older than in younger healthy women.

RECKER et al. (1988) showed a marked decline of the mineral apposition rate (the rate of addition of new layers of mineral at trabecular surfaces) with age in healthy postmenopausal women. However, this finding could not be confirmed in another study (KAJKENOVA et al. 1997).

Controversy also exists with respect to various markers of osteoclast activity in older age. An increased activation frequency has been observed in postmenopausal women compared to premenopausal women (MAKLUF et al. 2000). Other authors found reduced activity of bone-resorbing cells with advancing age, and no alteration of resorption depth (PALLE et al. 1989; CROUCHER et al. 1991)

To summarize, bone histomorphometric studies in humans consistently demonstrated an age-related decrease in trabecular bone volume. Most although not all authors found a decline of bone formation rate with aging. Also, data on the effect of age on osteoclastic bone resorption markers are inconsistent.

2.1.3
Aging of Bone Reflected by Biochemical Markers of Bone Turnover

In the past, bone turnover could only be assessed by laborious techniques such as calcium balance and isotope kinetic studies, or, as described above, by histomorphometric analysis of bone biopsies. The availability of biochemical markers of bone turnover constitutes an important methodological step forward: determining these markers in serum and urine is relatively inexpensive and also easy, because it is basically a noninvasive method. Currently available markers of bone formation include total and bone-specific alkaline phosphatase activity, osteocalcin, and type I collagen terminal extension peptides (PIETSCHMANN and PETERLIK 1999; DELMAS and GARNERO 1996). Bone resorption can be assessed by the urinary excretion or serum levels of bone type I collagen degradation products such as pyridinium crosslinks, and N- and C-telopeptide of collagen crosslinks.

A number of studies reported an increase in biochemical markers of bone resorption in postmenopausal women (UEBELHART et al. 1991; SCHLEMMER et al. 1994; KUSHIDA et al. 1995, PIETSCHMANN et al. 2003), reflecting the effect of estrogen deficiency on osteoclast generation and activity. Notably, as a result of bone formation/resorption coupling, higher levels of biochemical markers of bone formation, such as alkaline phosphatase or osteocalcin, are also observed in the postmenopausal period (PIETSCHMANN and PETERLIK 1999; RESCH et al. 1994).

In contrast to the data for women, data on age-related changes of markers of bone turnover in men are less consistent. In older men, serum osteocalcin levels have been reported to be increased (EPSTEIN et al. 1984), normal (DELMAS and GARNERO 1996; CATHERWOOD et al. 1985), or decreased (WORSFOLD et al. 1988; BLAIN et al. 2004). Levels of type I procollagen propeptide, another marker of bone formation, decline with age in men but increase in women (EBELING et al. 1992). In a population based study, SEIBEL et al. (1994) demonstrated progressive increases of bone resorption markers with age not only for women but also for men.

The determination of biochemical markers of bone turnover in studies on age-related alterations of bone metabolism has certainly expanded our knowledge in this field, although in certain cases meaningful interpretation of the respective findings is still difficult.

2.1.4
Hormones and Aging of Bone

Aging is associated with a decline in the secretion of a variety of hormones. These include hormones involved in the regulation of bone metabolism, such as estrogens, androgens, and growth hormone. It is well established that estrogen deficiency is a major determinant of the accelerated bone loss experienced by women in the postmenopausal period; on average, women loose between one-third and one-half of their bone within up to 10 years after the menopause (LEBOFF and GLOWACKI 1999). Although the rate of bone loss slows after that point, low estrogen levels continue to contribute to diminution of bone mass later in life, in addition to other factors which will be discussed in detail later in this chapter.

The existence of an "andropause," the male equivalent of the menopause, is highly questionable; most healthy aging men do not experience an abrupt cessation of gonadal functions. Nevertheless, although serum testosterone levels vary remarkably between individuals, it is generally accepted that androgen levels decline with aging. VERMEULEN (2000) noted subnormal testosterone levels in fewer than 1% of men below the age of 40 years, but in more than 20% of men older than 60 years. Of importance, the age-related decline of bioavailable testosterone is more pronounced than that of total testosterone (KHOSLA et al. 1998).

Androgens are important regulators of bone metabolism. This is best illustrated by the fact that osteoporosis is a main feature of overt hypogonadism (FINKELSTEIN et al. 1987; STEPAN et al. 1989; ORWOLL and KLEIN 1996). In a histomorphometric study, ERBEN et al. (2000) found that androgen deficiency induces high-turnover osteopenia in aged male rats. In castrated men, a study on biochemical markers of bone metabolism demonstrated that bone turnover following orchidectomy is increased (STEPAN et al. 1989).

It is less clear, however, whether androgen levels influence bone loss in healthy elderly men. MURPHY et al. (1993), studying elderly community-dwelling men, found a positive correlation between the free androgen index and femoral neck bone mineral density. KELLY and coworkers (1990) demonstrated that radial (but not lumbar spine or femoral neck) bone mineral density could be predicted by an index of free testosterone and weight. In contrast, RAPADO et al. (1999), studying 140 healthy elderly men, found no relationship between serum androgens or sex hormone-binding globulin and bone mineral density. KHOSLA et al. (1998) demonstrated by multivariate analysis that the bioavailable estrogen level, but not bioavailable testosterone, was a consistent independent predictor of bone mineral density in men and postmenopausal women. These data are in line with those reported by SLEMENDA et al. (1997) showing that in older men low serum testosterone levels within the normal range are not associated with low bone density; however, these authors consistently found a significant positive correlation between serum estradiol concentrations and bone density in men. Data from the Rancho Bernardo Study (GREENDALE et al. 1997) also indicate that, of various sex steroids tested in both men and women, bioavailable estrogen was most strongly associated with bone mineral density. In a longitudinal study 200 elderly men were followed for 4 years; measures of bioavailable estradiol – but not testosterone – were the most consistent predictors of bone turnover and bone loss (GENNARI et al. 2003). Altogether, it appears that androgen levels are not a major determinant of bone loss in healthy elderly men; recent data rather point to a major role of estrogens in the maintenance of homeostasis in the male skeleton.

A possible role in bone metabolism has been suggested for dehydroepiandrosterone (DHEA) and DHEA sulfate, two major androgens produced by the adrenal glands. Although DHEA levels decline with aging, nevertheless mean levels of these androgens are higher at all ages in men than in women. There is evidence that DHEA (sulfate) levels correlate with bone density in healthy women. Consequently, lower than normal levels have been observed in patients with osteoporosis (LEBOFF and GLOWACKI 1999).

In healthy individuals, spontaneous and stimulated growth hormone secretion as well as insulin-like growth factor I levels decrease with advancing age (LANG et al. 1987; HERMANN and BERGER 1999). The role of the growth hormone/insulin-like growth factor I axis in the regulation of bone turnover is demonstrated by the fact that bone density is decreased in patients with growth hormone deficiency (ROSEN et al. 1993) but increased in acromegaly (KOTZMANN et

al. 1993). Data from a cross sectional study suggested that in men insulin-like growth factor I accounted for 10% of femoral neck bone mineral density variance (BLAIN et al. 2004). However, further studies are necessary to establish that age-related bone loss is associated with defects in the growth hormone/insulin-like growth factor I axis.

1,25-dihydroxyvitamin D_3 is a central regulator of calcium and phosphorus homeostasis. Although some geographic variation exists, elderly subjects are frequently deficient in vitamin D. For example, although hypovitaminosis D is more common in elderly residents in Europe than in North America, nevertheless, a significant proportion of elderly Americans also have low levels of vitamin D (OMDAHL et al. 1982; MCKENNA 1992). Vitamin D deficiency is particularly common and severe in nursing home residents (TOSS et al. 1980; PIETSCHMANN et al. 1990; STEIN et al. 1996). The cause of vitamin D deficiency in the elderly is heterogeneous. Lack of sunlight exposure leading to depleted vitamin D stores is one major factor; other factors include inadequate dietary intake, medications that impair vitamin D metabolism, and medical conditions such as malabsorption or renal or severe hepatic disease. Consequences of vitamin D deficiency include secondary hyperparathyroidism (PIETSCHMANN et al. 1990; QUESADA et al. 1992), potentially leading to increased bone turnover and bone loss, muscle weakness, and pain. An age-related increase in serum PTH levels, causes of which, apart from a compromised vitamin D status (GALLAGHER et al. 1998), may be gender-related factors, poor nutritional calcium intake, or disturbances in calcium metabolism, has been documented by many authors (e.g., ORWOLL and MEIER 1986; ENDRES et al. 1987; SHERMAN et al. 1990; EASTELL et al. 1991).

To summarize, estrogen deficiency appears to be a major determinant of age-associated bone loss not only in women but also in men. 1,25-Dihydroxyvitamin D_3 is another factor of major importance for bone turnover in elderly subjects.

2.2
Pathophysiology of Osteoporosis

Osteoporosis is a multifactorial pathologic condition which affects the entire skeleton and is characterized by a low bone mass in combination with poor bone quality, particularly of cancellous but also of cortical bone, both adding to the fragility of bone at distinct sites of the axial as well as the appendicular skeleton. Osteoporosis is the most prevalent metabolic bone disease in developed countries. The prevalence of osteoporotic fractures increases with age; the incidence among woman is at least twice as high as that in men for all age-related fractures. Based on the WHO definition of osteoporosis, MELTON (1995) estimated that 30% of postmenopausal white women in the US have osteoporosis. Thus, osteoporosis is a very common disorder of postmenopausal women, and will become even more common as life expectancy increases further.

From a theoretical point of view, bone loss results from any imbalance of bone turnover when the rate of bone resorption exceeds that of bone formation. Moreover, individual bone mass is determined by two factors: (1) the peak bone mass (the amount of bone mass achieved at skeletal maturity), and (2) the subsequent rate of bone loss. Considering the pathogenesis of osteoporosis, it should be taken into account that, in addition to interindividual variations, there exists an important gender-related difference in peak bone mass achieved during adolescence, so that on average young females have a significantly lower peak bone mass than young males.

Although low bone mass is a very important determinant of osteoporotic fractures, poor bone quality also influences bone fragility. Currently there is no precise definition of "bone quality"; Mary Bouxsein suggested "the totality of features and characteristics that influence a bone's ability to resist fractures" as a working definition (BOUXSEIN 2003). Compromised trabecular architecture (Fig. 2.1) has

been identified as an independent causal factor in the pathogenesis of vertebral fractures (LEGRAND et al. 2000; DEMPSTER 2000). Alterations of cancellous bone architecture have also been reported in bone samples from hip fracture patients (CIARELLI et al. 2000). In addition to the microarchitecture of bone tissue further factors such as bone geometry, bone mineral density distribution or properties of collagen determine the resistance of bone to fracture (for review see BOUXSEIN 2003, SEEMAN 2003a,b). Complex age related alteration in bone geometry have been described. With aging both periosteal apposition and endocortical resorption of bone increases, these changes result in outward cortical displacement (AHLBORG et al. 2003; RIGGS et al. 2004). In contrast to endocortical resorption, enhanced periosteal bone apposition is beneficial to bone strength. Studies using quantitative backscattered electron imaging demonstrated that in osteoporotic women the relative calcium content of bone is significantly lower than that of healthy individuals (ROSCHGER et al. 2001).

2.2.1
Genetics of Osteoporosis

Several pieces of evidence strongly suggest that genetic factors are major determinants of peak bone mass. Bone mineral density is more highly correlated in monozygotic than in dizygotic twins (POCOCK et al. 1987). Moreover, family studies noted a significant correlation of bone mass in mother–daughter pairs (MATKOVIC et al. 1990; WOSJE et al. 2000). Although twin and family studies thus support a

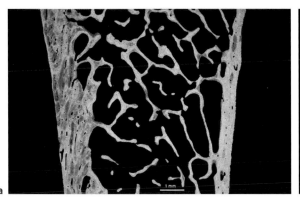 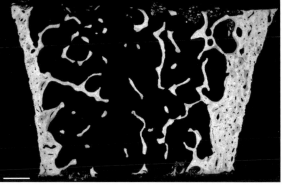

Fig. 2.1a,b. Backscattered electron images of transiliac bone biopsies (longitudinal section through biopsy cylinder). **a** Normal individual, female, aged 30 years. **b** Osteoporotic woman, aged 50 years. Note the compromised trabecular architecture of the osteoporotic bone sample. (Courtesy of Univ. Doz. Dr. P. Roschger, Ludwig Boltzmann Institute of Osteology, Vienna)

genetic effect on peak bone mass, it is less clear to what extent rates of bone loss after the menopause or with aging are also genetically determined. Studies on bone turnover markers in twins suggest a genetic influence on bone remodeling; for instance, it has been demonstrated that in adult twins 80% of the variance in serum osteocalcin, a marker of bone formation, is attributable to genetic factors (Kelly et al. 1991).

In 1992 Morrison and coworkers reported that serum osteocalcin levels in Australian women can be predicted from vitamin D receptor gene polymorphisms. In 1994 Morrison et al. demonstrated that bone density is also associated with the frequency of a certain vitamin D receptor allele. Since then the association between bone mineral density and vitamin D receptor polymorphisms has been studied extensively, albeit with disputed results (for review see Cooper 1999). Interestingly, vitamin D receptor polymorphisms appear to influence bone mineral density not only in primary but also in secondary osteoporosis such as in patients with ankylosing spondylitis (Obermayer-Pietsch et al. 2003). Moreover, associations between bone mineral density and other genes such as estrogen receptor α, collagen type 1_{a1}, insulin-like growth factor 1 and transforming growth factor-β as well as the genetic predisposition for adult lactose intolerance have been analyzed (Albaga and Ralston 2003; Zajickova and Zofkova 2003; Obermayer-Pietsch 2004, 2006). Nevertheless, many unresolved questions in the genetics of osteoporosis still exist and are currently under intensive investigation.

2.2.2
Peak Bone Mass

Data regarding the age at which peak bone mass is achieved are conflicting. Rodin et al. (1990), using dual photon absorptiometry, found that in young women peak spinal bone density is reached in the mid-30s, whereas loss at the femoral neck bone commenced in the late 20s. Recker et al. (1992) demonstrated by single and dual photon absorptiometry that in healthy young women gain in bone mass occurs during the third decade of life. In contrast, studies using dual energy X-ray absorptiometry instead of photon absorptiometry showed that peak bone mass is attained much earlier, namely in late adolescence (Kroger et al. 1993; Matkovic et al.

1994). Lu et al. (1994) found that bone mineral density of the total body and lumbar spine increased with age until 17.5 years of age in males and 15.8 years of age in females; femoral neck bone mineral density peaked in females at age 14.1 years. Males had a higher peak total body bone mineral density than females, which was attributed to greater weight and lean tissue mass.

As mentioned above, genetic factors are major determinants of peak bone mass. Interestingly, there also exist significant ethnic differences in bone mineral content, for example, between black and white women (Cohn et al. 1977). In addition, peak bone mass is also determined by nutritional factors (in particular calcium intake), hormonal factors, muscle mass, exercise and other environmental factors (Heaney et al. 2000; Parfitt 2004). In a review article, Tudor-Locke and McColl (2000) examined factors related to variation in premenopausal bone mineral status. The authors concluded that heredity and, possibly, age at menarche are unmodifiable determinative factors; amenorrhea, low body weight, eating disorders, and smoking were identified as modifiable risk factors. Protective factors for bone mass included higher body weight, calcium supplementation, and purposeful load-bearing exercise; positive effects of oral contraceptives were most apparent in women with menstrual irregularities.

2.2.3
The Riggs, Khosla and Melton Unitary Model of Involutional Osteoporosis

The term "involutional osteoporosis" refers to the common form of osteoporosis that begins in middle life and becomes increasingly more frequent with age (Melton and Riggs 1988). In 1983 Riggs and Melton proposed the existence of two distinct syndromes of involutional osteoporosis: type I ("postmenopausal") and type II ("senile"). Type I osteoporosis presents during the first 15–20 years after menopause and is characterized by excessive loss of trabecular bone, which causes the fractures typical of postmenopausal osteoporosis such as vertebral fractures and Colles' fractures. According to the original hypothesis of Riggs and Melton, type I osteoporosis results mainly from estrogen deficiency, which is responsible for the extent and duration of the rapid phase of postmenopausal bone loss.

Type II osteoporosis is characterized by loss of trabecular and cortical bone; the most frequent fractures thus involve the proximal femur and the vertebrae. The original hypothesis proposed that, in this slow phase of bone loss ("senile bone loss"), vitamin D insufficiency and the ensuing secondary hyperparathyroidism also contribute to increased net bone resorption.

In 1998 RIGGS and coworkers proposed a unitary model of involutional osteoporosis. In this model, too, the existence of two phases of involutional bone loss in women (an early rapid and a late slow phase) is emphasized, whereas aging men have only one slow phase of continuous bone loss. The accelerated phase of bone loss in women begins at the menopause, clearly results from estrogen deficiency, and involves a disproportionate loss of trabecular bone. Estrogen acts through specific estrogen receptors to inhibit the generation of osteoclasts (SCHILLER et al. 1997) and osteoclastic bone resorption (OURSLER et al. 1991). Recently, EGHBALI-FATOURECHI et al. (2003) demonstrated that in early postmenopausal women, upregulation of RANKL on bone marrow cells is an important determinant of increased bone resorption as a consequence of low estrogen levels. Women with (type 1) osteoporosis appear to have an enhanced responsiveness of bone resorption in the presence of estrogen deficiency (RIGGS et al. 2003). Estrogen insufficiency thus results in unrestrained bone resorption and an overall increase in bone turnover, with enhanced calcium mobilization from bone as a consequence. This leads on the one hand to an increase in urinary calcium excretion and on the other to mild suppression of PTH release and of renal 1,25-$(OH)_2D_3$ synthesis, which, in turn, has a negative effect on intestinal calcium absorption (HEANEY et al. 1978; KOH et al. 1997; PRINCE et al. 1995). In contrast, the late slow phase of bone loss is associated with a progressive rise in serum PTH levels. The significance of secondary hyperparathyroidism for slow bone loss in aging men and women can be deduced from several observations: serum PTH levels and indices of bone turnover increase in parallel with age; likewise, suppression of PTH secretion by intravenous calcium infusion abolished the differences in urinary markers of bone resorption between young and elderly women (KHOSLA et al. 1998). As described previously, in some elderly subjects, in particular those who are housebound or nursing home residents, vitamin D deficiency may further contribute to secondary hyperparathyroidism.

There is mounting evidence that not only vitamin D deficiency but also estrogen deficiency contributes to secondary hyperparathyroidism, and therefore the slow phase of bone loss is caused by a lack of estrogen effects on extraskeletal calcium homeostasis. HEANEY and coworkers suggested that approximately the negative calcium balance induced by menopause is due equally to reduced intestinal calcium absorption and to enhanced renal calcium excretion (HEANEY et al. 1978). A direct stimulating effect of estrogen on intestinal calcium absorption can be deduced from the observation that estrogen deficiency developing after oophorectomy blunted any 1,25$(OH)_2D_3$-related increment in intestinal calcium absorption (GENNARI et al. 1990). NORDIN et al. (1991) demonstrated evidence for a renal calcium leak in early postmenopausal women. Similarly, MCKANE and coworkers (1995) found a PTH-independent decrease in tubular calcium absorption in estrogen-deficient as compared with estrogen-replete women. Moreover, data from a study by COSMAN and coworkers (1994) strongly suggest that estrogen acts directly on the parathyroid gland to reduce PTH secretion. Thus, through its extraskeletal actions estrogen appears to have an indirect positive effect on bone mass and mineral density.

The importance of endogenous sex hormones as determinants of osteoporotic fractures is also demonstrated by the observation that older postmenopausal women with undetectable serum estradiol concentrations and high serum concentrations of sex hormone binding globulin have an increased risk of hip and vertebral fracture (CUMMINGS et al. 1998). Similar findings were obtained by the Rotterdam Study (GODERIE-PLOMP et al. 2004). Moreover, in a recently published study, elderly women with hip fractures were found to exhibit an increased RANKL/OPG ratio mRNA content of iliac bone (ABDALLAH et al. 2005). Interestingly, the effect of increased RANKL/OPG ratio was additive to that of hip BMD.

In the original type I/II model of osteoporosis, the slow phase of bone loss was suggested to result from a combination of enhanced osteoclastic resorption due to secondary hyperparathyroidism and decreased bone formation (RIGGS and MELTON 1983). The notion that it is mainly bone formation that is compromised in type II osteoporosis was derived from histomorphometric studies: for instance, LIPS et al. (1978) found a reduced wall thickness of trabecular packets in late postmenopausal women, indicating a reduced rate of bone formation at the cellular level.

However, the concept that a low rate of bone formation is the only cause of senile osteoporosis has not
been confirmed by the many studies analyzing biochemical parameters of bone metabolism. GARNERO
et al. (1994) demonstrated that several markers of
bone formation are higher in late postmenopausal
osteoporotic women than in healthy premenopausal
women. In a population of elderly women characterized by serum levels of the bone formation marker
osteocalcin above the median, bone loss at the hip
was significantly faster than in women with levels
below the median (BAUER et al. 1999).

In their unitary model, RIGGS et al. (1998) propose that estrogen deficiency also substantially contributes to typical continuous slow bone loss in men.
Although castrated men rapidly lose bone (STEPAN et
al. 1989), there is no abrupt decline of serum testosterone levels in normal aging men. Several data suggest that estrogen deficiency could be a major cause
of bone loss in (aging) men. In 1989 BOURDEL et al.
found a positive correlation between serum estradiol levels and bone mineral content in men with
idiopathic osteoporosis. SMITH et al. (1994) reported
the occurrence of a mutated estrogen receptor gene
in a patient with severe osteopenia. As mentioned,
SLEMENDA et al. (1997) found that in men over age 65,
bone density is significantly associated with serum
estradiol levels. In the Rancho Bernardo Study a
positive relation between bioavailable estradiol and
bone mineral density was found in both men and
women (GREENDALE et al. 1997). Likewise, in a large
population based study KHOSLA and coworkers
(1998) identified serum bioavailable estrogen levels
as consistent independent predictors of bone mineral density in men and postmenopausal women. An
intervention study revealed that in normal elderly
men estrogen is the dominant sex steroid regulating
bone resorption whereas both estrogen and testosterone are important in maintaining bone formation (FALAHATI-NINI et al. 2000). An association
of a particular estrogen receptor polymorphism
with bone mineral density has been reported in
Thai men (ONGPHIPHADHANAKUL et al. 1998). Data
from our laboratory demonstrated decreased serum
estradiol levels in men with idiopathic osteoporosis
(PIETSCHMANN et al. 2001). Similar findings were
reported by GILLBERG and coworkers (1999).

To summarize, RIGGS et al. (1998) propose estrogen deficiency as the cause of both the early, accelerated and the late, slow phases of bone loss in postmenopausal women and as a contributing cause of
the continuous phase of bone loss in aging men.

2.2.4
Further Determinants of Osteoporosis and Osteoporotic Fractures

All factors which exert a negative influence on the
achievement of an adequate peak bone mass and/or
are likely to accelerate the rate of involutional bone
loss must be considered risk factors for osteoporotic bone disease. In addition to genetic disposi-
tion, the aging process per se, and hormonal imbal-
ances, particularly estrogen deficiency, a number of
other markers can be used to predict an increased
fracture risk. In a comprehensive prospective study
of more than 9,500 white women over 65 years of
age, CUMMINGS and coworkers (1995) identified
the following risk factors for hip fracture: mater-
nal history of hip fracture, history of any fracture
since the age of 50 years, tallness at the age of
25 years, fair or poor self-reported health status,
previous hyperthyroidism, treatment with long-
acting benzodiazepines or anticonvulsants, high
caffeine intake, spending 4 h or less on one's feet
per day. Physical examination findings associated
with an increased risk were the inability to rise
from a chair, poor depth perception, poor contrast
sensitivity, and tachycardia at rest. Women who
had gained weight since the age of 25 years had
a lower risk of hip fracture. Women with multiple risk factors who also had low calcaneal bone
density had a particularly high risk. In the Dubbo
osteoporosis epidemiology study, independent predictors of rate of femoral neck bone loss in elderly
women included age, baseline bone mineral density, weight, weight change, and physical activity;
collectively these factors accounted for 13% of total
bone loss by multiple regression analysis (NGUYEN
et al. 1998).

Cigarette smoking has been identified as another
risk factor for low bone mineral density. The negative effect on the skeleton may be explained in part
by reduced body mass in smokers; moreover, low
levels of 25-OH vitamin D and osteocalcin have been
found in smokers (HERMANN et al. 2000). KRALL
and DAWSON-HUGHES (1999) demonstrated that in
elderly men and women smoking accelerates bone
loss as measured at several skeletal sites including
the femoral neck. Impairment of intestinal calcium
absorption may contribute to the observed bone
loss.

In a prospective population based study the relationship between the risk of nontraumatic fractures
and serum levels of RANKL was determined (SCHETT

et al. 2004). Noteworthy, a low level of RANKL was found to be an independent parameter of nontraumatic fracture.

Finally – in particular in the elderly – falls and other nonskeletal factors are very important determinants of fracture risk (GEUSENS et al. 2003; SUH and LYLES 2003).

2.2.5
Secondary Osteoporosis

Although a great number of diseases or conditions are associated with low bone mass and mineral density, only a few selected examples of secondary osteoporosis will be discussed.

Glucocorticoid-induced osteoporosis is among the most frequent forms of secondary osteoporosis. Even low doses of oral glucocorticoids and endogenous hypercortisolism (Cushing's syndrome) may be associated with bone loss and fractures (SHAKER and LUKERT 2005). The mechanism by which glucocorticoids induce osteoporosis appears to be different from that of postmenopausal osteoporosis. Of particular importance in glucocorticoid-induced osteoporosis is a direct effect of the steroids on osteoblasts, resulting in reduced bone matrix synthesis and a shorter life span of active osteoblasts (EASTELL et al. 1998). Moreover, glucocorticoids impair the differentiation of stromal cells toward osteoblasts (CANALIS et al. 2004). Glucocorticoids have a dual effect on osteoclasts. Whereas at physiologic concentrations they promote late-stage osteoclast differentiation and function, high doses of, for example, dexamethasone have been reported to stimulate the formation of osteoclast-like cells (LUKERT 1999; SHUTO et al. 1994). Moreover, glucocorticoids inhibit intestinal calcium absorption, enhance renal calcium excretion, and reduce the secretion of gonadal hormones (CANALIS 2004).

In patients with hyperthyroidism several alterations of bone and mineral metabolism that may lead to the development of osteoporotic fractures can be observed (LAKATOS 2003). These alterations include an increase in bone remodeling with excessive bone degradation, hypercalciuria, and decreased intestinal calcium absorption (SUWANWALAIKORN and BARAN 1996). In organ cultures thyroid hormones stimulate bone resorption (KLAUSHOFER et al. 1989); data from our laboratory indicate that triiodothyronine augments $1,25\text{-}(OH)_2D_3$-induced osteoclastogenesis (SCHILLER et al. 1998). In osteoblasts triio-

dothyronine acts as a differentiation factor (VARGA et al. 1997).

Alcohol abuse appears to confer a high risk for osteoporotic fractures in particular in men. Measurements of biochemical markers of bone turnover demonstrate that alcohol-induced bone loss is due to a reduction in bone formation; other pathogenetic factors related to excess alcohol consumption include gonadal dysfunction (in men) and vitamin D deficiency (SEEMAN 1996; TURNER 2000).

Several inflammatory rheumatic diseases are associated with osteoporosis; rheumatoid arthritis provides an excellent example of both local and systemic consequences of inflammatory processes on bone remodeling. In patients with rheumatoid arthritis, juxtaarticular osteopenia adjacent to inflamed joints and radiographically detectable bone erosions can be found as well as generalized axial and appendicular osteopenia (GOLDRING 1999; LERNBASS et al. 2002; INABA 2004). Bone loss may also constitute a significant clinical problem in patients with systemic lupus erythematosus (REDLICH et al. 2000) or ankylosing spondylitis (GRISAR et al. 2002; EL MAGHRAOUI 2004).

The pathogenesis of post-transplantation bone disease (which is observed after kidney, heart, bone marrow, liver, or lung transplantation) is complex and incompletely understood (CUNNINGHAM 2005; KERSCHAN-SCHINDL et al. 2004). Many patients who are candidates for transplantation either have disease-associated risk factors for osteoporosis, and/or are treated with drugs potentially resulting in bone loss e.g., glucocorticoids, anticoagulants, or loop diuretics, or a have preexisting bone disease, such as renal osteodystrophy. Bone loss after organ transplantation is caused primarily by the effects of glucocorticoids and other immunosuppressive drugs (in particular cyclosporin A), as well as of hypogonadism and vitamin D deficiency (ARINGER et al. 1998; SHANE 1999; KERSCHAN-SCHINDL et al. 2003).

2.2.6
Osteoporosis in Men

Traditionally osteoporosis has been viewed as a disease of postmenopausal women; nevertheless, a significant number of men may present with this disorder. In the European Vertebral Osteoporosis Study vertebral deformities were detected in 12% of the men studied (O'NEILL et al. 1996); one-third

of hip fractures occur in men. In contrast to osteoporosis in women, osteoporosis in men frequently
is a secondary condition; only about half of male
osteoporosis cases are diagnosed as idiopathic/pri-
mary osteoporosis (FRANCIS et al. 1989; RESCH et
al. 1992; GRANINGER et al. 1998). Chronic alcohol
abuse, glucocorticoid treatment, and hypogonadism
are among the most frequent secondary causes of
osteoporosis in men.

In studies on bone histomorphometry in idiopathic osteoporosis in men, some authors described
impaired bone formation (DEVERNEJOUL et al. 1983;
JACKSON et al. 1986; HILLS et al. 1989; ZERWEKH et
al. 1992; CHAVASSIEUX and MEUNIER 2001), while
others found that bone resorption is increased
(PERRY et al. 1982; NORDIN et al. 1984). Thus, at
least from the point of view of histomorphometry,
the syndrome of idiopathic osteoporosis in men
appears to be quite heterogeneous. In two independent studies we found increased biochemical
markers of bone resorption in men with idiopathic
osteoporosis (RESCH et al. 1992; PIETSCHMANN et
al. 2001).

As discussed above, several data suggest that
estrogen deficiency contributes to bone loss in
aging men. In addition, several other aspects of the
pathophysiology of idiopathic osteoporosis in men
have been described in the literature. Several independent studies found increased serum levels of sex
hormone binding globulin in men with idiopathic
osteoporosis (GILLBERG et al. 1999; PIETSCHMANN
et al. 2001; LORMEAU et al. 2004). LJUNGHALL and
coworkers (1992) found low plasma levels of insulin-
like growth factor 1 in male patients with idiopathic
osteoporosis. NEED et al. (1998) demonstrated that
calcium absorption is low in men with osteoporosis; about half of this deficit was due to low serum
1,25-dihydroxyvitamin D_3 levels, but there
appeared to be some intestinal resistance to the
effect of 1,25-dihydroxyvitamin D_3 on calcium
absorption. Renal calcium loss and hypercalciuria
may be further pathogenetic aspects of osteoporosis in men. In some series of patients with idiopathic osteoporosis, a significant number have
associated hypercalciuria (PERIS and GUANABENS
1996). Moreover, decreased bone mineral density has been reported in patients with idiopathic
renal stone formation (PIETSCHMANN et al. 1992).
Finally, PACIFICI et al. (1987) showed increased
release of IL-1 from blood monocytes in a group
of male and female patients with idiopathic osteoporosis.

2.2.7
Osteoporosis in Premenopausal Women

In relatively rare cases, osteoporosis also occurs in
premenopausal women. Most young women with
osteoporosis have an identifiable cause such as glucocorticoid treatment, eating disorders or pregnancy
(MITRINGER and PIETSCHMANN 2002). There are
only few studies on the pathogenesis of idiopathic
osteoporosis in premenopausal women; a recent histomorphometric investigation demonstrated osteoblast dysfunction with uncoupling of resorption and
formation of bone (DONOVAN et al. 2005).

2.3
Pathophysiology of Metabolic Bone Diseases Other than Osteoporosis

In the final part of this chapter some aspects of the
pathophysiology of selected metabolic bone diseases
will be discussed. For a more detailed description of
these and other bone disorders (such as neoplastic,
infectious or ischemic bone diseases) the reader is
referred elsewhere.

2.3.1
Paget's Disease

Paget's disease of bone is a localized disorder of bone
remodeling (Fig. 2.2). The disease process is initiated
by increases in osteoclast-mediated bone resorption,
with subsequent compensatory increases in new
bone formation, resulting in a disorganized mosaic
of woven and lamellar bone at affected skeletal sites
(SIRIS 1999; SIEGHART 2004). Paget's disease appears
to have a significant genetic component; 15%–30%
of patients with Paget's disease have family histories
of the disorder.

Osteoclasts in Paget's disease are increased both
in number and in size; osteoclast-like multinucleated cells form more rapidly in marrow cultures from
patients with Paget's disease and produce increased
levels of IL-6 (REDDY et al. 1999). Moreover, osteoclast precursors from patients with Paget's disease
are hypersensitive to 1,25-dihydroxyvitamin D3
and RANKL (MENAA et al. 2000; NEALE et al. 2000).
There are data that support a viral etiology of Paget's
disease (SINGER 1999; ROODMAN and WINDLE 2005).

Fig. 2.2. Whole body bone scan of a 40-year-old woman with Paget's disease of the right tibia showing intense activity of the involved bone. (Courtesy of Univ. Doz. Dr. P Mikosch 2nd Department of Medicine, State Hospital Klagenfurt, Klagenfurt.) [Reproduced from MIKOSCH (2004)]

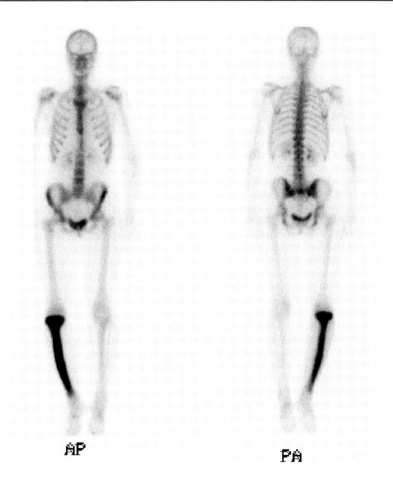

AP   PA

For instance, MEE and coworkers (1998) were able to detect canine distemper virus by in situ reverse transcriptase polymerase chain reaction in 100% of Paget's disease samples.

2.3.2
Primary Hyperparathyroidism

Primary hyperparathyroidism is a relatively frequent endocrine disease and is one of the most common causes of hypercalcemia. In the majority of cases the disease is caused by a benign, solitary parathyroid adenoma; less frequently it is due to hyperplasia of all four parathyroid glands (BILEZIKIAN 1999). While severe primary hyperparathyroidism is classically associated with a condition called osteodystrophia fibrosa generalisata cystica v. Recklinghausen, it remained uncertain whether mild, asymptomatic primary hyperparathyroidism adversely affects the skeleton. KHOSLA and coworkers (1999), however, clearly demonstrated that primary hyperparathy-

roidism among unselected patients in the community is associated with a significant increase in the risk of vertebral, Colles', rib, and pelvic fractures. Primary hyperparathyroidism is generally associated with an increased bone turnover; this can be assessed by biochemical markers and bone histomorphometry (PIETSCHMANN et al. 1991; CHRISTIANSEN et al. 1999; ERIKSEN 2002).

2.3.3
Osteomalacia and Rickets

Osteomalacia is characterized by impaired bone mineralization (Fig. 2.3). The term "rickets" applies to the defective mineralization of bone and the cartilaginous growth plate in children. Rickets or osteomalacia may result from reduced availability of vitamin D as a consequence of insufficient intake or ultraviolet light exposure or malabsorption. Moreover, alterations in the metabolism of vitamin D, such as in severe hepatic disease or in renal insufficiency,

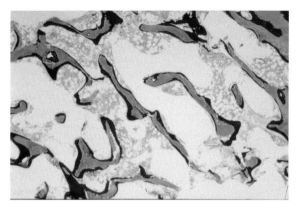

Fig. 2.3. Microscopic appearance of osteomalacia showing abnormally wide osteoid seams covering the trabecular surfaces (Goldner's stain). (Courtesy of Univ. Prof. Dr. I Sulzbacher, Clinical Institute of Pathology, Medical University of Vienna, Vienna)

may result in osteomalacia. Other causes of rickets/osteomalacia are phosphate deficiency, acidosis, hypophosphatasia, drugs that inhibit mineralization (e.g., fluoride or etidronate) and tumors (oncogenic osteomalacia) (LeBoff 1997; Carpenter 2003).

2.3.4
Renal Osteodystrophy

Renal osteodystrophy is a multifactorial disorder of bone remodeling observed in patients with end-stage renal disease. Histologically renal osteodystrophy is classified as osteitis fibrosa, osteomalacia, mixed disease, mild disease, or adynamic renal bone disease; the most common histologic diagnosis is osteitis fibrosa (Hutchinson et al. 1993). Factors contributing to renal osteodystrophy include 1,25-dihydroxyvitamin D3 deficiency, hypocalcemia, secondary hyperparathyroidism, skeletal resistance to PTH, hyperphosphatemia, and aluminum intoxication (Hruska and Teitelbaum 1995; Elder 2002).

2.4
Conclusion

This chapter has reviewed mechanisms responsible for the aging of bone and the pathogenesis of osteoporosis and other metabolic bone diseases.

A variety of alterations of the local as well as the systemic regulation of bone turnover that result in an uncoupling of bone resorption and bone formation has been suggested to account for these conditions. In postmenopausal women and older men estrogen deficiency and vitamin D insufficiency appear to be major determinants of bone loss.

Acknowledgement. The authors are grateful to Ms. Maria Steiner and Ms. Brigitte Freudhofmeier for her help with the preparation of the manuscript.

References

Abdallah BM, Stilgren LS, Nissen N, Kassem M, Jorgensen HRI, Abrahamsen B (2005) Increased RANKL/OPG mRNA ratio in iliac bone biopsies from women with hip fractures. Calcif Tissue Int 76:90–97

Ahlborg HG, Johnell O, Turner CH, Rannevik G, Karlsson MK (2003) Bone loss and bone size after menopause. N Engl J Med 349:327–334

Albaga OM, Ralston SH (2003) Genetic determinants of susceptibility to osteoporosis. Endocrinol Metab Clin North Am 32:65–81

Aringer M, Kiener HP, Koeller MD, Artemiou O, Zuckermann A, Wieselthaler G, Klepetko W, Seidl G, Kainberger F, Bernecker P, Smolen JS, Pietschmann P (1998) High turnover bone disease following lung transplantation. Bone 23:485–488

Ballanti P, Bonucci E, Della-Rocca C, Milani S, Lo-Cascio V, Lo-Imbibo B (1990) Bone histomorphometric reference values in 88 normal Italian subjects. Bone Miner 11:187–197

Battmann A, Battmann A, Jundt G, Schulz A (1997) Endosteal human bone cells (EBC) show age-related activity in vitro. Exp Clin Endocrinol Diabetes 105:98–102

Bauer DC, Sklarin PM, Stone KL, Black DM, Nevitt MC, Ensrud KE, Arnaud CD, Genant HK, Garnero P, Delmas PD, Lawaetz H, Cummings SR (1999) Biochemical markers of bone turnover and prediction of hip bone loss in older women: the study of osteoporotic fractures. J Bone Miner Res 14:1404–1410

Bergmann RJ, Gazit D, Kahn AJ, Gruber H, McDougall S, Hahn TJ (1996) Age-related changes in osteogenic stem cells in mice. J Bone Miner Res 11:568–577

Bilezikian JP (1999) Primary hyperparathyroidism. In: Favus MJ (ed) Primer on the metabolic bone diseases and disorders of mineral metabolism. Lippincott Williams and Wilkins, Philadelphia, pp 187–192

Blain H, Vuillemin A, Blain A, Guillemin F, De Talance N, Doucet B, Jeandel C (2004) Age-related femoral bone loss in men: evidence for hyperparathyroidism and insulin-like growth factor-1 deficiency. J Gerontol A Biol Sci Med Sci 59:1285–1289

Bourdel A, Mahoudeau JA, Guadyier-Souquières, Leymarie P, Sabatier JP, Loyau G (1989) Étude de la fonction gonadique au cours de l'ostéoporose masculine en apparence primitive. Presse Med 34:1691–1694

Bouxsein ML (2003) Bone quality: where do we go from here? Osteoporos Int 14:118–127

Brockstedt H, Kassem M, Eriksen EF, Mosekilde L, Melsen F (1993) Age- and sex-related changes in iliac cortical bone mass and remodeling. Bone 14:681–691

Canalis E, Bilezikian JP, Angeli A, Giustina A (2004) Perspectives on glucocorticoid-induced osteoporosis. Bone 34:593–598

Cao J, Venton L, Sakata T, Halloran BP (2003) Expression of RANKL and OPG correlates with age-related bone loss in male C57BL/6 mice. J Bone Miner Res 18:270–277

Carpenter TO (2003) Oncogenic osteomalacia – a complex dance of factors. N Engl J Med 348:1705–1708

Catherwood BD, Marcus R, Madvig P, Cheung AK (1985) Determinants of bone gamma-carboxyglutamic acid containing protein in plasma of healthy aging subjects. Bone 6:9–13

Chavassieux P, Meunier PJ (2001) Histomorphometric approach of bone loss in men. Calcif Tissue Int 69:209–213

Christiansen P, Steiniche T, Brixen K, Hessov I, Melsen F, Heickendorff L, Mosekilde Le (1999) Primary hyperparathyroidism: short-term changes in bone remodeling and bone mineral density following parathyroidectomy. Bone 25:237–244

Ciarelli TE, Fyhrie DP, Schaffler MB, Goldstein SA (2000) Variations in three-dimensional cancellous bone architecture of the proximal femur in female hip fractures and in controls. J Bone Miner Res 15:32–40

Clarke BL, Ebeling PR, Jones JD, Wahner HW, O'Fallon WM, Riggs BL, Fitzpatrick LA (1996) Changes in quantitative bone histomorphometry in aging healthy men. J Clin Endocrinol Metab 81:2264–2270

Cohn SH, Abesamis C, Yasumura S, Aloia JF, Zanzi I, Ellis KJ (1977) Comparative skeletal mass and radial bone mineral content in black and white women. Metabolism 26:171–178

Cooper GS (1999) Genetic studies of osteoporosis: what have we learned? J Bone Miner Res 14:1646–1648

Cosman F, Nieves J, Horton J, Shen V, Lindsay R (1994) Effects of estrogen on response to edetic acid infusion in postmenopausal osteoporotic women. J Clin Endocrinol Metab 78:939–943

Croucher PI, Garrahan NJ, Mellish RW, Compston JE (1991) Age-related changes in resorption cavity characteristics in human trabecular bone. Osteoporosis Int 4:257–261

Cummings SR, Browner WS, Bauer D, Stone K, Ensrud K, Jamal S, Ettinger B (1998) Endogenous hormones and the risk of hip and vertebral fractures among older women. N Engl J Med 339:733–738

Cummings SR, Nevitt MC, Browner WS, Stone K, Fox KM, Ensrud KE, Cauley J, Black D, Vogt TM (1995) Risk factors for hip fracture in white women. N Engl J Med 332:767–773

Cunningham J (2005) Posttransplantation bone disease. Transplantation 79:629–634

Delmas PD, Garnero P (1996) Utility of biochemical markers of bone turnover in osteoporosis. In: Marcus R, Feldman D, Kelsey J (eds) Osteoporosis. Academic, San Diego, pp 1075–1088

Dempster DW (2000) The contribution of trabecular architecture to cancellous bone quality. J Bone Miner Res 15:20–23

DeVernejoul MC, Bielakoff J, Herve M, Gueris J, Hott M, Modrowski D, Kuntz D, Miravet L, Ryckewaert A (1983) Evidence for defective osteoblastic function. Clin Orthop Rel Res 179:107–115

Donovan MA, Dempster D, Zhou H, McMahon DJ, Fleischer J, Shane E (2005) Low bone formation in premenopausal women with idiopathic osteoporosis. J Clin Endocrinol Metab 90:3331–3336

Eastell R, Delmas PD, Hodgson SF, Eriksen EF, Mann KG, Riggs BL (1988) Bone formation rate in older normal women: concurrent assessment with bone histomorphometry, calcium kinetics, and biochemical markers. J Clin Endocrinol Metab 67:741–748

Eastell R, Yergey AL, Vieira NE, Cedel SL, Kumar R, Riggs BL (1991) Interrelationship among vitamin D metabolism, true calcium absorption, parathyroid function, and age in women; evidence of an age-related intestinal resistance to 1,25-dihydroxyvitamin D action. J Bone Miner Res 6:125–132

Eastell R, Reid DM, Compston J, Cooper C, Fogelman I, Francis RM, Hosking DJ, Purdie DW, Ralston SH, Reeve J, Russell RGG, Stevenson JC, Torgerson DJ (1998) A UK consensus group on management of glucocorticoid-induced osteoporosis: an update. J Intern Med 244:271–292

Ebeling PR, Peterson JM, Riggs BL (1992) Utility of type I procollagen propeptide assays for assessing abnormalities in metabolic bone diseases. J Bone Miner Res 7:1243–1250

Eghbali-Fatourechi G, Khosla S, Sanyal A, Boyle WJ, Lacey DL, Riggs BL (2003) Role of RANK ligand in mediating increased bone resorption in early postmenopausal women. J Clin Invest 111:1120–1122

Elder G (2002) Pathophysiology and recent advances in the management of renal osteodystrophy. J Bone Miner Res 17:2094–2105

Endres DB, Morgan CH, Garry PJ, Omdahl JL (1987) Age-related changes in serum immunoreactive parathyroid hormone and its biological action in healthy men and women. J Clin Endocrinol Metab 65:724

El Maghraoui A (2004) Osteoporosis and ankylosing spondylitis. Joint Bone Spine 71:291–295

Epstein H, Poser J, Mc Clintock R, Johnston CC, Bryce G, Hui S (1984) Differences in serum bone GLA protein with age and sex. Lancet i:307–310

Erben RG, Eberle J, Stahr K, Goldberg M (2000) Androgen deficiency induces high turnover osteopenia in aged male rats: a sequential histomorphometric study. J Bone Miner Res 15:1085–1098

Eriksen EF (2002) Primary hyperparathyroidism: lessons from bone histomorphometry. J Bone Miner Res 17:N95–N97

Falahati-Nini A, Riggs BL, Atkinson EJ, O'Fallon WM, Eastell R, Khosla S (2000) Relative contributions of testosterone and estrogen in regulating bone resorption and formation in normal elderly men. J Clin Invest 106:1553–1560

Finkelstein JS, Klibanski A, Neer RM, Greenspan SL, Rosenthal DI, Crowley WF (1987) Osteoporosis in men with idiopathic hypogonadotropic hypogonadism. Ann Intern Med 106:354–361

Francis RM, Peacock M, Marshall DH, Horsman A, Aaron JE (1989) Spinal osteoporosis in men. Bone Miner 5:347–357

Gallagher JC, Kinyamu HK, Fowler SE, Dawson-Hughes B, Dalsky GP, Sherman SS (1998) Calciotropic hormones and bone markers in the elderly. J Bone Miner Res 13:475–482

Garnero P, Shih WJ, Gineyts E, Karpf DB, Delmas PD (1994) Comparison of new biochemical markers of bone turnover in late postmenopausal osteoporotic women in response to alendronate treatment. J Clin Endocrinol Metab 79:1693–1700

Gennari C, Agnusdei D, Nardi P, Civitelli R (1990) Estrogen preserves a normal intestinal responsiveness to 1,25-dihydroxyvitamin D₃ in oophorectomized women. J Clin Endocrinol Metab 71:1288–1293

Gennari L, Merlotti D, Martini G, Gonnelli S, Franci B, Campagna S, Lucani B, Dal Canto N, Valenti R, Gennari C, Nuti R (2003) Longitudinal association between sex hormone levels, bone loss, and bone turnover in elderly men. J Clin Endocrinol Metab 88:5327–5333

Geusens P, Milisen K, Dejaeger E, Boonen S (2003) Falls and fractures in postmenopausal women: a review. J Br Menopause Soc 9:101–106

Gillberg P, Johansson AG, Ljunghall S (1999) Decreased estradiol levels and free androgen index and elevated sex hormone-binding globulin levels in male idiopathic osteoporosis. Calcif Tissue Int 64:209–213

Glowacki J (1999) Cellular models of human aging. In: Rosen CJ, Glowacki J, Bilezikian JP (eds) The aging skeleton. Academic, San Diego, pp 59–73

Goderie-Plomp HW, van der Klift M, de Ronde W, Hofman A, de Jong FH, Pols HAP (2004) Endogenous sex hormones, sex hormone-binding globulin, and the risk of incident vertebral fractures in elderly men and women: the Rotterdam study. J Clin Endocrinol Metab 89:3261–3269

Goldring SR (1999) Osteoporosis and rheumatic diseases. In: Favus MJ (ed) Primer on the metabolic bone diseases and disorders of mineral metabolism. Lippincott Williams and Wilkins, Philadelphia, pp 313–315

Graninger M, Dirnberger E, Kainberger F, Bernecker P, Graninger W, Smolen J, Pietschmann P (1998) Comparison of spinal and femoral dual energy X-ray absorptiometry (DXA) in men with primary and secondary osteoporosis. Osteologie 7:48–52

Greendale GA, Edelstein S, Barrett-Connor E (1997) Endogenous sex steroids and bone mineral density in older women and men: the Rancho Bernardo Study. J Bone Miner Res 12:1833–1843

Grisar J, Bernecker PM, Aringer M, Redlich K, Sedlak M, Wolozcszuk W, Spitzauer S, Grampp S, Kainberger F, Ebner W, Smolen JS, Pietschmann P (2002) Ankylosing spondylitis, psoriatic arthritis, and reactive arthritis show increased bone resorption, but differ with regard to bone formation. J Rheumatol 29:1430–1436

Heaney RP, Recker RR, Saville PD (1978) Menopausal changes in calcium balance performance. J Lab Clin Med 92:953–963

Heaney RP, Abrams S, Dawson-Hughes B, Looker A, Marcus R, Matkovic V, Weaver C (2000) Peak bone mass. Osteoporos Int 11:985–1009

Hermann M, Berger P (1999) Hormone replacement in the aging male? Exp Gerontol 34:923–933

Hermann AP, Brot C, Gram J, Kolthoff N, Mosekilde L (2000) Premenopausal smoking and bone density in 2015 perimenopausal women. J Bone Miner Res 15:780–787

Hills E, Dunstan CR, Wong SYP, Evans RA (1989) Bone histology in young adult osteoporosis. J Clin Pathol 42:391–397

Hruska KA, Teitelbaum SL (1995) Renal osteodystrophy. N Engl J Med 333:166–174

Hutchinson AJ, Whitehouse RW, Boulton HF, Adams JE, Mawer EB, Freemont TJ, Gokal R (1993) Correlation of bone histology with parathyroid hormone, vitamin D3, and radiology in end-stage renal disease. Kidney Int 44:1071–1077

Inaba M (2004) Secondary osteoporosis: thyrotoxicosis, rheumatoid arthritis, and diabetes mellitus. J Bone Miner Metab 22:287–292

Jackson JA, Kleerekoper M, Parfitt M, Rao DS, Villanueva AR, Frame B (1986) Bone histomorphometry in hypogonadal and eugonadal men with spinal osteoporosis. J Clin Endocrinol Metab 65:53–58

Jilka RL, Weinstein RS, Takahashi K, Parfitt AM, Manolagas SC (1996) Linkage of decreased bone mass with impaired osteoblastogenesis in a murine model of accelerated senescence. J Clin Invest 97:1732–1740

Kahn A, Gibbons R, Perkins S, Gazit D (1995) A hypothesis and initial assessment in mice. Clin Orthop 313:69–75

Kajkenova O, Lecka-Czernik B, Gubrij I, Hauser SP, Takahashi K, Parfitt AM, Jilka RL, Manolagas SC, Lipschitz DA (1997) Increased adipogenesis and myelopoiesis in the bone marrow of SAMP6, a murine model of defective osteoblastogenesis and low turnover osteopenia. J Bone Miner Res 12:1772–1779

Kelly PJ, Pocock NA, Sambrock PN, Eisman JA (1990) Dietary calcium, sex hormones, and bone mineral density in men. Br Med J 300:1361–1364

Kelly PJ, Hopper LJ, Macaskill NA, Pocock PN, Sambrook PN, Eisman JA (1991) Genetic determinants of collagen synthesis and degradation: further evidence of genetic regulation of bone turnover. J Clin Endocrinol Metab 78:1461–1466

Kerschan-Schindl K, Strametz-Juranek J, Heinze G, Grampp S, Bieglmayer C, Pacher R, Maurer G, Fialka-Moser V, Pietschmann P (2003) Pathogenesis of bone loss in heart transplant candidates and recipients. J Heart Lung Transplant 22:843–850

Kerschan-Schindl K, Mitterbauer M, Fureder W, Kudlacek S, Grampp S, Bieglmayer C, Fialka-Moser V, Pietschmann P, Kalhs P (2004) Bone metabolism in patients more than five years after bone marrow transplantation. Bone Marrow Transplant 34:491–496

Khosla S, Melton LJ III, Atkinson EJ, O'Fallon WM, Klee GG, Riggs BL (1998) Relationship of serum sex steroid levels and bone turnover markers with bone mineral density in men and women: a key role for bioavailable estrogen. J Clin Endocrinol Metab 83:2266–2274

Khosla S, Melton LJ III, Wermers RA, Crowson CS, O'Fallon WM, Riggs BL (1999) Primary hyperparathyroidism and the risk of fracture: a population-based study. J Bone Miner Res 14:1700–1707

Klaushofer K, Hoffmann O, Gleispach H, Leis HJ, Czerwenka E, Koller K, Peterlik M (1989) Bone resorbing activity of thyroid hormones is related to prostaglandin production in neonatal mouse calvaria. J Bone Miner Res 4:305

Koh LKH, Bauer DC, Forsyth BA, Gore LR, Vogt MT, Cummings SR (1997) PTH in postmenopausal osteoporotic women. J Bone Miner Res 12:S166

Kotzmann H, Bernecker P, Hübsch T, Pietschmann P, Wolo-szczuk W, Svoboda T, Geyer G, Luger A (1993) Bone mineral density and parameters of bone metabolism in patients with acromegaly. J Bone Miner Res 8:459–465

Krall EA, Dawson-Hughes B (1999) Smoking increases bone loss and decreases intestinal calcium absorption. J Bone Miner Res 14:215–220

Kroger H, Kotaniemi A, Kroger L, Alhava E (1993) Development of bone mass and bone density of the spine and femoral neck – a prospective study of 65 children and adolescents. Bone Miner 23:171–182

Kushida K, Takahashi M, Kawana K (1995) Comparison of markers for bone formation and resorption in premeno-pausal and postmenopausal subjects, and osteoporosis patients. J Clin Endocrinol Metab 80:2447–2450

Lakatos P (2003) Thyroid hormones: beneficial or deleterious for bone? Calcif Tissue Int 73:205–209

Lang I, Schernthaner G, Pietschmann P, Kurz R, Stephenson JM, Templ H (1987) Effects of sex and age on growth hor-mone response to growth hormone-releasing hormone in healthy individuals. J Clin Endocrinol Metab 65:535–540

LeBoff MS (1997) Metabolic bone disease. In: Kelley WN, Harry ED, Ruddy S, Sledge CB (eds) Textbook of rheu-matology. Saunders, Philadelphia, pp 1563–1580

LeBoff MS, Glowacki J (1999) Sex steroids, bone and aging. In: Rosen CJ, Glowacki J, Bilezikian JP (eds) The aging skeleton. Academic, San Diego, pp 159–174

Legrand E, Chappard D, Pascaretti C, Duquenne M, Krebs S, Rohmer V, Basle MF, Audran M (2000) Trabecular bone microarchitecture, bone mineral density, and ver-tebral fractures in male osteoporosis. J Bone Miner Res 15:13–19

Lernbass I, Wutzl A, Grisar J, Schett G, Redlich K, Spitzauer S, Grampp S, Imhof H, Peterlik M, Pietschmann P (2002) Quantitative ultrasound in the assessment of bone status of patients suffering from rheumatic diseases. Skeletal Radiol 31:270–276

Lips P, Courpron P, Meunier PJ (1978) Mean wall thickness of trabecular bone packets in the human iliac crest: changes with age. Calcif Tissue Res 26:13–17

Ljunghall S, Johansson AG, Burman P, Kämpe O, Lindh E, Karlsson FA (1992) Low plasma levels of insulin-like growth factor (IGF-I) in male patients with idiopathic osteoporosis. J Intern Med 232:59–64

Lormeau C, Soudan B, d'Herbomez M, Pigny P, Duquesnoy B, Cortet B (2004) Sex hormone-binding globulin, estra-diol, and bone turnover markers in male osteoporosis. Bone 34:933–939

Lu PW, Briody JN, Ogle GD, Morley K, Humphries IR, Allen J, Howman-Giles R, Sillence D, Cowell CT (1994) Bone mineral density of total body, spine, and femoral neck in children and young adults: a cross-sectional and longitu-dinal study. J Bone Miner Res 9:1451–1458

Lukert BP (1999) Glucocorticoid-induced osteoporosis. In: Favus MJ (ed) Primer on the metabolic bone diseases and disorders of mineral metabolism. Lippincott Williams and Wilkins, Philadelphia, pp 292–296

Makluf HA, Mueller SM, Mizuno S, Glowacki J (2000) Age-related decline in osteoprotegerin expression by human bone marrow cells cultured in three dimensional collage sponges. Biochem Biophys Res Commun 268:669–672

Matkovic V, Fontana D, Tominac C, Goel P, Chesnut CH III (1990) Factors that influence peak bone mass formation:

a study of calcium balance and the inheritance of bone mass in adolescent females. Am J Clin Nutr 52:878–888

Matkovic V, Jelic T, Wardlaw GM, Ilich JZ, Goel PK, Wright JK, Andon MB, Smith KT, Heaney RP (1994) Timing of peak bone mass in Caucasian females and its implica-tion for the prevention of osteoporosis. Inference from a cross-sectional model. J Clin Invest 93:799–808

Matsushita M, Tsuboyama T, Kasai R, Okumura H, Yama-muro T, Higuchi K, Higuchi K, Kohno A, Yonezu T, Utani A, et al. (1986) Age-related changes in bone mass in the senescence-accelerated mouse (SAM). SAM-R/3 and SAM-P/6 as new murine models for senile osteoporosis. Am J Pathol 125:276–283

McKane WR, Khosla S, Burritt MF, Kao PC, Wilson DM, Ory SJ, Riggs BL (1995) Mechanism of renal conserva-tion with estrogen replacement therapy in women in early postmenopause – a clinical research center study. J Clin Endocrinol Metab 80:3458–3464

McKenna MJ (1992) Differences in vitamin D status between countries in young adults and the elderly. Am J Med 93:69–77

Mee AP, Dixon JA, Hoyland JA, Davies M, Selby PL, Mawer EB (1998) Detection of canine distemper virus in 100% of Paget's disease samples by in situ-reverse transcriptase-polymerase chain reaction. Bone 23:171–175

Melton LJ III, Riggs BL (1988) Clinical spectrum. In: Riggs BL, Melton LJ III (eds) Osteoporosis: etiology, diagnosis and management. Raven Press, New York, pp 155

Melton LJ III (1995) How many women have osteoporosis now? J Bone Miner Res 10:175–177

Menaa C, Barsony J, Reddy SV, Cornish J, Cundy T, Roodman GD (2000) 1,25-Dihydroxyvitamin D_3 hypersensitivity of osteoclast precursors from patients with Paget's disease. J Bone Miner Res 15:228–236

Mikosch P (2004) Die Knochenszintigraphie in der Diag-nostik metabolischer Knochenerkrankungen. Wien Med Wochenschr 154:119–126

Mitringer A, Pietschmann P (2002) Osteoporose bei prä-menopausalen Frauen. Wien Med Wochenschr 152:586–590

Morrison NA, Yeoman R, Kelly PJ, Eisman JA (1992) Con-tribution of trans-acting factor alleles to normal physi-ological variability: vitamin D receptor gene polymor-phisms and circulating osteocalcin. Proc Natl Acad Sci USA 89:6665–6669

Morrison NA, Qi JC, Tokita A, Kelly PJ, Crofts TV, Nguyen TV, Sambrook PN, Eisman JA (1994) Prediction of bone density by vitamin D receptor alleles. Nature 367:284–287

Murphy S, Khaw K, Cassidy A, Compston JE (1993) Sex hor-mones and bone mineral density in elderly men. Bone Miner 20:133–140

Neale SD, Smith R, Wass JA, Athanasou NA (2000) Osteoclast differentiation from circulating mononuclear precursors in Paget's disease is hypersensitive to 1,25-dihydroxyvi-tamin D(3) and RANKL. Bone 27:409–416

Need AG, Morris HA, Horowitz M, Scopacasa F, Nordin BEC (1998) Intestinal calcium absorption in men with spinal osteoporosis. Clin Endocrinol (Oxf) 48:163–168

Nguyen TV, Sambrook PN, Eisman JA (1998) Bone loss, phys-ical activity, and weight change in elderly women: the Dubbo osteoporosis epidemiology study. J Bone Miner Res 13:1458–1467

Nordin BEC, Aaron J, Speed R, Francis RM, Makins N (1984) Bone formation and resorption as the determinants of trabecular bone volume in normal osteoporotic men. Scott Med J 29:171–175

Nordin BEC, Need AG, Morris HA, Horowitz M, Robertson WG (1991) Evidence for a renal calcium leak in postmenopausal women. J Clin Endocrinol Metab 72:401–407

Obermayer-Pietsch BM, Lange U, Tauber G, Fruhauf G, Fahrleitner A, Dobnig H, Hermann J, Aglas F, Teichmann J, Neeck G, Leb G (2003) Vitamin D receptor initiation codon polymorphism, bone density and inflammatory activity of patients with ankylosing spondylitis. Osteoporos Int 14:995–1000

Obermayer-Pietsch BM, Bonelli CM, Walter DE, Kuhn RJ, Fahrleitner-Pammer A, Berghold A, Goessler W, Stephan V, Dobnig H, Leb G, Renner W (2004) Genetic predisposition for adult lactose intolerance and relation to diet, bone density, and bone fractures. J Bone Miner Res 19:42–47

Obermayer-Pietsch BM (2006) Genetics of osteoporosis. Wien Med Wochenschr 156:162–167

Omdahl JL, Garry PJ, Hunsaker LA, Hunt WC, Goodwin JS (1982) Nutritional status in a healthy elderly population: vitamin D. Am J Clin Nutr 36:1225–1233

O'Neill TW, Felsenberg D, Varlow J, Cooper C, Kanis JA, Silman AJ (1996) The prevalence of vertebral deformity in European men and women: the European vertebral osteoporosis study. J Bone Miner Res 11:1010–1018

Ongphiphadhanakul B, Rajatanavin R, Chanprasertyothin S, Piaseu N, Chailurkit L (1998) Serum oestradiol and oestrogen-receptor gene polymorphism are associated with bone mineral density independently of serum testosterone in normal males. Clin Endocrinol (Oxf) 49:803–809

Orwoll ES, Klein RF (1996) Osteoporosis in men: epidemiology, pathophysiology, and clinical characterization. In: Marcus R, Feldman D, Kelsey J (eds) Osteoporosis. Academic, San Diego, pp 745–784

Orwoll ES, Meier DE (1986) Alterations in calcium, vitamin D, and parathyroid hormone physiology in normal men with aging: relationship to the development of senile osteopenia. J Clin Endocrinol Metab 63:1262

Oursler MJ, Osodoby P, Pyfferoen J, Riggs PL, Spelsberg TC (1991) Avian osteoclasts as estrogen target cells. Proc Natl Acad Sci USA 88:6613–6617

Pacifici R, Rifas L, Teitelbaum S, Slaptopolsky E, McCracken R, Bergfeld M, Lee W, Avioli LV, Peck WA (1987) Spontaneous release of interleukin 1 from human blood monocytes reflects bone formation in idiopathic osteoporosis. Proc Natl Acad Sci USA 84:4616–4620

Palle S, Chappard D, Vico L, Riffat G, Alexandre C (1989) Evaluation of the osteoclastic population in iliac crest biopsies from 36 normal subjects: a histoenzymologic and histomorphometric study. J Bone Miner Res 4:501–506

Parfitt AM (2004) The attainment of peak bone mass: what is the relationship between muscle growth and bone growth? Bone 34:767–770

Peris P, Guanabens N (1996) Male osteoporosis. Curr Opin Rheumatol 8:357–364

Perkins SL, Gibbons R, Kling S, Kahn AJ (1994) Age-related bone loss in mice is associated with an increased osteoclast progenitor pool. Bone 15:65–72

Perry HM III, Fallon MD, Bergfeld M, Teitelbaum SL, Avioli LV (1982) Osteoporosis in young men: a syndrome of hypercalciuria and accelerated bone turnover. Arch Intern Med 142: 1295–1298

Pfeilschifter J, Diel I, Pilz U, Brunotte K, Naumann A, Ziegler R (1993) Mitogenic responsiveness of human bone cells in vitro to hormone and growth factors decreases with age. J Bone Miner Res 8:707–717

Pietschmann P, Peterlik M (1999) Pathophysiologie der Osteoporose. Wien Med Wochenschr 16/17:454–462

Pietschmann P, Woloszcuzk W, Pietschmann H (1990) Increased serum osteocalcin levels in elderly females with vitamin D deficiency. Exp Clin Endocrinol 95:275–278

Pietschmann P, Niederle B, Anvari A, Woloszczuk W (1991) Serum osteocalcin levels in primary hyerparathyroidism. Klin Wochenschr 69:351–353

Pietschmann F, Breslau NA, Pak CY (1992) Reduced vertebral bone density in hypercalciuric nephrolithiasis. J Bone Miner Res 7:1383–1388

Pietschmann P, Kudlacek S, Grisar J, Spitzauer S, Woloszczuk W, Willvonseder R, Peterlik M (2001) Bone turnover markers and sex hormones in men with idiopathic osteoporosis. Eur J Clin Invest 31:444–451

Pietschmann P, Gollob E, Brosch S, Hahn P, Kudlacek S, Willheim M, Woloszczuk W, Peterlik M, Tragl KH (2003) The effect of age and gender on cytokine production by human peripheral blood mononuclear cells and markers of bone metabolism. Exp Gerontol 38:1119–1127

Pocock NA, Eisman JA, Hopper JL, Yeates MG, Sambrook PN, Eberl S (1987) Genetic determinants of bone mass in adults. A twin study. J Clin Invest 80:706–710

Prince R, Dick I, Devine A, Price R, Gutteridge D, Kerr D, Criddle A, Garcia-Webb P, St John A (1995) The effects of menopause and age on calcitropic hormones: a cross-sectional study of 655 healthy women aged 35–90. J Bone Miner Res 10:835–842

Quarto R, Thomas D, Linag CT (1995) Bone progenitor cell deficits and the age-associated decline in bone repair capacity. Calcif Tissue Int 56:123–129

Quesada JM, Coopmans W, Ruiz B, Aljama P, Jans I, Bouillon R (1992) Influence of vitamin D on parathyroid function in the elderly. J Clin Endocrinol Metab 75:494–501

Rapado A, Hawkins F, Sobrinho L, Diaz-Curiel M, Galvao-Telles A, Arver S, Melo Gomes J, Mazer N, Garcia e Costa J, Horcajada C, Lopez-Gavilanes E, Mascarenhas M, Papapietro K, Lopez Alvarez MB, Pereira MC, Martinez, G, Valverde I, Garcia JJ, Carballal JJ, Garcia I (1999) Bone mineral density and androgen levels in elderly males. Calcif Tissue Int 65:417–21

Recker RR, Kimmel DB, Parfitt AM, Davies KM, Keshawarz N, Hinders S (1988) Static and tetracycline-based bone histomorphometric data from 34 normal postmenopausal females. J Bone Miner Res 3:133–144

Recker RR, Davies KM, Hinders SM, Heaney RP, Stegman MR, Kimmel DB (1992) Bone gain in young adult women. JAMA 268:2403–2408

Reddy SV, Menaa C, Singer FR, Demulder A, Roodman GD (1999) Cell biology of Paget's disease. J Bone Miner Res 14:3–8

Redlich K, Ziegler S, Kiener HP, Spitzauer S, Stohlawetz P, Bernecker P, Kainberger F, Grampp S, Kudlacek S, Woloszczuk W, Smolen JS, Pietschmann P (2000) Bone mineral density and biochemical parameters of bone metabolism in female patients with systemic lupus erythematosus. Ann Rheum Dis 59:308–310

Resch H, Pietschmann P, Woloszczuk W, Krexner E, Bernecker P, Willvonseder R (1992) Bone mass and biochemical parameters of bone metabolism in men with spinal osteoporosis. Eur J Clin Invest 22:542–545

Resch H, Pietschmann P, Kudlacek P, Woloszczuk W, Krexner E, Bernecker P, Willvonseder R (1994) Influence of sex and age on biochemical bone metabolism parameters. Miner Electrolyte Metab 20:117–121

Riggs BL, Melton LJ III (1983) Evidence for two distinct syndromes of involutional osteoporosis. Am J Med 75:899–901

Riggs BL, Khosla S, Melton LJ III (1998) A unitary model for involutional osteoporosis: estrogen deficiency causes both type I and type II osteoporosis in postmenopausal women and contributes to bone loss in aging men. J Bone Miner Res 13:763–773

Riggs BL, Khosla S, Atkinson EJ, Dunstan CR, Melton LJ III (2003) Evidence that type I osteoporosis results from enhanced responsiveness of bone to estrogen deficiency. Osteoporos Int 14:728–733

Riggs BL, Melton Iii LJ 3rd, Robb RA, Camp JJ, Atkinson EJ, Peterson JM, Rouleau PA, McCollough CH, Bouxsein ML, Khosla S (2004) Population-based study of age and sex differences in bone volumetric density, size, geometry, and structure at different skeletal sites. J Bone Miner Res 19:1945–1954

Rodin A, Murby B, Smith MA, Caleffi M, Fentiman I, Chapman MG, Fogelman I (1990) Premenopausal bone loss in the lumbar spine and neck of femur: a study of 225 Caucasian women. Bone 11:1–5

Roholl PJM, Blauw E, Zurcher C, Dormans JAMA, Theuns HM (1994) Evidence for a diminished maturation of proteoblasts into osteoblasts during aging in rats: an ultrastructural analysis. J Bone Miner Res 9:355–366

Roodman GD, Windle JJ (2005) Paget disease of bone. J Clin Invest 115:200–208

Roschger P, Rinnerthaler S, Yates J, Rodan GA, Fratzl P, Klaushofer K (2001) Alendroante increases degree and uniformity of mineralization in cancellous bone and decreases the porosity in cortical bone of osteoporotic women. Bone 29(2): 185–91

Rosen T, Hansson T, Granhed H, Szucs J, Bengtson BA (1993) Reduced bone mineral content in adult patients with growth hormone deficiency. Acta Endocrinol (Copenh) 129:201–206

Schett G, Kiechl S, Redlich K, Oberhollenzer F, Weger S, Egger G, Mayr A, Jocher J, Xu Q, Pietschmann P, Teitelbaum S, Smolen J, Willeit J (2004) Soluble RANKL and risk of nontraumatic fracture. JAMA 291:1108–1113

Schiller C, Gruber R, Redlich K, Ho GM, Gober HJ, Katzgraber F, Willheim M, Hoffmann O, Pietschmann P, Peterlik M (1997) 17β-estradiol antagonizes effects of 1α,25-dihydroxyvitamin D3 on interleukin-6 production and osteoclast-like cell formation in mouse bone marrow primary cultures. Endocrinology 138:4567–4571

Schlemmer A, Hassager C, Pedersen BJ, Christiansen C (1994) Posture, age, menopause, and osteopenia do not influence the circadian variation in the urinary excretion of pyridinium crosslinks. J Bone Miner Res 9:1883–1888

Seeman E (1996) The effects of tobacco and alcohol use on the bone. In: Marcus R, Feldman D, Kelsey J (eds) Osteoporosis. Academic, San Diego, pp 577–597

Seeman E (2003a) Periosteal bone formation – a neglected determinant of bone strength. N Engl J Med 349:4

Seeman E (2003b) Bone quality. Osteoporos Int 14:3–7

Seibel MJ, Woitge H, Scheidt-Nave C, Leidig-Bruckner G, Duncan A, Nicol P, Ziegler R, Robins SP (1994) Urinary hydroxypyridinium crosslinks of collagen in population-based screening for overt vertebral osteoporosis: results of a pilot study. J Bone Miner Res 9:1433–1440

Shaker JL, Lukert BP (2005) Osteoporosis associated with excess glucocorticoids. Endocrinol Metab Clin North Am 34:341–356

Shane E (1999) Transplantation osteoporosis. In: Favus MJ (ed) Primer on the metabolic bone diseases and disorders of mineral metabolism. Lippincott Williams and Wilkins, Philadelphia, pp 296–301

Sherman SS, Hollis BW, Tobin JD (1990) Vitamin D status and related parameters in a healthy population: the effects of age, sex, and season. J Clin Endocrinol Metab 71:405–413

Shuto T, Kukita T, Hirata M, Jimi E, Koga T (1994) Dexamethasone stimulates osteoclast-like cell formation by inhibiting granulocyte-macrophage colony-stimulating factor production in mouse bone marrow cultures. Endocrinology 134:1121–1126

Sieghart S (2004) Osteitis deformans–Paget's disease. Wien Med Wochenschr 154:97–101

Silva MJ, Brodt MD, Ko M, Abu-Amer Y (2005) Impaired marrow osteogenesis is associated with reduced endocortical bone formation but does not impair periosteal bone formation in long bones of SAMP6 mice. J Bone Miner Res 20:419–427

Singer FR (1999) Update on the viral etiology of Paget's disease of bone. J Bone Miner Res 14:29–33

Siris E (1999) Paget's disease of bone. In: Favus MJ (ed) Primer on the metabolic bone diseases and disorders of mineral metabolism. Lippincott Williams and Wilkins, Philadelphia, pp 415–425

Slemenda CW, Longcope C, Zhou L, Hui, SL, Peacock M, Johnston CC (1997) Sex steroids and bone mass in older men. J Clin Invest 100:1755–1759

Smith EP, Boyd J, Frank GR, Takahashi H, Cohen RM, Specker B, Williams TC, Lubahn DB, Korach KS (1994) Estrogen resistance caused by a mutation in the estrogen-receptor gene in man. N Engl J Med 331:1056–1061

Stein MS, Scherer SC, Walton SL, Gilbert RE, Ebeling PR, Flicker L, Wark JD (1996) Risk factors for secondary hyperparathyroidism in a nursing home population. Clin Endocrinol (Oxf) 44:375–383

Stepan JJ, Lachmann M, Zverina J, Pacovsky V, Baylink DJ (1989) Castrated men exhibit bone loss: effect of calcitonin treatment on biochemical indices of bone remodeling. J Clin Endocrinol Metab 69:523–527

Suh TT, Lyles KW (2003) Osteoporosis considerations in the frail elderly. Curr Opin Rheumatol 15:481–486

Suwanwalaikorn S, Baran D (1996) Thyroid hormone and the skeleton. In: Marcus R, Feldman D, Kelsey J (eds) Osteoporosis. Academic, San Diego, pp 855–861

Toss G, Almqvist S, Larsson L, Zetterqvist H (1980) Vitamin D deficiency in welfare institutions for the aged. Acta Med Scand 208:87–89

Tudor-Locke C, McColl RS (2000) Factors related to variation in premenopausal bone mineral status: a health promotion approach. Osteoporosis Int 11:1–24

Turner RT (2000) Skeletal response to alcohol. Alcohol Clin Exp Res 24:1693–1701

Uebelhart D, Schlemmer A, Johansen JS, Gineyts E, Christiansen K, Delmas PD (1991) Effect of menopause and hormone replacement therapy on the urinary excretion of pyridinium cross-links. J Clin Endocrinol Metab 72:367–373

Varga F, Rumpler M, Luegmayr E, Fratzl-Zelman N, Glantschnig H, Klaushofer K (1997) Triiodothyreonine, a regulator of osteoblastic differentiation: depression of histone H4, attenuation of c-fos/c-jun, and induction of osteocalcin expression. Calif Tissue Int 61:404–411

Vedi S, Compston JE, Webb A, Tighe JR (1982) Histomorphometric analysis of bone biopsies from the iliac crest of normal British subjects. Metab Bone Dis Relat Res 4:231 236

Vermeulen A (2000) Der senile Hypogonadismus beim Mann und seine hormonelle Substitutionstherapie. Acta Med Aust 27:11–17

Worsfold M, Sharp CA, Davie MJ (1988) Serum osteocalcin and other indices of bone formation: an 8-decade population study in healthy men and women. Clin Chim Acta 178:225–236

Wosje KS, Binkley TL, Fahrenwald NL, Specker BL (2000) High bone mass in a female Hutterite population. J Bone Miner Res 15:1429–1436

Zajickova K, Zofkova I (2003) Osteoporosis: genetic analysis of multifactorial disease. Endocr Regul 37:31–44

Zerwekh JE, Sakhaee K, Breslau NA, Gottschalk F, Park CYC (1992) Impaired bone formation in male idiopathic osteoporosis: further reduction in the presence of concomitant hypercalciuria. Osteoporosis Int 2:128–134

Pathophysiology of Rheumatoid Arthritis and Other Disorders

Heinrich Resch

CONTENTS

H. RESCH, MD
Professor of Medicine, University of Vienna (Rheumatology, Osteology); Head, Department of Internal Medicine II, St. Vincent Hospital, Vienna, Ludwig Boltzmann-Institut für Altersforschung, Stumpergasse 13, 1060 Vienna, Austria

3.1 Introduction

Rheumatoid arthritis (RA) is a chronic systemic disorder of unknown cause. There are many manifestations, but the typical feature of RA is chronic inflammatory synovitis, usually involving peripheral joints in a symmetric pattern. Although family studies indicate a clear genetic predisposition, it must be considered that this genetic risk does not fully account for the incidence of the disease, suggesting that environmental factors also play a role in the etiology of RA. The findings in the pathophysiology and production of cytokines allow the suggestion that RA is an event mediated by immunologic factors although the initiating stimulus has not yet been characterized. The most typical characteristics of the disease are inflammatory processes in the synovia, which cause cartilage damage and bone erosions and subsequent changes in joint integrity. Despite its destructive potential, the pattern of RA can be quite variable (Table 3.1). Some patients may experience only a mild oligoarticular illness of brief duration with minimal joint damage, whereas others will have progressive polyarthritis with severe functional impairment and also systemic manifestations.

The basic medical approach is to use nonsteroidal anti-inflammatory drugs (NSAIDs) and simple analgesics to control the clinical symptoms and the local inflammation. The second line of therapy involves using steroids. The third line of substances includes agents that have been classified as disease-modifying drugs. These agents seem to decrease elevated levels of acute-phase reactants in treated patients and therefore to modify the capacity of the disease to cause damage. Other agents are the immunosuppressive and cytotoxic drugs that have been shown to ameliorate the disease process in some patients. The increased mortality rate associated with these drugs seems to be limited to patients with more severe articular disease and can be attributed largely to infection and gastrointestinal bleeding. Drug

Table 3.1. The 1987 revised criteria for the classification of rheumatoid arthritis (ARNETT et al. 1988)

1. Guidelines for classification
a. Four of seven criteria are required to classify a patient as having rheumatoid arthritis.
b. Patients with two or more clinical diagnoses are not excluded.
2. Criteria[a]
a. Morning stiffness: Stiffness in and around the joints lasting 1 h before maximum improvement.
b. Arthritis of three or more joint areas: At least three joint areas, observed by a physician simultaneously, have soft tissue swelling or joint effusions, not just bony overgrowth. The 14 possible joint areas involved are the right and left proximal interphalangeal, metacarpophalangeal, wrist, elbow, knee, ankle, and metatarsophalangeal joints.
c. Arthritis of hand joints: Arthritis of wrist, metacarpophalangeal joint, or proximal interphalangeal joint.
d. Symmetric arthritis: Simultaneous involvement of the same joint areas on both sides of the body.
e. Rheumatoid nodules: Subcutaneous nodules over bony prominences, extensor surfaces, or juxtaarticular regions observed by a physician.
f. Serum rheumatoid factor: Demonstration of abnormal amounts of serum rheumatoid factor by any method for which the result has been positive in less than 5% of normal control subjects.
g. Radiographic changes: Typical changes of RA on posteroanterior hand and wrist radiographs which must include erosions or unequivocal bony decalcification localized in or most marked adjacent to the involved joints.

[a] Criteria a–d must be present for at least 6 weeks.
Criteria b–e must be observed by a physician

therapy may also play a role in the increased mortality rate seen in these individuals. Factors correlated with early death include disability, disease duration or severity, glucocorticoid use, age at onset, and low socioeconomic or educational status.

3.2
Epidemiology

The prevalence of RA is approximately 0.8% of the population (range 0.3%–2.1%); females are affected about three times more often than males. There is a clear relationship between prevalence and increasing age, and sex differences diminish in the older age group. RA is seen throughout the world and affects all races. The economic and social costs of musculoskeletal conditions in rheumatoid arthritis are substantial. These conditions are responsible for a sizable amount of health care use and disability, and they significantly affect the psychological status of the individuals with the conditions as well as their families (YELIN and CALLAHAN 1995). Onset during the fourth and fifth decades of life is most frequent, with 80% of all patients developing the disorder between the ages of 35 and 50. The incidence (VAN SCHAARDENBURG and BREEDVELD 1994) of RA is more than six times as great in 60- to 64-year-old women as in 18- to 29-year-old women.

3.3
Genetics

Family studies indicate a clear genetic predisposition (WEYAND et al. 1995; WINCHESTER and GREGERSEN 1988). For example, severe RA is found at approximately four times the expected rate in first-degree relatives of individuals with disease associated with the presence of the autoantibody rheumatoid factor; approximately 10% of patients with RA will have an affected first-degree relative. Moreover, monozygotic twins are at least four times more likely to be concordant for RA than dizygotic twins, who have a similar risk of developing RA as nontwin siblings (JAWAHEER et al. 1994). One of the major genetic factors in the etiology of RA is the class II major histocompatibility complex (MHC) gene product HLA-DR4 (NEPOM et al. 1987), which is expressed by as many as 70% of RA patients compared with 28% of control individuals. An association with HLA-DR4 has been noted in many populations (MOXLEY 1989); however, there is no association between the development of RA and HLA-DR4 in Israeli Jews, Asian Indians, and Yakima Indians of North America (MCDANIEL et al. 1995). In these individuals, there is an association between RA and HLA-DR1 and HLA-Dw16. Molecular analysis of HLA-DR antigens has provided insight into these apparently disparate findings. Additional genes in the HLA-D complex may also convey altered susceptibility to RA. Certain HLA-DR alleles (ZANELLI et al. 1995), including HLA-DR5 (DRb1*1101), HLA-DR2 (DRb*1501), HLA-DR3 (DRb*0301), and HLA-DR7 (DRb*0701) may protect against the development of RA in that they tend to be found at lower frequency in RA patients than in controls. Disease manifestations have also been associated with HLA phenotype. Thus, early aggressive disease and extraarticular manifestations are more frequent in patients with DRb*0401 or DRb*0404 (WEYAND et al. 1992), and more slowly progressive disease with DRb*0101. The presence of both DRb*0401 and DRb*0404 appears to increase the risk of both aggressive articular and extraarticular disease. It has been estimated that HLA genes contribute only a portion of the genetic susceptibility to RA. Thus, genes outside the HLA complex also contribute. These include genes controlling the expression of the antigen receptor on T cells (FIRESTEIN and ZVAIFLER 1990) and both immunoglobulin heavy and light chains.

It must be considered that genetic risk factors do not fully account for the incidence of RA, suggesting that environmental factors also play a role in the etiology of the disease. This is emphasized by epidemiologic studies in Africa (MCDANIEL et al. 1995) that have indicated that climate and urbanization have a major impact on the incidence and severity of RA in groups of similar genetic background.

3.4 Etiology

The cause of RA remains unknown and is still to be clarified. It has been suggested that RA might be a manifestation of the immune response to an infectious agent in a genetically susceptible host. A number of possible inductive agents have been suggested (ALBANI et al. 1995; TAKAHASHI et al. 1998), including *Mycoplasma*, Epstein–Barr virus, cytomegalovirus, parvovirus, and rubella virus, but convincing evidence that these or other infectious agents cause RA has not emerged. Furthermore, the mechanism by which an infectious agent might induce chronic inflammatory arthritis with a characteristic distribution also remains a matter of debate. Whether there is persistent infection of structures in the joints or retention of microbial products in the synovial tissues which induces an inflammatory response, or whether the microorganism itself might induce an immune response to components of the joint, is still a matter of discussion. In this connection, reactivity to type II collagen and heat shock proteins has been demonstrated

(WOOLEY et al. 1977). Another possible mechanism is that the infecting microorganism might prime the host to cross-reactive determinants expressed within the joint as a result of "molecular mimicry." Recent evidence of similarity between products of certain gram-negative bacteria and the HLA-DR molecule itself has supported this possibility. Finally, products of infecting microorganisms might induce the disease (ALBANI et al. 1995). Recent work has focused on the possible role of "superantigens" produced by a number of microorganisms, including staphylococci, streptococci, and *M. arthritidis*; however, the role of superantigens in the etiology of RA remains speculative.

3.5 Pathophysiology

Microvascular damage and an increase in the number of synovial lining cells (CUSH and LIPSKY 1991) appear to be the earliest lesions in rheumatoid synovitis. In addition, an increased number of synovial lining cells is seen along with perivascular infiltration with mononuclear cells (COLVILLE-NASH and SCHOTT 1992). As the process continues, the synovium becomes edematous and protrudes into the joint cavity as villous projections (ZVAIFLER and FIRESTEIN 1994; FIRESTEIN 1992).

Light microscopic examination shows endothelial cells of the rheumatoid synovium having the appearance of high endothelial venules (HEV) of lymphoid organs and having been altered by cytokine exposure. Rheumatoid synovial endothelial cells express increased amounts of various adhesion molecules involved in this process. This pathologic picture, which is typical of RA, can also be seen in other forms of chronic inflammatory arthritis. The predominant infiltrating cell is the T lymphocyte. CD4+ T cells predominate over CD8+ T cells and are frequently found in close proximity to HLA-DR+ macrophages and dendritic cells. The major population of T cells in the rheumatoid synovium is composed of CD4+ memory T cells, which form most of the cells aggregated around postcapillary venules. Analysis of T cell receptors expressed by CD4+ T cells (from the synovial fluid and blood of patients with RA) suggests that a significant proportion of CD4+ T cells in the synovium have been selected and expanded in response to conventional antigen(s) (STRIEBICH et al. 1998). Besides the accumulation of T cells, rheumatoid synovitis is also characterized by the infiltration of large numbers of B cells that differentiate locally into antibody-producing plasma cells. These cells produce both polyclonal immunoglobulin and the autoantibody rheumatoid factor, resulting in the local formation of immune complexes. Finally, the synovial fibroblasts in RA seem to produce enzymes such as collagenase and cathepsins. These can degrade components of the articular matrix. These activated fibroblasts are particularly prominent in the lining layer and at the interface with bone and cartilage (BROMLEY et al. 1984). Osteoclasts are also prominent at sites of bone erosion.

The rheumatoid *synovium* is characterized (COPE et al. 1992) by the presence of a number of secreted products of activated lymphocytes, macrophages, and fibroblasts, and the activity of these cytokines (LIPSKY et al. 1989) seems to be responsible for many of the features of rheumatoid synovitis (CUSH and LIPSKY 1991). These effector molecules include those derived from T lymphocytes such as interleukin (IL)-2, interferon (IFN), IL-6, IL-10, granulocyte-macrophage colony-stimulating factor (GM-CSF), tumor necrosis factor (TNF), and transforming growth factor (TGF); those originating from activated macrophages, including IL-1, TNF, IL-6, IL-8, IL-10, GM-CSF, macrophage CSF, platelet-derived growth factor, insulin-like growth factor, and TGF; as well as those secreted by other cell types in the synovium, such as fibroblasts and endothelial cells, including IL-1, IL-6, IL-8, GM-CSF, and macrophage CSF. The activity of these chemokines and cytokines appears to account for many of the features of rheumatoid synovitis, including the synovial tissue inflammation, synovial fluid inflammation, synovial proliferation, and cartilage and bone damage, as well as the systemic manifestations of RA (YANNI et al. 1993). In addition to the production of effector molecules that propagate the inflammatory process, local factors are produced that tend to slow the inflammation, such as TGFa, which inhibits T cell activation and proliferation, B cell differentiation, and migration of cells into the inflammatory site. These findings suggest that RA is an event mediated by immunologic factors, although the initiating stimulus has not been characterized.

There is some evidence that the inflammatory process is directed by the CD4+ T cells which are predominant in the synovium; in this connection, there is also an increase in soluble IL-2 receptors, a product of activated T cells. Furthermore, the disease is ameliorated by removal of T cells by peripheral lymphapheresis or suppression of their function by cyclosporine. T lymphocytes also produce a variety of cytokines that lead to activation of macrophages and promote B cell proliferation and differentiation into antibody-forming cells, and therefore also may promote local B cell stimulation. The resultant production of immunoglobulin and rheumatoid factor can lead to immune-complex formation with consequent complement activation and exacerbation of the inflammatory process by the production of anaphylatoxins and chemotactic factors. It remains unclear whether the persistent T cell activity represents a response to a persistent exogenous antigen or to altered autoantigens such as collagen, immunoglobulin, or one of the heat shock proteins. Alternatively, it could represent persistent responsiveness to activated autologous cells such as might occur as a result of Epstein–Barr virus infection or persistent response to a foreign antigen or superantigen in the synovial tissue. Finally, rheumatoid inflammation could reflect persistent stimulation of T cells by synovium-derived antigens that cross-react with determinants introduced during antecedent exposure to foreign antigens or infectious microorganisms.

A number of mechanisms play a role in stimulating the exudation of *synovial fluid*. Locally produced immune complexes can activate complement and generate anaphylatoxins and chemotactic factors. Local production by mononuclear phagocytes of factors such as IL-1, TNF, and leukotriene B_4, as well as products of complement activation, can stimulate the endothelial cells of postcapillary venules to become more efficient at binding circulating cells, whereas TNF, IL-8, C5a, and leukotriene B_4 stimulate the migration of polymorphonuclear leukocytes into the synovial site. In addition, vasoactive mediators such as histamine produced by the mast cells that infiltrate the rheumatoid synovium may also facilitate the exudation of inflammatory cells into the synovial fluid. Finally, the vasodilatory effects of locally produced prostaglandin E_2 also may facilitate entry of inflammatory cells into the inflammatory site. Locally produced cytokines and chemokines such as TNFa, IL-8, and GM-CSF can additionally stimulate polymorphonuclear leukocytes. The production of large amounts of cyclooxygenase and lipoxygenase pathway products of arachidonic acid metabolism by cells in the synovial fluid and tissue further accentuates the signs and symptoms of inflammation.

The precise mechanism by which bone and *cartilage destruction* occurs has not been completely resolved (FASSBENDER 1983). Although the synovial fluid contains a number of enzymes potentially able to degrade cartilage, the majority of destruction occurs in juxtaposition to the inflamed synovium, or pannus, that spreads to cover the articular cartilage. This vascular granulation tissue is composed of proliferating fibroblasts, small blood vessels, and a variable number of mononuclear cells, and produces a large amount of degradative enzymes, including collagenase and stromelysin, that may facilitate tissue damage. The cytokines IL-1 and TNFa play an important role by stimulating the cells of the pannus to produce collagenase and other neutral proteases. These same two cytokines also activate chondrocytes in situ, stimulating them to produce proteolytic enzymes that can degrade cartilage locally.

Finally, IL-1, TNF, and prostaglandin E_2 produced by fibroblasts and macrophages may contribute to the local bone demineralization by activating osteoclasts (KOTAKE et al. 1999)

Systemic manifestations of RA including malaise, fatigue, and elevated levels of serum acute-phase reactants can be accounted for by release of IL-1, TNF, and IL-6 from the synovium. In addition, immune complexes produced within the synovium and entering the circulation may account for other features of the disease, such as systemic vasculitis.

3.6
Clinical Manifestations

In approximately 60% of patients, RA begins with fatigue, anorexia, generalized weakness, and diffuse musculoskeletal complaints until synovitis appears. This early stage may persist for months and make diagnosis complicated. Specific symptoms usually become apparent gradually as joints of the hands, wrists, knees, and feet, become affected in a symmetric fashion. In approximately 10% of the patients, the onset is more acute, with progressive development of polyarthritis, often accompanied by systemic reactions including fever, swelling of lymph nodes, and splenomegaly. Although the pattern of joint involvement may remain asymmetric in 25%–30% of the individuals, a symmetric pattern is more typical.

3.6.1
Clinical Signs of Articular Disease

Pain, swelling, and tenderness may be localized to the joints in the initial stages of the disease, but this is rare. Pain in affected joints, aggravated by movement, is, however, the most common manifestation of established RA. Generalized stiffness is frequent and pronounced after periods of inactivity and immobilization. Morning stiffness is a most typical feature of inflammatory arthritis and may help to distinguish it from other noninflammatory arthropathies. Elevated temperature of 38°C is unusual and suggests the presence of an intercurrent infectious problem.

Clinically, inflammation of the synovia causes swelling, tenderness, and limitation of motion. Pain originates predominantly in the pain fibers of the joint capsule, which are sensitive to stretching or distention. Joint swelling results from accumulation of synovial fluid and thickening of the joint capsule. Initially, motion is limited by pain. RA most often causes symmetric arthritis with characteristic involvement of certain specific joints such as the proximal interphalangeal and metacarpophalangeal joints. Synovitis of the wrist joints is a nearly uniform feature of RA and may lead to limitation of motion, deformity, and median nerve entrapment (carpal tunnel syndrome). The knee joint is commonly involved, with synovial hypertrophy, chronic effusion, and, frequently, ligamentous laxity. Arthritis in the forefoot, ankles, and subtalar joints can produce severe pain with ambulation as well as a number of deformities. Axial involvement is usually limited to the upper cervical spine and there is no evidence of rheumatoid inflammation of the lumbar region. On occasion, the inflammatory process causes atlantoaxial subluxation, which may lead to compression of the spinal cord.

With persistent inflammation, a variety of characteristic deformities develop including (1) radial deviation at the wrist with ulnar deviation of the digits, often with palmar subluxation of the proximal phalanges ("Z" deformity), (2) hyperextension of the proximal interphalangeal joints, with compensatory flexion of the distal interphalangeal joints (swan-neck deformity), (3) flexion deformity of the proximal interphalangeal joints and extension of the distal interphalangeal joints (boutonnière deformity), and (4) hyperextension of the first interphalangeal joint and flexion of the first metacarpophalangeal joint, with a consequent loss of thumb mobility and pinch. In addition, characteristic deformities may develop in the feet, including eversion at the hindfoot (subtalar joint), plantar subluxation of the metatarsal heads, widening of the forefoot, hallux valgus, and lateral deviation and dorsal subluxation of the toes.

3.6.2
Extraarticular Manifestations

Since RA is a systemic disease, a variety of extraarticular manifestations may occur, not all of them being of clinical significance. *Rheumatoid nodules* of different sizes on periarticular structures, extensor surfaces, or other areas subjected to mechanical pressure – very seldom in the pleura or meninges – develop in 20%–30% of the patients, preferentially in those with circulating rheumatoid factor (VOLLERSTEN 1986). Histologically, rheumatoid nodules consist of a central zone of necrotic material including collagen fibrils, noncollagenous filaments, and cellular debris; a midzone of palisading macrophages that express HLA-DR antigens; and an outer zone of granulation tissue. Examination of early nodules has suggested that the initial event may be focal vasculitis.

Rheumatoid vasculitis affecting almost all organ systems is seen in patients with high titers of circulating rheumatoid factor. Eventually vasculitis can cause polyneuropathy and mononeuritis multiplex, cutaneous ulceration and dermal necrosis, digital gangrene, and visceral infarction. Cutaneous vasculitis usually presents as crops of small brown spots in the nail beds, nail folds, and digital pulp. Larger ischemic ulcers, especially in the lower extremity, also may develop.

Pleuropulmonary manifestations, which are more commonly observed in men, include pleural disease, interstitial fibrosis, pleuropulmonary nodules, pneumonitis, and arteritis (JURIK et al. 1982). Pulmonary fibrosis can produce impairment of the diffusing capacity of the lung. Pulmonary nodules may appear singly or in clusters.

Clinically apparent heart disease attributed to the rheumatoid process is rare, but evidence of asymptomatic pericarditis is found. Between 15% and 20% of the patients with RA may develop keratoconjunctivitis sicca (Sjögren's syndrome). The combination of splenomegaly, neutropenia, and on occasion anemia and thrombocytopenia is called *Felty's syndrome* (ROSENSTEIN and KRAMER

1991) and is most common in individuals with long-standing disease and high titers of rheumatoid factor. The leukopenia is a selective neutropenia with counts of sometimes less than 1000 cells per microliter. Splenomegaly has been proposed as one of the causes of leukopenia together with increased frequency of infections. The cause of the increased susceptibility to infection in patients with Felty's syndrome is related to the defective function of polymorphonuclear leukocytes as well as the decreased number of cells.

Osteoporosis secondary to rheumatoid involvement is common and may be aggravated by glucocorticoid therapy. Glucocorticoid treatment may cause significant loss of bone mass, especially early in the course of therapy, even when low doses are employed.

3.6.3
Clinical Course

Remissions of the disease activity are most likely to occur during the first year. A number of features are correlated with a greater likelihood of developing joint abnormalities or disability, including the presence of more than 20 inflamed joints, an elevated erythrocyte sedimentation rate, typical radiologic changes, the presence of rheumatoid nodules, high titers of serum rheumatoid factor, and the presence of functional disability. The presence of one or more of these implies the presence of more aggressive disease with a greater likelihood of developing progressive joint abnormalities and disability (VAN ZEBEN et al. 1992). Several features of patients with RA appear to have prognostic significance. White females tend to have more persistent synovitis and more progressively erosive disease than males. Persons who present with high titers of rheumatoid factor, C-reactive protein, and haptoglobin also have a worse prognosis, as do individuals with subcutaneous nodules or radiographic evidence of erosions at the time of initial evaluation. Indeed, the rate of progression of joint damage is greater during the first year of observation compared with the second and third years. Within 3 years of disease, as many as 70% of patients will have some radiographic evidence of damage to joints; more than 50% of these persons will have had evidence of erosions in the first year of disease. Foot joints are affected more frequently than hand joints.

3.7
Laboratory Findings

Although not specific for diagnosing RA, rheumatoid factors, which are autoantibodies that react with the Fc portion of IgG, are found in more than 60% of adults with the disease (BAUM 1993). Most widely utilized tests detect IgM rheumatoid factors. The prevalence of rheumatoid factor in the general population (SHIMERLING and DELBANCO 1991) increases with age, and 10%–20% of individuals over 65 years old have a positive test. In addition, a number of related disorders are associated with the presence of rheumatoid factor. These include systemic lupus erythematosus, Sjögren's syndrome, chronic liver disease, sarcoidosis, interstitial pulmonary fibrosis, infectious mononucleosis, hepatitis B, tuberculosis, leprosy, syphilis, subacute bacterial endocarditis, visceral leishmaniasis, schistosomiasis, and malaria.

Although the presence of rheumatoid factor does not establish the diagnosis of RA, it can be of prognostic significance because patients with high titers tend to have more severe and progressive disease with extraarticular manifestations. Rheumatoid factor is uniformly found in patients with nodules or vasculitis. The test is not useful as a screening procedure but can be employed to confirm a diagnosis in individuals with a suggestive clinical presentation and, if present in high titer, to designate patients at risk of severe systemic disease.

Normochromic, normocytic anemia is frequently present in active RA. It is thought to reflect ineffective erythropoiesis; large stores of iron are found in the bone marrow. In general, anemia and thrombocytosis correlate with disease activity. The white blood cell count is usually normal, but a mild leukocytosis may be present.

Sedimentation rate is increased in nearly all patients with active RA. The levels of a variety of other acute-phase reactants including ceruloplasmin and C-reactive protein are also elevated. Synovial fluid analysis confirms the presence of inflammatory arthritis, although none of the findings is specific.

3.8
Treatment

The basic medical approach is the use of NSAIDs and simple analgesics to control the clinical symptoms and the local inflammation. The second line of therapy involves the use of steroids. The third line of substances includes agents that have been classified as disease-modifying drugs. These agents seem to reduce elevated levels of acute-phase reactants in treated patients and therefore to modify the damaging capacity of the disease . Other agents are the immunosuppressive and cytotoxic drugs that have been shown to ameliorate the disease process in some patients. The fourth approach involves the use of intraarticular glucocorticoids, which can provide transient relief when systemic medical therapy has failed to resolve the inflammation. A final approach involves the use of a variety of investigational therapies, including combinations of disease-modifying antirheumatic drugs (DMARDs) and other more experimental agents (anti TNF-a Rc).

3.8.1
Nonsteroidal Anti-inflammatory Drugs

NSAIDs block the activity of the enzyme cyclooxygenase and therefore the production of prostaglandins, prostacyclin, and thromboxanes; they have analgesic, anti-inflammatory, and antipyretic properties (BROOKS and DAY 1991). However, these agents are all associated with a wide spectrum of side effects. Some, such as gastric irritation, azotemia, platelet dysfunction, and exacerbation of allergic rhinitis and asthma, are related to the inhibition of cyclooxygenase activity. None of the newer NSAIDs appears to show significant therapeutic advantages over the other available agents. Recent evidence indicates that two separate enzymes, cyclooxygenase 1 and 2, are responsible for the initial metabolism of arachidonic acid into various inflammatory mediators. The former is constitutively present in many cells and tissues, including the stomach and the platelet, whereas the latter is specifically induced in response to inflammatory stimuli. Inhibition of cyclooxygenase 2 accounts for the anti-inflammatory effects of NSAIDs, and suppression of cyclooxygenase 1 induces much of the mechanism-based toxicity. As the currently available NSAIDs inhibit both enzymes, additional therapeutic benefit and less toxicity is expected from newer, specific cyclo-oxygenase 2 inhibitors (SIMON et al. 1998).

Celecoxib is a NSAID that inhibits prostaglandin synthesis by inhibition of cyclooxygenase-2. The ability of celecoxib to decrease joint pain, tenderness, and swelling is comparable to that of other available NSAIDs that inhibit both cyclooxygenase 1 and cyclooxygenase 2. Consistent with the selectivity of celecoxib for cyclooxygenase 2 inhibition, the incidence of endoscopically observed gastroduodenal ulceration during celecoxib therapy is similar to that observed with placebo and significantly lower than that observed with other NSAIDs. (SIMON et al. 1998).

3.8.2
Disease-Modifying Antirheumatic Drugs

This group of agents includes gold compounds, D-penicillamine, the antimalarials, and sulfasalazine. Despite having no chemical similarities, in practice these agents share a number of characteristics (KAVANAUGH and LIPSKY 1992). They exert minimal direct nonspecific anti-inflammatory or analgesic effects, and therefore NSAIDs must be continued during their administration. In addition to a somewhat delayed clinical improvement, there is frequently an improvement in serologic evidence of disease activity, and titers of rheumatoid factor and C-reactive protein and the blood sedimentation rate frequently decline. Each of these drugs is associated with considerable toxicity, and therefore careful patient monitoring is necessary. Which DMARD should be the drug of first choice remains controversial (BOERS and RAMSDEN 1991).

The folic acid antagonist methotrexate, given in an intermittent low dose (7.5–20 mg once weekly), is currently a frequently utilized DMARD (KREMER et al. 1994). Recent trials have documented the efficacy of methotrexate and have indicated that its onset of action is more rapid than that of other DMARDs (WEINBLATT et al. 1992), and patients tend to remain on therapy with methotrexate longer than they remain on other DMARDs because of better clinical responses and less toxicity. The maximum improvement is observed after 6 months of therapy, with little additional improvement seen thereafter. Major toxicity includes gastrointestinal upset, oral ulceration, and dose-related liver function abnormalities that appear to be reversible (KREMER et al. 1994). Drug-induced pneumonitis also has been reported.

Leflunomide, an isoxazol derivative, has recently been approved for the treatment of RA. Leflunomide is a cytostatic agent due to its inhibition of dihydro-orotate dehydrogenase and tyrosine kinases (FOX 1998). The drug slows progression of the disease and is therefore considered a DMARD. Responses to leflunomide and sulfasalazine were comparable in one trial (SMOLEN et al. 1999). Responses to leflunomide versus methotrexate were compared in two other clinical trials. In one of these trials, responses to both drugs were comparable; however, in the second study, a significantly higher response rate to methotrexate was found. Improvement was generally noted by 1 month, with maximum responses by 3–6 months that were sustained throughout the 12-month study period. The most common adverse events associated with the use of leflunomide include gastrointestinal symptoms, weight loss, allergic reactions, rash, reversible alopecia, and transient elevation in liver function studies (MLADENOVIC et al. 1998). The drug also is potentially teratogenic; women of childbearing age must not become pregnant while taking leflunomide. Women who wish to become pregnant after discontinuing leflunomide can speed elimination of the drug (which is concentrated in tissues) by taking a 10-day course of cholestyramine.

3.8.3
Glucocorticoid Therapy

Systemic glucocorticoid therapy can provide effective symptomatic therapy in patients with RA. Low-dose (less than 7.5 mg/day) prednisone has been advocated as a useful additive therapy to control symptoms (KIRWAN 1995). Monthly pulses with high-dose glucocorticoids may be useful in some patients and may hasten the response when therapy with a DMARD is initiated.

3.8.4
Immunosuppressive Therapy

The immunosuppressive drugs azathioprine and cyclophosphamide have been shown to be effective in the treatment of RA and to exert therapeutic effects similar to those of the DMARDs. Moreover, they cause a variety of toxic side effects, and cyclophosphamide appears to predispose the patient to the development of malignant neoplasms. Therefore, these drugs have been reserved for patients who have clearly failed to respond to therapy with DMARDs. Recent trials have suggested that cyclosporine may also be effective in the treatment of RA. Although high-dose therapy may induce rapid improvement, it is associated with frequent renal and gastrointestinal toxicity. Lower doses (TUGWELL et al. 1995) of cyclosporine (<5 mg/kg per day), however, appear to cause slower but nonetheless significant improvement in disease activity (DOUGADA et al. 1988) with fewer toxic side effects, which are reversed upon lowering the dose further. In addition, concomitant use of methotrexate and cyclosporine may afford additional benefit (TUGWELL et al. 1995).

Tumor necrosis factor (TNF) is an important mediator of the inflammatory pathology associated with RA. Therapies aimed at blocking the effects of TNF are now available (O'DELL 1999). Infliximab is a chimeric IgG anti-TNF-a antibody that in combination with methotrexate has shown clinical benefit in RA and Crohn's disease (MAINI et al. 1998). Another approach to TNF blockade is represented by etanercept, a fusion protein composed of two recombinant p75 TNF receptors fused with the Fc portion of human IgG1. Etanercept has shown clinical benefit in RA, alone or in combination with methotrexate (WEINBLATT et al. 1999).

References

Albani S, Keystone EC, Nelson JL, Ollier WER, La Cava A, Montemayor AC, Weber DA, Montecucco C, Martini A, Carson DA (1995) Positive selection in autoimmunity: abnormal immune responses to a bacterial dnaJ antigenic determinant in patients with early rheumatoid arthritis. Nat Med 1:448–452

Arnett FC, Edworthy St M, Bloch DA, et al (1988) The American Rheumatism Association 1987 revised criteria for the classification of rheumatoid arthritis. Arthritis Rheum 31:315–324

Baum J (1993) Laboratory tests in rheumatoid arthritis. J Musculoskel Med 10:55

Boers M, Ramsden M (1991) Long-acting drug combinations in rheumatoid arthritis: a formal overview. J Rheumatol 18:316–324

Bromley M, Fischer WD, Wooley DE (1984) Mast cells at sites of cartilage erosions in the rheumatoid joint. Ann Rheum Dis 43:76–79

Brooks PM, Day RO (1991) Nonsteroidal anti-inflammatory drugs: differences and similarities. N Engl J Med 324:1716

Colville-Nash PR, Schott DL (1992) Angiogenesis and rheumatoid arthritis: pathogenic and therapeutic implications. Ann Rheum Dis 51:919–925

Cope AP, Aderka D, Doherty M, et al (1992) Increased levels of soluble tumor necrosis factor receptors in the sera and synovial fluid of patients with rheumatic diseases. Arthritis Rheum 35:1160

Cush J, Lipsky PE (1991) Cellular basis for rheumatoid inflammation. Clin Orthop 265:9–22

Dougada M, Awada H, Amor B (1988) Cyclosporine in rheumatoid arthritis: a double-blind placebo controlled study in 52 patients. Ann Rheum Dis 47:127–113

Fassbender HG (1983) Histomorphic basis of articular cartilage destruction in rheumatoid arthritis. Coll Relat Res 3:141–155

Firestein GS (1992) Mechanisms of tissue destruction and cellular activation in rheumatoid arthritis. Curr Opin Rheumatol 4:348–354

Firestein GS, Zvaifler NJ (1990) How important are T cells in chronic rheumatoid synovitis? Arthritis Rheum 33:768–773

Fox RI (1998) Mechanism of action of leflunomide in rheumatoid arthritis. J Rheumatol Suppl 53:20–26

Jawaheer D, Thomson W, MacGregor AJ, Carthy D, Davidson J, Dyer PA, Silman AJ, Ollier WER (1994) "Homozygosity" for the HLA-DR shared epitope contributes the highest risk for rheumatoid arthritis concordance in identical twins. Arthritis Rheum 37:681–686

Jurik AG, Davidsen D, Graudal H (1982) Prevalence of pulmonary involvement in rheumatoid arthritis and its relationship to some characteristics of the patients. Scand J Rheumatol 11:217–224

Kavanaugh AF, Lipsky PE (1992) Gold, penicillamine, antimalarials, and sulfasalazine. In: Gallin JI, Goldstein IM, Snyderman R (eds) Inflammation: basic principles and clinical correlates, 2nd edn. Raven, New York, pp 1083–1101

Kirwan JR (1995) The effect of glucocorticoids on joint destruction in rheumatoid arthritis. N Engl J Med 333:142–146

Kotake S, Udagawa N, Takahashi N et al (1999) IL-17 in synovial fluids from patients with rheumatoid arthritis is a potent stimulator of osteoclastogenesis. J Clin Invest 103:1345–1352

Kremer JM, Alarcon GS, Lightfoot RW Jr, Willkens RF, Furst DE, Williams HJ, Dent PB, Weinblatt ME (1994) Methotrexate for rheumatoid arthritis: suggested guidelines for monitoring liver toxicity. Arthritis Rheum 37:316–328

Lipsky PE, Davis LS, Cush JJ, Oppenheimer-Marks N (1989) The role of cytokines in the pathogenesis of rheumatoid arthritis. Springer Semin Immunopathol 11:123–162

Maini RN, Breedveld FC, Kalden JR et al (1998) Therapeutic efficacy of multiple intravenous infusions of anti-tumor necrosis factor alpha monoclonal antibody combined with low dose weekly methotrexate in rheumatoid arthritis. Arthritis Rheum 41:1552–1563

McDaniel DO, Alarcon GS, Pratt PW, Reveille (1995) Most African-American patients with rheumatoid arthritis do not have the rheumatoid antigenic determinant (epitope). Ann Intern Med 123:181–187

Mladenovic V, Domljan Z, Rozman B et al (1998) Safety and effectiveness of leflunomide in the treatment of patients with active rheumatoid arthritis. Results of a randomized, placebo-controlled, phase II study. Arthritis Rheum 38:1595–1603

Moxley G (1989) Immunoglobulin kappa genotype confers risk of rheumatoid arthritis among HLA-DR4 negative individuals. Arthritis Rheum 32:1365–1370

Nepom GT, Hansen JA, Nepom BS (1987) The molecular basis for HLA class II associations with rheumatoid arthritis. J Clin Immunol 7:1–7

O'Dell JR (1999) Anticytokine therapy: a new era in the treatment of rheumatoid arthritis? N Engl J Med 340:310–312

Rosenstein ED, Kramer N (1991) Felty's and pseudo-Felty's syndromes. Semin Arthritis Rheum 21:129–142

Shimerling RH, Delbanco TH (1991) The rheumatoid factor: an analysis of clinical utility. Am J Med 91:528

Simon LS, Lanza FL, Lipsky PE, et al (1998) Preliminary study of the safety and efficacy of SC-58635, a novel cyclooxygenase 2 inhibitor: efficacy and safety in two placebo-controlled trials in osteoarthritis and rheumatoid arthritis, and studies of gastrointestinal and platelet effects. Arthritis Rheum 41:1591–1602

Smolen JS, Kalden JR, Scott DL, et al (1999) Efficacy and safety of leflunomide compared with placebo and sulphasalazine in active rheumatoid arthritis: a double-blind, randomised, multicentre trial. Lancet 353:259–266

Striebich CC, Falta MT, Wang Y, et al (1998) Selective accumulation of related CD4+ T cell clones in the synovial fluid of patients with rheumatoid arthritis. J Immunol 161:4428–4436

Takahashi Y, Murai C, Shibata S, et al (1998) Human parvovirus B19 as a causative agent for rheumatoid arthritis. Proc Natl Acad Sci USA 95:8227–8232

Tugwell P, Pincus T, Yocum D, Stein M, Gluck O, Kraag G, McKendry R, Tesser J, Baker P, Wells G (1995) Combination therapy with cyclosporine and methotrexate in severe rheumatoid arthritis. N Engl J Med 333:137–141

van Schaardenburg D, Breedveld FC (1994) Elderly-onset rheumatoid arthritis. Semin Arthritis Rheum 23:367–378

van Zeben D, Hazes JM, Zwinderman AH, et al (1992) Clinical significance of rheumatoid factors in early rheumatoid arthritis: results of a follow up study. Ann Rheum Dis 51:1029–1035

Vollersten RS (1986) Rheumatoid vasculitis: survival and associated risk factors. Medicine (Baltimore) 65:365–375

Weinblatt ME, Weissmann BN, Holdsworth DE, et al (1992) Long-term prospective study of methotrexate in the treatment of rheumatoid arthritis: 84-month update. Arthritis Rheum 35:129–137

Weinblatt ME, Kremer JM, Bankhurst AD, et al (1999) A trial of etanercept, a recombinant tumor necrosis factor receptor:Fc fusion protein, in patients with rheumatoid arthritis receiving methotrexate. N Engl J Med 340:253–259

Weyand CM, Hicok KC, Conn DL, Goronzy JJ (1992) The influence of HLA-DRB1 genes on disease severity in rheumatoid arthritis. Ann Intern Med 117:801–806

Weyand CM, McCarthy TG, Goronzy JJ (1995) Correlation between disease phenotype and genetic heterogeneity in rheumatoid arthritis. J Clin Invest 95:2120–2126

Winchester RJ, Gregersen PK (1988) The molecular basis of susceptibility to rheumatoid arthritis: the conformational equivalence hypothesis. Springer Semin Immunopathol 10:119–139

Wooley DE, Crossley MJ, Evanson JM (1977) Collagenase at sites of cartilage erosion in the rheumatoid joint. Arthritis Rheum 20:1231–1239

Yanni G, Whelan A, Feighery C, Fitzgerald O, Bresnihan B (1993) Morphometric analysis of synovial membrane blood vessels in rheumatoid arthritis: associations with the immunohistochemical features, synovial fluid cytokine levels and the clinical course. J Rheumatol 20:634–638

Yelin E, Callahan LF (1995) The economic costs and social and psychological impact of musculoskeletal conditions. Arthritis Rheum 38:1351–1362

Zanelli E, Gonzalez-Gay MA, David CS (1995) Could HLA-DRB1 be the protective locus in rheumatoid arthritis? Immunol Today 16:274–278

Zvaifler NJ, Firestein GS (1994) Pannus and pannocytes: alternative models of joint destruction in rheumatoid arthritis. Arthritis Rheum 37:783–789

Therapeutic Approaches and Mechanisms of Drug Action

PETER M. BERNECKER

CONTENTS

P. M. BERNECKER, MD
Baumgarten Geriatric Center, Hütteldorferstrasse 188,
1010 Vienna, Austria

Therapeutic strategies in osteoporosis are aimed at the prevention of osteoporotic fractures. Since osteoporosis develops gradually over the course of years, therapy has to be matched to the stage of the disease and underlying risk factors. During the early postmenopausal years, prophylactic measures such as hormone replacement therapy (HRT) seem adequate, whereas in old age and in persons with very low bone mass more aggressive means of treatment should be initiated.

As of today, several drugs have been clearly shown to exert positive effects on the skeleton and to prevent osteoporotic fractures. A critical point is still the delay until the diagnosis is made and treatment started, but the widespread use of accurate diagnostic tools such as densitometry and the increase in public awareness may be expected to shorten this period and allow physicians to start specific treatment early enough to reduce the burden of osteoporotic fractures on society and on the individual.

4.1 Principles of Therapy

Since the pathophysiologic mechanisms that cause the loss of bone involve increased resorption as well as diminished bone formation, both of these mechanisms, which are usually coupled together, can be targeted by therapeutic intervention. However, the current status of the skeleton – which changes over time – must also be assessed and taken into account when selecting the right drug for the individual patient.

In respect of their actions on bone metabolism, drugs are usually divided into those with antiresorptive capabilities – i.e., that inhibit bone resorption by influencing osteoclast activity – and those that are able to stimulate osteoblastic bone formation.

Again, the ultimate goal in treating patients with osteoporosis is to prevent new fractures. However, in the case of some drugs, such as estrogen, their possible fracture-preventing capabilities have never been studied in large, prospective, placebo-controlled trials; circumstantial evidence certainly indicates positive effects, but no proof has ever been established. Since HRT and estrogen are not bone-specific therapies, their characteristics are described under basic therapeutic measures.

4.2
Basic Therapeutic Measures

4.2.1
Calcium and Vitamin D Supplementation

The basic therapeutic and also prophylactic measure in osteoporosis is adequate calcium and vitamin D supplementation.

Intestinal calcium absorption declines with increasing age; however, this can be overcome by increasing the intake of calcium (IRELAND and FORDTRAN 1973). The possible connection between intestinal calcium absorption and incidence of fractures has been investigated in a new prospective study (ENSRUD et al. 2000). In this study, which enrolled over 5,000 patients, low intestinal calcium intake associated with low fractional intestinal calcium absorption correlated with a high prevalence of fractures. Patients with low intestinal calcium absorption and a high calcium intake had a risk for fractures that was not significantly higher than that of subjects with high intestinal calcium absorption; the lowest risk for fractures was in the group with both high calcium intake and high intestinal calcium absorption. High calcium intake can definitely lessen the postmenopausal decline in bone density (ALOIA et al. 1994).

Vitamin D deficiency is common in Europe and the United States of America, especially during wintertime (BETTICA et al. 1999). Vitamin D deficiency and secondary hyperparathyroidism are associated with low bone mass and high bone turnover (MEZQUITA-RAYA et al. 2001). In addition to their actions on bone, calcium and vitamin D also seem to exert actions on muscle strength and coordination; in geriatric patients, the propensity to fall is highly associated with low levels of vitamin D and increased parathyroid hormone (PTH) (STEIN et al. 1999). In a prospec-

tive study in geriatric patients, short-term (8 weeks) oral supplementation of 1200 mg calcium and 800 IU vitamin D per day significantly reduced body sway and also reduced the cumulative number of falls by 40% (PFEIFER et al. 2000) over a period of 1 year.

The strongest evidence of beneficial effects of calcium and vitamin D supplementation is found in geriatric patients. CHAPUY et al. (1992) investigated the incidence of hip fractures in a prospective, placebo-controlled study with more than 3,000 participating women with a mean age of 84 years. In this study, daily supplementation of 1200 mg calcium and 800 IU vitamin D led to a drastic reduction in fracture risk (a 42% drop in the number of hip fractures and a 32% drop in other nonvertebral fractures) after 18 months of observation. These findings were confirmed by DAWSON-HUGHES et al. (1997); although in this study a dose of 500 mg calcium and 700 IU vitamin D daily was used, the patients were considerably younger (mean age: 71 years), a third of the patients were men, and the observation period was double the length (36 months), the results showed very similar reductions in fracture rates. On the basis of these findings, to prevent falling and associated fractures in geriatric patients, giving supplementary calcium and vitamin D is an therapeutic intervention that meets evidence-based medical criteria.

4.2.2
Physical Exercise

Physical exercise is a necessary part of every therapeutic approach to osteoporosis. Without physical exercise, drug therapy for osteoporosis may be in vain; the negative effects of prolonged bed rest (UEBELHART et al. 1995; HOLM and HEDRICKS 1989; SCHOUTENS et al. 1989; KROLNER and TOFT 1983) or reduced gravity during space flights (HUGHES-FULFORD et al. 1998; BIKLE et al. 1997; OGANOV et al. 1991; VICO et al. 2000) on bone are very well documented. Immobility causes rapid bone loss which may exceed the potential of drugs to strengthen bone. There are many reports in the literature testifying that exercise is able to increase bone mass and balance skills (e.g., MAYOUX-BENHAMOU et al. 1997; HEINONEN et al. 1996; ETHERINGTON et al. 1996; KRONHED and MOLLER 1998); however, solid evidence that exercise alone is able to reduce fracture risk is lacking (PREISINGER et al. 2001).

Nevertheless, the additional benefit of exercise on bone seems evident, and physical exercise training in addition to drug therapy should be strongly recommended in the treatment of patients with osteoporosis.

4.2.3
Estrogen and HRT

For a long time, estrogen was the agent of choice for the prevention and treatment of postmenopausal osteoporosis. Estrogen can prevent bone loss when started at the menopause (PEPI Trial 1996), and increases bone mass by 5%–10% when given after the age of 65 years (LINDSAY and TOHME 1990). Once estrogen administration is stopped, bone mass decreases quickly (LINDSAY et al. 1978), so that estrogen treatment has to be maintained for a long time to keep the achieved skeletal benefits.

Despite these positive effects, however, long-term HRT has been strongly associated with an increased risk of breast cancer, coronary heart disease, stroke, and thromboembolic events since the Women's Health Initiative (WHI) Study has been published in 2002.

4.2.3.1
Mechanisms of Action

Although the relationship between estrogen deficiency and osteoporosis has been well known for some 40 years, the mechanisms by which estrogen acts on bone are still not fully elucidated. Estrogen binds with the receptor in nuclei of target cells and activates response genes (TURNER et al. 1994). It suppresses osteoclastic bone resorption, possibly through multiple pathways, e.g., by influencing cytokine and growth factor production. It shows also effects on osteoblasts; however, there is no clear evidence about a proposed stimulation of bone formation. Estrogen influences calcium homeostasis by acting on kidney and bowel and possibly altering their responsiveness to calcitropic hormones (Prince 1994); moreover, it seems to sensitize remodeling units in bone to mechanical forces (SCHIESSL et al. 1998).

The optimal dose of estrogen, the method of delivery, and the required plasma levels for optimal effects on bone are still unclear.

4.2.3.2
Therapeutic Effects

Estrogen increases bone density as stated above. A large meta-analysis showed that the gain in bone mass was considerably greater with concomitant calcium supplementation (NIEVES et al. 1998), underlining the necessity of adequate calcium intake (see above).

Lack of estrogen in the menopause is associated with an increase in bone turnover. In women 6 months to 3 years after menopause, HRT lowered biochemical markers of bone resorption by 25%–50% and markers of bone formation by 15%–25% after 1 year of treatment (LUFKIN et al. 1992; CHESNUT et al. 1997).

Several studies have examined the effects of HRT on fracture incidence. In 100 women who had undergone oophorectomy, estrogen was able to reduce height loss and vertebral fracture incidence during a 10 year intervention period (LINDSAY et al. 1980). Another controlled study showed no fractures in 164 women receiving HRT and 7 fractures in the control group during a 10 year observation period (NACHTIGALL et al. 1979); a study on transdermal estrogen treatment in 75 women with prior vertebral fractures showed a reduction in the incidence of new fractures after 1 year (LUFKIN et al. 1992). There is more evidence from large longitudinal cohort studies to confirm the efficacy of HRT with regard to fractures. In more than 9,000 postmenopausal women over 65 years of age, current use of estrogen was associated with a significant risk reduction for wrist and other nonspinal fractures (CAULEY et al. 1995). The WHI Study (2002) with more than 16,000 participants was the first prospective study demonstrating the ability of HRT to decrease the risk of hip fracture and colon cancer; on the other hand, the risk ratios for breast cancer, stroke, coronary heart disease and thromboembolic events were elevated. Since then, regulation authorities in many countries have restricted the use of HRT. The risk-benefit ratio of HRT does not make its use currently advisable for the prevention and treatment of osteoporosis

4.3
Antiresorptive Drugs

4.3.1
Calcitonins

4.3.1.1
Chemical Properties

Calcitonins are peptide hormones usually produced by C cells of the thyroid gland in mammals, birds, amphibians, and fish; however, calcitonins have also been found in many tissues and even in unicellular organisms such as E. coli or Candida albicans (MCINTYRE and CRAIG 1982), underlining the important role of calcium homeostasis in all cell systems and at all stages of evolution. Calcitonins are usually about 3.5 kDa in size and are composed of 32 amino acid residues; typically there is a disulfide bridge between cysteine residues in positions 1 and 7, forming a ring of 7 amino acid residues at the N-terminal end and a proline amide group at the C-terminal end of the chain. Midchain structure varies considerably from species to species, and these variations are mainly responsible for the formation of specific antibodies.

Endogenous calcitonin levels in man are primarily influenced by the blood level of ionized calcium, secretion and release being stimulated by a rise in serum calcium, whereas a fall in ionized calcium levels has an inhibitory effect. Other factors such as food intake (AUSTIN and HEATH 1981), pregnancy (WHITEHEAD et al. 1981), lactation (TOVERUD et al. 1978), and estrogen deficiency (GREENBERG et al. 1986) can elevate endogenous calcitonin levels.

Currently, calcitonins of the human, eel, and salmon variety are used for therapy; to avoid injections, a salmon calcitonin that can be nasally administered has been developed. Human calcitonin seems to have a shorter time of action than salmon calcitonin (NEWSOME et al. 1973).

4.3.1.2
Mechanism of Action

Calcitonins inhibit osteoclastic bone resorption by acting directly on the osteoclastic cells (CHAMBERS and DUNN 1983) and countering the osteolytic effects of endogenous PTH, thus slowing accelerated bone remodeling. Calcitonins reduce the activity and motility of the osteoclasts and the number

and the rate at which new ones are formed; these changes are associated with alterations of the internal structure of the cells, namely inhibiting the cytoplasmic motility and thereby affecting the mechanisms essential to bone resorption (CHAMBERS and DUNN 1983). The suppression of bone resorption is long-lasting; however, an escape phenomenon can be observed which occurs in vitro after 12–48 h in culture (WENER et al. 1972). Another possible factor diminishing the effect of calcitonin therapy on bone may be the formation of antibodies in secondary nonresponders. Primary lack of response to the drug also occurs but is infrequent.

In therapeutic doses, the calcitonins show effects on other cell systems besides bone; they have a pronounced analgesic effect in the central nervous system, probably by modulating the serotoninergic system, an action at specific central receptors, and an increase in b-endorphin levels (LAURIAN et al. 1986; ORMAZABAL et al. 1999, 2001; FISCHER et al. 1981), and show anti-inflammatory properties (STRETTLE et al. 1980). They also cause vasodilatation, leading to side effects such as dizziness or vertigo; some reports state that symptoms from venous insufficiency may be worsened by calcitonin injections.

4.3.1.3
Therapeutic Effects

Calcitonin has been used for treatment of osteoporosis since the 1970s (JOWSEY et al. 1978), mostly using subcutaneous injections at a dose range from 200 IU per day to 120 IU per week. During the 1980s, the first prospective placebo-controlled studies were published (e.g., MAZZUOLI et al. 1986; CIVITELLI et al. 1988) and showed mild to moderate gains in bone mass, commonly assessed by dual-photon absorptiometry or dual-energy X-ray absorptiometry, and measuring changes in biochemical markers of bone metabolism, indicating a slowdown of high-turnover remodeling. Calcitonins have been investigated in various therapeutic combinations, such as with human growth hormone (ALOIA et al. 1985), vitamin D (PALMIERI et al. 1989; USHIROYAMA et al. 2001), estrogen (MESCHIA et al. 1993), and PTH (HESCH et al. 1989; HODSMAN et al. 1997). Other prospective studies report calcitonin to be effective in glucocorticoid-induced osteoporosis (LUENGO et al. 1994) and in other forms of secondary osteoporosis.

Almost all these findings are based on bone density measurements and assessment of biochemical markers of bone metabolism; there are only a few studies in the literature that offer prospective fracture data. The work by Palmieri and coworkers cited above was one of the first to report fractures; however, the case numbers were far too small to give hard evidence. In 2000, the first long-term, double-blind, placebo-controlled study (the PROOF study) to use fractures as a clinical endpoint was published (Chesnut et al. 2000). This report shows that giving nasal salmon calcitonin at a dose of 200 IU per day – in combination with 1,000 mg calcium and 400 IU vitamin D daily – can significantly reduce the occurrence of new vertebral fractures in postmenopausal osteoporotic women over a 5 year period. However, nonvertebral fractures such as those of the hip or wrist were not significantly reduced, and the risk reduction was definitely less than in studies using bisphosphonates or selective estrogen receptor modulators (SERMs), leaving the calcitonins as second-line drugs in the treatment of osteoporosis.

4.3.2
Bisphosphonates

4.3.2.1
Chemical Properties

Bisphosphonates are analogs of pyrophosphate, consisting of two phosphonic acid groups joined to a carbon, resulting in a central P–C–P structure. This structure makes them bind to bone surfaces via the phosphonic groups, whereas the central carbon prevents enzymatic degradation of the drug. The side chains attached to the central carbon atom are variable and can be modified to change the antiresorptive potency and adsorption to bone surfaces (Fleisch 1998). For example, the second-generation bisphosphonate alendronate, which contains an amino-terminal group, shows a relative antiresorptive potency of 100–1,000 compared to the first-generation drug etidronate. Third-generation drugs like risedronate and ibandronate with cyclical side chains show an even higher relative potency of 1,000–10,000 compared to etidronate, reducing side effects and enhancing tolerability. Bisphosphonates are poorly absorbed by the gastrointestinal tract when administered orally; typically, less than 5% of the given dose is found in circulation. Furthermore, absorption is almost annihilated when the drug is taken together with calcium or food or drink other than plain

water. Oral bisphosphonates have to be taken on an empty stomach with plain water and no oral intake of food or drink for at least the next 30 min, preferably longer. Since bisphosphonates can cause esophageal irritation (deGroen 1996), it is advisable to remain sitting or standing upright after taking the drug orally.

Up to 24 h after administration, between 30%–50% of the drug found in circulation is bound to bone surfaces, where it exerts its actions on osteoclasts; any of the drug not bound to bone is not metabolized but excreted by the kidney. After binding to the surface, the drug becomes buried in bone, where it is retained for a long time (months to years) but is no longer active until it is released again by bone resorption processes (Kasting and Francis 1992). Kasting and Francis (1992) also estimate the amount of bisphosphonates that would be released from the skeleton after 10 years of continuous therapy to be about 25% of the absorbed amount of a daily oral dose.

As of today, alendronate, risedronate and ibandronate are available in oral forms (ibandronate can also be given intravenously) and are in widespread therapeutic use; the combination of their effectiveness and the very low incidence of associated side effects makes them safe and useful drugs for long-term treatment of osteoporosis.

4.3.2.2
Mechanism of Action

Bisphosphonates quickly and effectively reduce bone resorption by acting on cells of the osteoclastic lineage. The drug binds to the bone surface, preferentially at a remodeling site, where it is released locally and interferes with the resorption process first by binding protons and diminishing the amount of lysosomal enzymes produced by the ruffled border of the osteoclast (Rodan and Fleisch 1996). Next, it is incorporated into the osteoclast and exerts a cytotoxic effect, causing the osteoclast to undergo apoptosis. Other effects of the drug have also been described, such as inhibiting differentiation of osteoclast precursors into mature osteoclasts and interference with osteoclast attachment to bone surfaces, (Lowik et al. 1986; Van Beek et al. 2002). Bisphosphonates may also have indirect effects on bone resorption mediated by osteoblasts (Vitte et al. 1996) or direct effects on osteoblasts, causing an increase in osteoblastic differentiation and number (Giuliani et al. 1998).

Because of their antiresorptive properties, bisphosphonates reduce the rate at which new bone remodeling units are formed (the activation frequency), thus reducing bone turnover. The most useful effect of this class of compounds is to maintain a positive bone balance at individual remodeling sites; since the activated osteoclasts are not able to dig deep resorption lacunae, the amount of newly formed bone exceeds the amount of bone resorbed (MILLER et al. 1997).

4.3.2.3
Therapeutic Use

Bisphosphonates are the most comprehensively studied drugs for the clinical treatment of osteoporosis today. Etidronate was the first bisphosphonate used for treatment, but due to its poor antiresorptive potency it is rarely used nowadays and may soon be regarded as obsolete.

Alendronate has been shown to be effective in postmenopausal osteoporosis when combined with calcium and vitamin D at standard doses. Alendronate is able to increase bone density, to reduce bone turnover, and to significantly lower fracture risk at all skeletal sites (LIBERMAN et al. 1995; BLACK et al. 1996). The so-called FIT study (Fracture Intervention Trial) was originally carried out in 2,027 postmenopausal women and showed the drug was able to reduce fractures of the spine, hip, and wrist by 50% after 3 years of treatment when given in doses between 5 and 10 mg. The study was then modified by the inclusion of another group of patients with preexisting fractures, and since the results concerning the reduction of incidence of new fractures were similar, the two groups were pooled and a total of 3,658 patients were studied (BLACK et al. 1996, 2000). Alendronate has also been studied in postmenopausal women younger than 60 years and compared to HRT, with results showing that the drug was able to prevent the accelerated bone loss that follows the menopause; however, the bisphosphonate group showed less gain in bone density than the group receiving HRT (HOSKING et al. 1998).

The studies testing the third-generation bisphosphonate risedronate show similar outcomes. Risedronate has been shown to enhance bone density and reduce fracture rates to a very similar extent as alendronate (MORTENSEN et al. 1998; HARRIS et al. 1999). Risedronate was also tested in (a) a large population with either preexisting hip fractures or very low bone density in conjunction with a high propensity for falls versus (b) women over 80 years of age (McCLUNG et al. 2001). The results obtained from this trial are still under discussion, since in the 3,886 patients over 80 years of age no significant reduction of fracture incidence could be observed, whereas in the 5,445 patients aged 70–79 years a 30% risk reduction was found after 3 years of treatment with 5 mg risedronate daily. Alendronate has not been tested in similar populations, i.e., in women over 80 years of age.

Both drugs have been shown to successfully prevent bone loss and reduce fractures in patients receiving glucocorticoid treatment (WALLACH et al. 2000; REID et al. 2000; COHEN et al. 1999; ADACHI et al. 2001). Additionally, risedronate has been shown to reduce fracture risk and enhance bone density in male patients receiving medium to high doses of glucocorticoids (REID et al. 2001).

Alendronate has also been showed to be efficient in male idiopathic osteoporosis (ORWOLL et al. 2000); since data on therapy of osteoporosis in men are scarce, this study was of great clinical interest. Although fractures were not a primary endpoint in this study, data showed an increase in bone density and an impressive 80% reduction in fracture risk – although the statistical power of this finding is not great enough to declare it hard evidence.

Bisphosphonates can be given daily, weekly, monthly; ibandronate has been shown to be effective even when given in a three months interval intravenously. Zoledronat is expected to be available soon – the drug is designed to be administered intravenously only once a year.

As of today, bisphosphonates in combination with calcium and vitamin D supplementation are the treatment of choice for established osteoporosis (defined by a T score lower than –2.5 or preexisting fractures), although these drugs are also effective in prophylaxis of osteoporosis in younger postmenopausal patients.

4.3.3
Selective Estrogen Receptor Modulators

4.3.3.1
Chemical Properties

Selective estrogen receptor modulators (SERMs) are not new compounds; tamoxifen, formerly called an "antiestrogen," has been in widespread clinical use for adjuvant treatment of estrogen receptor-positive breast cancer for many years.

Raloxifene is the first selective SERM to be approved for the treatment of postmenopausal osteoporosis. Another similar substance, lasofoxifene, is currently in clinical testing. Chemically raloxifene is a nonsteroidal benzothiophene compound with tissue-specific agonist and antagonist actions. In the skeletal system raloxifene acts as an estrogen agonist, whereas in the uterus and breast antagonistic effects can be observed.

At the approved dosage of 60 mg/day raloxifene is able to lower serum LDL cholesterol by approximately 10%; total cholesterol levels are reduced by 6% (Delmas et al. 1997). Serum levels of triglycerides are not affected, even in diabetic patients (Mosca et al. 2001). Unlike estrogen, raloxifene does not affect HDL cholesterol levels; however, a somewhat weaker but similar reduction of cardiovascular risk factors has been reported in patients using raloxifene instead of estrogen over a period of 2 years (de Valk-de Roo et al. 1999). Moreover, raloxifene has been shown to stimulate nitric oxide release by endothelial cells by directly influencing the enzymatic activity of nitric oxide synthase, perhaps causing a vasoprotective effect (Simoncini and Genazzani 2000).

Raloxifene seems to reduce the incidence of breast cancer impressively – the results of the MORE (multiple outcomes of raloxifene evaluation) study which enrolled over 7,500 postmenopausal women suggest a risk reduction of more than 80% for development of invasive estrogen receptor-positive breast cancer after 4 years. The authors calculate that 93 osteoporotic women would need to be treated for 4 years with raloxifene to prevent one case of invasive breast cancer. These findings are promising; however, more time is needed to confirm this preliminary observation (Cauley et al. 2001).

Raloxifene does not cause endometrial thickening and therefore does not cause vaginal bleeding. Establishing whether there is a reduction in endometrial cancer incidence compared to that seen with HRT needs further observation, but the properties of the drug and its lack of effect on the uterus make that a logical expectation.

Like estrogen, raloxifene is associated with a higher incidence of thromboembolic events and should therefore not be used at times of prolonged bed rest or in patients with a history of deep vein thrombosis or pulmonary embolism (Ettinger et al. 1999).

The most common side effect of the drug is a high incidence (up to 25%) of hot flushes, even in patients who are years beyond the menopause and have not been receiving HRT.

4.3.3.2
Mechanisms of Action

Like estrogen, the mechanisms of action of the SERMs on bone tissue and bone cells are not fully understood; since the SERMs bind to the estrogen receptor, molecular mechanisms similar to those of estrogen are postulated.

4.3.3.3
Therapeutic Effects

In combination with calcium and vitamin D, raloxifene prevented bone loss in early postmenopausal women and induced a 2%–3% gain in bone mineral density. The drug was able to lower biochemical parameters of bone resorption and formation (Delmas et al. 1997) but – in contrast to estrogen – did not reduce activation frequency. The gain in bone mineral density was significantly lower than in patients using estrogen or alendronate (Ettinger et al. 1999; Prestwood et al. 2000).

Fracture data from the MORE trial show a significant reduction in the incidence of new vertebral fractures. After 3 years, patients receiving 60 mg/day raloxifene showed a relative risk reduction of about 30%–40%; in another group of patients receiving 120 mg/day, fracture risk decreased by approximately 50%. Nonvertebral fracture rates were not influenced by raloxifene treatment and showed the same – though very low – incidence as in the placebo group. These fracture data are certainly significant, but should be interpreted with caution as the population studied was relatively young and the total fracture incidence was clearly lower than in a population at high risk.

More data are expected to be reported since the MORE trial has now been going on for over 5 years; since the beneficial effects on bone (assessed by bone densitometry and biochemical changes) appear to be smaller in magnitude than in patients undergoing estrogen therapy, the current status of raloxifene is that of an alternate drug for younger postmenopausal women in whom HRT is not indicated and skeletal status reveals a moderate risk for developing fractures. The promising data regarding breast cancer and cardiovascular risk factors may alter this valuation soon.

4.4
Drugs That Stimulate Bone Formation

4.4.1
Sodium Fluoride

Sodium fluoride is not approved in the USA, but in Europe in particular it has long been used to treat osteoporosis. Sodium fluoride is a potent stimulator of bone formation, sometimes causing undermineralization and osteomalacia-like symptoms such as intratrabecular fractures, similar to stress fractures. A slow-release preparation of fluoride was endorsed for treatment of postmenopausal osteoporosis by the FDA advisory committee in 1995 but is still under review because of questions about its effectiveness in strengthening bone.

In countries where fluoride treatment of osteoporosis is approved, fluoride is usually available as slow-release, enteric-coated tablets of sodium fluoride or as effervescent tablets containing disodium monofluorophosphate. Dosage seems to be a major problem; most studies show increases in bone mass with doses of 20–30 mg fluoride ion daily. However, the therapeutic window appears to be small and individual resorption rates are highly variable (RESCH and BERNECKER, data on file).

4.4.1.1
Mechanism of Action

Fluoride is rapidly absorbed by the stomach; in the presence of food or calcium the bioavailability of sodium fluoride is reduced by 20%–50%, but no such effect is seen on the bioavailability of monofluorophosphate. Fluoride is eliminated by the kidney with a half-life of approximately 3 h. The remainder is stored in bone, mostly in the form of hydroxyfluoroapatite crystals.

Fluoride is a potent mitogenic agent for osteoblasts, perhaps through alteration of tyrosine phosphorylation (CAVERZASIO et al. 1997). In contrast to antiresorptive agents, which produce an initial gain in bone density that plateaus over time, fluoride produces sustained linear increases in spinal bone density, averaging 9% per year for 4 years (RIGGS et al. 1990). While the gains in spinal bone mineral density are impressive, some studies suggest that cortical bone density at other skeletal sites seems to be diminished, which could eventually result in an increase in peripheral fractures (RIGGS et al. 1990,

1994). This "shift" from cortical to trabecular bone density could possibly be reduced by administration of calcium and vitamin D, or by intermittent treatment incorporating fluoride-free intervals; however, this matter is still under discussion.

In the studies by RIGGS and coworkers, sodium fluoride doses below 30 mg/day have no measurable effects on bone, whereas doses above 80 mg/day produce grossly abnormal bone, sometimes presenting as "fluorosis" in radiographs (Fig. 4.1).

4.4.1.2
Therapeutic Use

Currently, fluoride is not used very often even in countries even where it was formerly a standard therapy. The reason for this change is the availability of newer and safer drugs such as bisphosphonates on the one hand, coinciding with the rise of serious doubts about the effectiveness of fluoride therapy with regard to nonvertebral fractures on the other. Although there is no doubt about the effectiveness of fluoride in reducing vertebral fractures (RUBIN et al. 2001; PAK et al. 1996), a significant increase in nonvertebral fractures was found in the above-cited studies by RIGGS et al. These findings are still the subject of discussion. Riggs and coworkers used a relatively high dose of standard sodium fluoride (75 mg/day), whereas the study by PAK and coworkers used a slow-release preparation of sodium fluoride with a lower dosage (50 mg/day) and did not confirm the findings of the Riggs study.

The mechanical properties of bone produced under the influence of fluoride are still not clear. FRATZL et al. (1994, 1996) reported grossly abnormal structures at the crystalline level in humans and minipigs treated with sodium fluoride; the crystal structures are not directionally orientated and a loss of biomechanical properties is postulated. Another study reports increased bone fragility in fluoride-treated patients (SOGAARD et al. 1994).

Side effects in fluoride therapy are common; gastric irritation is often observed when using sodium fluoride and is caused by gastric formation of hydrofluoric acid. These side effects appear to be less common when monofluorophosphate or enteric-coated preparations are used. High doses or longer use may cause lower-extremity pain syndrome, typically in the ankles, which is related to stress microfractures or rapid bone remodeling (O'DUFFY et al. 1986) As mentioned before, the main problem with fluoride lies in the narrow therapeutic window: low

Fig. 4.1. a Lateral radiograph of the lumbar spine showing discrete signs of osteoporosis. **b** Lateral spine radiograph of the same patient after 3 years of high-dosed fluoride therapy, showing manifest fluorosis. Note the coarse structure of the trabeculae and the high density sometimes mimicking osteomalacia. (Photographs kindly supplied by Dr. G. Seidl, Vienna)

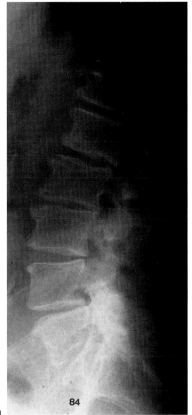
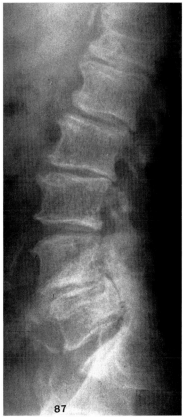

a   b

doses seem to be ineffective and toxic doses lead to production of bone that is histologically abnormal, undermineralized, and more dense but apparently of poor quality with regard to the biomechanical properties, which may result in an increase in hip and wrist fractures.

Until the questions of safety, optimal dose regimen, and biomechanical properties are sufficiently answered, fluoride treatment of osteoporosis seems inadvisable.

4.4.2
Exogenous Parathyroid Hormone or Active Fragment (PTH; PTH 1–34)

Almost 75 years ago, positive effects on bone mass were reported in rats treated once daily with PTH (BAUER et al. 1929; SELYE 1932). Since these findings were in contrast to the newly elucidated role of PTH as a bone-resorbing agent and contradicted the clinical findings in hyperparathyroidism, this report was largely ignored for decades.

In the 1980s, a German group restarted the idea of using possible anabolic effects of PTH for treatment of osteoporosis (HESCH et al. 1989), since the active fragment, recombinant PTH 1–34, was commercially available. As a safety measure, the protocols of the Hesch studies contained an antiresorptive agent, calcitonin or etidronate, given additionally to prevent possible PTH-induced bone loss. Today, in pulsatile PTH treatment, we see a new and potent agent to treat osteoporosis.

4.4.2.1
Mechanism of Action

Continuously elevated PTH levels lead to demineralization of the skeleton and can cause fractures, as can be seen in cases of persisting untreated hyperparathyroidism.

However, PTH is also an anabolic agent on bone cells, exerting its anabolic power when given in low doses in a pulsatile manner The primary target cell of PTH in bone is the osteoblast, since osteoclasts do not express PTH receptors. Pulsatile rPTH(1–

34) treatment is able to increase the number of osteoblasts in bone by actions on osteoblast progenitor cells and also by initiating redifferentiation of lining cells into their formerly active osteoblastic phenotype (Schmidt et al. 1995; Dobnig et al. 1995). It was also reported that this form of treatment was able to activate de novo bone formation on formerly quiescent bone surfaces (Hodsman and Steer 1993). Since histomorphometric studies showed no cortical thinning, but rather revealed a tremendous increase in the size and thickness of newly formed trabeculae (Bradbeer et al. 1992) as well as a rise in cortical thickness in women receiving PTH plus HRT (Dempster et al. 2001), it can be assumed that the biomechanical properties are improved. Moreover, the study by Dempster and coworkers showed an increase in trabecular connectivity; therefore, PTH treatment might actually improve bone microarchitecture and not only bone mass.

Recombinant human PTH(1–34) is used for treatment, dose-finding studies suggesting that the best effective dose is between 20 and 40 µg given by subcutaneous injection once daily. Calcium and vitamin D supplementation is not contraindicated and hypercalcemia not a common event in the trials performed so far. Common side effects are dizziness and leg cramps. In a long-term toxicologic study in rats, a higher incidence of osteosarcoma was found in the treatment group; however, the doses used were considerably higher than in clinical trials. Nevertheless, this point needs further clarification.

4.4.2.2
Therapeutic Efficacy

Neer et al. (2001) investigated over 1,600 postmenopausal women with at least one vertebral osteoporotic fracture; women with a history of urolithiasis within the last 5 years were excluded. All women received 1000 mg elementary calcium and 400–1200 IU vitamin D daily. rhPTH(1–34) was self-administered by subcutaneous injection at doses of 20 or 40 µg daily. Serum and urinary calcium concentrations were closely monitored and calcium supplementation adjusted accordingly if mild hypercalcemia or hypercalciuria developed. Mean testing time was 21 months. Bone density in the lumbar spine increased by 9%–13% and in the femoral neck by 3%–6%. With the 40 µg dose, a cor-

tical bone loss of 2% was observed in the midshaft of the radius, whereas the 20 µg dose resulted in no cortical changes. The reduction of fracture risk was highly significant: about 70% risk reduction for vertebral fractures and approximately 50% for nonvertebral fractures. Nausea, headache, and leg cramps were the adverse events most commonly observed.

Another study (Cosman et al. 2001) investigated the effects of rhPTH(1–34) when given additionally to premedicated estrogen (ongoing HRT for at least 2 years; plus calcium and vitamin D) in postmenopausal women with osteoporosis. Dosage was 25 µg/day for 3 years, then PTH medication was terminated but HRT continued for 1 more year. PTH in combination with HRT increased bone density in the lumbar spine by 13% and in the hip by 4.5%. In the PTH group, serum markers of bone metabolism rose until they peaked at 6 months, then remained elevated until 30 months after start of PTH therapy, when they returned to baseline values. Fracture incidence was clearly reduced by 75%–100% compared to HRT alone. Furthermore, HRT was able to maintain the gain in BMD after cessation of PTH over 1 year.

Impressive results were obtained in a trial conducted in postmenopausal women with corticoid-induced osteoporosis (Lane et al. 1998). All women were receiving HRT, and a subgroup was additionally given PTH at a dose of 25 µg daily, similar to the protocol in the study by Cosman described above. The endpoint was a change in BMD; fractures were not assessed. BMD rose in the PTH/HRT group by more than 35% in only 1 year, compared to approximately 4% in the group receiving HRT alone.

The Treatment of Osteoporosis with Parathyroid Hormone (TOP) Study (Greenspan et al. 2007) showed similar positive results using the intact hormone rhPTH(1–84).

Recombinant human parathyroid hormon is an interesting addition to established therapy, perhaps diminishing the risk of fractures in patients with very low bone mass or severe osteoporosis with multiple preexistent vertebral fractures; it is a potent anabolic agent on bone when administered in low dose pulses; however, costs of PTH therapy are very high and side effects (especially nausea) are observed frequently. Monitoring blood calcium and urinary calcium excretion levels seems advisable in patients with PTH therapy.

4.4.3
Synthetic Analogues of Vitamin D
(Calcitriol, Alfacalcidol)

Analogues of vitamin D – containing a hydroxyl group in the 1, a position – have been used for therapy of osteomalacia and renal osteopathy with secondary hyperparathyroidism for more than two decades.

With regard to osteoporosis, no hard evidence exists that these compounds are really effective. Some studies have investigated the effects in osteoporosis, but sample numbers and study designs were usually weak. The active forms of vitamin D are regarded as stimulators of bone formation, but in vitro both anabolic actions and stimulation of bone resorption can be observed. Since the role of these compounds is not clear, they cannot be recommended as a validated osteoporosis therapy and must still be considered experimental.

In 1987, ORIMO et al. studied 61 patients with senile osteoporosis treated with alfacalcidol (1 μg/day) with or without calcium (1000 mg/day). Mean duration of treatment was about 1.75 years. In this study, a reduction of spinal crush fractures in the alfacalcidol plus calcium group was found versus calcium alone.

OTT and CHESNUT (1989) studied 86 postmenopausal women with vertebral fractures. The patients received calcitriol or placebo and dietary calcium intake was set to 1000 mg/day. Calcium and calcitriol medication was adjusted according to hypercalcemia or hypercalciuria; mean dose of calcitriol was 0.43 μg/day. After 2 years, bone density did not differ between the two groups; fractures were 10% higher in the calcitriol group than in the placebo group, and bone biopsies showed no difference. The authors concluded that calcitriol is not effective in postmenopausal osteoporosis.

In 1990, GALLAGHER and GOLDGAR (1990) studied 50 postmenopausal women with vertebral fractures and treated with calcitriol plus calcium versus placebo. The design was prospective and double-blind, placebo-controlled. After 2 years, the BMD of the lumbar spine had decreased by almost 4% in the placebo group and risen by 1.9% in the calcitriol group. The authors reported no difference in fractures between the two groups, but the calcitriol and calcium dose had to be reduced by almost 40% to prevent hypercalcemia or hypercalciuria.

TILYARD et al. (1992) examined over 600 female postmenopausal patients with pre-existing vertebral fractures in a prospective, single-blinded setting. Incidence of new fractures was the primary endpoint. Patients received either calcitriol (0.25 μg twice daily) or calcium (100 mg/day) over 3 years. The authors found a significant reduction in new vertebral fractures in patients receiving calcitriol; however, this effect was only observed in patients who had less than five vertebral fractures at baseline. Nonvertebral fractures were also reduced.

ORIMO et al. (1994) presented another trial using 1 μg alfacalcidol plus 300 mg calcium in 80 postmenopausal Japanese osteoporotic women for 1 year. BMD in the lumbar spine increased by 0.65% in the treatment group versus a reduction of 1.14% in the placebo group. BMD at the femoral neck showed no differences. Vertebral fracture incidence was lower in the alfacalcidol group (2 patients vs 7 patients).

Two years later, the same group published a study (SHIKARI et al. 1996) with similar design enrolling 113 female osteoporotic patients; this time the alfacalcidol dosage amounted to 0.75 μg per day, and the observation period was 2 years. BMD increased again slightly in the alfacalcidol group, whereas in the placebo group BMD decreased. Fracture data showed no difference between the two groups.

REGINSTER et al. (1999) published a study regarding the effects of alfacalcidol in the prevention of glucocorticoid-induced osteoporosis. In 145 patients, a beneficial effect on bone density was demonstrated.

In post-transplantational osteoporosis, SAMBROOK et al. (2000) showed benefits of calcitriol medication. In 65 patients who had undergone cardiac or lung transplantation, BMD was studied after 1 and 2 years. Patients received either calcitriol in doses from 0.5 μg to 0.75 μg plus 600 mg calcium per day. The study was placebo-controlled; the authors conclude that calcitriol reduces post-transplantational bone loss at the femoral neck, but state that the fracture data are not realistic because of the small sample size.

EBELING et al. (2001) studied 42 men with osteoporosis. They received either calcitriol (0.25 μg twice daily) or calcium (1000 mg /day) for 2 years. After 2 years, the number of vertebral fractures did not differ between the groups. The authors state that calcitriol as a single therapeutic agent is not effective in male osteoporosis.

From these data, it is clear that further studies are needed to elucidate the therapeutic potential of vitamin D analogues.

4.4
Drugs With Dual Action on Bone Formation and Bone Resorption

4.4.1
Strontiumranelate

Strontiumranelate has been licensed in Europe for the treatment of postmenopausal osteoporosis; it is not available in the United States. Strontium – a bivalent cation like calcium – is the active agent, administered as a salt of ranelic acid. Strontium is believed to exert actions on bone by influencing resorption and formation simultaneously.

4.4.1.1
Mechanism of Action

Strontium has been shown to stimulate bone formation in growing rats (ARLOT et al. 1995), and to enhance osteoprogenitor cell formation (CANALIS et al. 1996). Bone resorption is inhibited by strontium in ovarectomized rats, whereas bone formation remains on a high level (MARIE et al. 1993); strontium also seems to increase bone mass in osteopenic animals and bone strength in normal animals (MARIE et al. 2001). The molecular mechanisms of these actions are still not fully understood. Anabolic actions of strontium on bone are probably owing to an increase in osteoblast differentiation and activity. Inhibition of bone resorption is probably mediated by an increase in osteoprotegerin (OPG) expression by the osteoblasts.

Strontium is embedded in the bone matrix to a certain extent in the form of strontium – hydroxyapatite crystals. Since strontium with its greater molecular weight shows higher X-ray attenuation than calcium, bone density measurements are not accurate in strontium – treated patients and measured values higher than in reality; densitometry cannot be used for follow up of these patients.

4.4.1.2
Therapeutic Use

Strontiumranelate has been tested in two large clinical trials. In the Spinal Osteoporosis Therapeutic Intervention Study (SOTI) (MEUNIER et al. 2005), a 49% decrease in vertebral fractures was observed after only one year of treatment; at completion of the study after three years, the relative risk for (new)

vertebral fractures was 41% lower in the strontium group. In the Treatment of Peripheral Osteoporosis Study (TROPOS – REGINSTER et al. 2005) a significant effect of strontium on non – vertebral fractures could be shown; with regard to hip fractures, strontium proved to be effective in a high – risk population (especially in women over 80 years old) and reduced the relative risk for hip fracture by more than 30%.

During the clinical tests, an increase in the number of thromboembolic events was noticed in the strontium group; patients with a history of deep venous thrombosis or pulmonary emboly should not be treated with strontiumranelate until new data on this side effect are available.

References

Adachi JD, Saag KG, Delmas PD, Liberman UA, Emkey RD, Seeman E, Lane NE, Kaufman JM, Poubelle PE, Hawkins F, Correa-Rotter R, Menkes CJ, Rodriguez-Portales JA, Schnitzer TJ, Block JA, Wing J, McIlwain HH, Westhovens R, Brown J, Melo-Go mes JA, Gruber BL, Yanover MJ, Leite MO, Siminoski KG, Nevitt MC, Sharp JT, Malice M P, Dumortier T, Czachur M, Carofano W, Daifotis A (2001) Two-year effects of alendronate on bone mineral density and vertebral fracture in patients receiving glucocorticoids: a randomized, double-blind, placebo-controlled extension trial. Arthritis Rheum 44:202–211

Aloia JF, Vaswani A, Kapoor A, Yeh JK, Cohn SH (1985) Treatment of osteoporosis with calcitonin, with and without growth hormone. Metabolism 34:124–129

Aloia JF, Vaswani A, Yeh JK, Ross PL, Flaster E, Dilmanian FA (1994) Calcium supplementation with and without hormone replacement therapy to prevent postmenopausal bone loss. Ann Intern Med 120:97–103

Arlot ME, Roux JP, Boivin G, Perrat B, Tsouderos Y, Deloffre P, Meunier PJ (1995) Effects of strontium salt (S 12911) in both tibial metaphysis and epiphysis in normal growing rats. J Bone Miner Res 10 (S1):M415

Austin LA, Heath H (1981) Calcitonin: physiology and pathophysiology. N Engl J Med 304:269–278

Bauer W, Aub JC, Albright F (1929) Studies of calcium phosphorus metabolism. V. A study of the bone trabeculae as a readily available reserve supply of calcium. J Exp Med 49:145–162

Bettica P, Bevilacqua M, Vago T, Norbiato G (1999) High prevalence of hypovitaminosis D among free-living postmenopausal women referred to an osteoporosis outpatient clinic in northern Italy for initial screening. Osteoporos Int 9:226 229

Bikle DD, Halloran BP, Morey-Holton E (1997) Space flight and the skeleton: lessons for the earthbound. Endocrinologist 7:10–22

Black DM, Cummings SR, Karpf DB, Cauley JA, Thompson DE, Nevitt MC, Bauer DC, Genant HK, Haskell WL, Marcus R, Ott SM, Torner JC, Quandt SA, Reiss TF, Ensrud

KE (1996) Randomised trial of effect of alendronate on risk of fracture in women with existing vertebral fractures. Fracture Intervention Trial Research Group. Lancet 348:1535–1541

Black DM, Thompson DE, Bauer DC, Ensrud K, Musliner T, Hochberg MC, Nevitt MC, Suryawanshi S, Cummings SR (2000) Fracture Intervention Trial: fracture risk reduction with alendronate in women with osteoporosis: the Fracture Intervention Trial. FIT Research Group. J Clin Endocrinol Metab 85:4118–4124

Bradbeer JN, Arlot ME, Meunier PJ, Reeve J (1992) Treatment of osteoporosis with parathyroid peptide (hPTH 1-34) and oestrogen: increase in volumetric density of iliac cancellous bone may depend on reduced trabecular spacing as well as increased thickness of packets of newly formed bone. Clin Endocrinol (Oxf) 37:282–289

Canalis E, Hott M, Deloffre P, Tsouderos Y, Marie PJ 1996 The divalent salt S 12911 enhances bone cell replication and bone formation in vitro. Bone 18:517–523

Cauley JA, Seeley DG, Ensrud K, Ettinger B, Black D, Cummings SR (1995) Estrogen replacement therapy and fractures in older women. Study of Osteoporotic Fractures Research Group. Ann Intern Med 122:9–16

Cauley JA, Norton L, Lippman ME, Eckert S, Krueger KA, Purdie DW, Farrerons J, Karasik A, Mellstrom D, Ng KW, Stepan JJ, Powles TJ, Morrow M, Costa A, Silfen SL, Walls EL, Schmitt H, Muchmore DB, Jordan VC (2001) Continued breast cancer risk reduction in postmenopausal women treated with raloxifene: 4-year results from the MORE trial. Multiple outcomes of raloxifene evaluation. Breast Cancer Res Treat 65:125–134

Caverzasio J, Palmer G, Suzuki A, Bonjour JP (1997) Mechanism of the mitogenic effect of fluoride on osteoblast-like cells: evidences for a G protein-dependent tyrosine phosphorylation process. J Bone Miner Res 12:1975–1983

Chambers TJ, Dunn CJ (1983) Pharmacologic control of osteoclast mobility. Calcif Tissue Int 35:566–570

Chapuy MC, Arlot ME, Duboeuf F, Brun J, Crouzet B, Arnaud S, Delmas PD, Meunier PJ (1992) Vitamin D3 and calcium to prevent hip fractures in the elderly women. N Engl J Med 327:1637–1642

Chesnut CH III, Bell NH, Clark GS, Drinkwater BL, English SC, Johnson CC Jr, Notelovitz M, Rosen C, Cain DF, Flessland KA, Mallinak NJ (1997) Hormone replacement therapy in postmenopausal women: urinary N-telopeptide of type I collagen monitors therapeutic effect and predicts response of bone mineral density. Am J Med 102:29–37

Chesnut CH III, Silverman S, Andriano K, Genant H, Gimona A, Harris S, Kiel D, LeBoff M, Maricic M, Miller P, Moniz C, Peacock M, Richardson P, Watts N, Baylink D (2000) A randomized trial of nasal spray salmon calcitonin in postmenopausal women with established osteoporosis: the prevent recurrence of osteoporotic fractures study. PROOF Study Group. Am J Med 109:267–276

Civitelli R, Gonnelli S, Zacchei F, Bigazzi S, Vattimo A, Avioli LV, Gennari C (1988) Bone turnover in postmenopausal osteoporosis. Effect of calcitonin treatment. J Clin Invest 82:1268–1274

Cohen S, Levy RM, Keller M, Boling E, Emkey RD, Greenwald M, Zizic TM, Wallach S, Sewell KL, Lukert BP, Axelrod DW, Chines AA (1999) Risedronate therapy prevents corticosteroid-induced bone loss: a twelve-month, mul-

ticenter, randomized, double-blind, placebo-controlled, parallel-group study. Arthritis Rheum 42:2309–2318

Cosman F, Nieves J, Woelfert L, Formica C, Gordon S, Shen V, Lindsay R (2001) Parathyroid hormone added to established hormone therapy: effects on vertebral fracture and maintenance of bone mass after parathyroid hormone withdrawal. J Bone Miner Res 16:925–931

Dawson-Hughes B, Harris SS, Krall EA, Dallal GE (1997) Effect of calcium and vitamin D supplementation on bone density in men and women 65 years of age or older. N Engl J Med 337:670–676

De Groen PC, Lubbe DF, Hirsch LJ, Daifotis A, Stephenson W, Freedholm D, Pryor-Tillotson S, Seleznick MJ, Pinkas H, Wang KK (1996) Esophagitis associated with the use of alendronate. N Engl J Med 335:1016–1021

De Valk-de Roo GW, Stehouwer CD, Meijer P, Mijatovic V, Kluft C, Kenemans P, Cohen F, Watts S, Netelenbos C (1999) Both raloxifene and estrogen reduce major cardiovascular risk factors in healthy postmenopausal women: a 2-year, placebo-controlled study. Arterioscler Thromb Vasc Biol 19:2993–3000

Delmas PD, Bjarnason NH, Mitlak BH, Ravoux AC, Shah AS, Huster WJ, Draper M, Christiansen C (1997) Effects of raloxifene on bone mineral density, serum cholesterol concentrations, and uterine endometrium in postmenopausal women. N Engl J Med 337:1641–1647

Dempster DW, Cosman F, Kurland ES, Zhou H, Nieves J, Woelfert L, Shane E, Plavetic K, Muller R, Bilezikian J, Lindsay R (2001) Effects of daily treatment with parathyroid hormone on bone microarchitecture and turnover in patients with osteoporosis: a paired biopsy study. J Bone Miner Res 16:1846–1853

Dobnig H, Turner RT (1995) Evidence that intermittent treatment with parathyroid hormone increases bone formation in adult rats by activation of bone lining cells. Endocrinology 136:3632–3638

Ebeling PR, Wark JD, Yeung S, Poon C, Salehi N, Nicholson GC, Kotowicz MA (2001) Effects of calcitriol or calcium on bone mineral density, bone turnover, and fractures in men with primary osteoporosis: a two-year randomized, double blind, double placebo study. J Clin Endocrinol Metab 86:4098–4103

Ensrud KE, Duong T, Cauley JA, Heaney RP, Wolf RL, Harris E, Cummings SR (2000) Low fractional calcium absorption increases the risk for hip fracture in women with low calcium intake. Study of Osteoporotic Fractures Research Group. Ann Intern Med 132:345–353

Etherington J, Harris PA, Nandra D, Hart DJ, Wolman RL, Doyle DV, Spector TD (1996) The effect of weight-bearing exercise on bone mineral density: a study of female ex-elite athletes and the general population. J Bone Miner Res 11:1333–1338

Ettinger B, Black DM, Mitlak BH, Knickerbocker RK, Nickelsen T, Genant HK, Christiansen C, Delmas PD, Zanchetta JR, Stakkestad J, Gluer CC, Krueger K, Cohen FJ, Eckert S, Ensrud KE, Avioli LV, Lips P, Cummings SR (1999) Reduction of vertebral fracture risk in postmenopausal women with osteoporosis treated with raloxifene: results from a 3-year randomized clinical trial. Multiple Outcomes of Raloxifene Evaluation (MORE) Investigators. JAMA 282:637–645

Fischer JA, Sagar SM, Martin JB (1981) Characterization and regional distribution of calcitonin binding sites in the rat brain. Life Sci 29:663–671

Fleisch H (1998) Bisphosphonates. Mechanisms of action. J Clin Endocrinol Metab 19:80–100

Fratzl P, Roschger P, Eschberger J, Abendroth B, Klaushofer K (1994) Abnormal bone mineralization after fluoride treatment in osteoporosis: a small-angle X-ray-scattering study. J Bone Miner Res 9:1541–1549

Fratzl P, Schreiber S, Roschger P, Lafage MH, Rodan G, Klaushofer K (1996) Effects of sodium fluoride and alendronate on the bone mineral in minipigs: a small-angle X-ray scattering and backscattered electron imaging study. J Bone Miner Res 11:248–253

Gallagher JC, Goldgar D (1990) Treatment of postmenopausal osteoporosis with high doses of synthetic calcitriol. A randomized controlled study. Ann Intern Med 113:649–655

Giuliani N, Pedrazzoni M, Negri G, Passeri G, Impicciatore M, Girasole G (1998) Bisphosphonates stimulate formation of osteoblast precursors and mineralized nodules in murine and human bone marrow cultures in vitro and promote early osteoblastogenesis in young and aged mice in vivo. Bone 22:455–461

Greenberg C, Kukreja SC, Bowser EN, Hargis GK, Henderson WJ, Williams GA (1986) Effects of estradiol and progesterone on calcitonin secretion. Endocrinology 118:2594–2598

Greenspan SL, Bone HG, Ettinger MP, Hanley DA, Lindsay R, Zanchetta JR, Blosch CM, Mathisen AL, Morris SA, Marriott TB; Treatment of Osteoporosis with Parathyroid Hormone Study Group (2007) Effect of recombinant human parathyroid hormone (1–84) on vertebral fracture and bone mineral density in postmenopausal women with osteoporosis: a randomized trial. Ann Intern Med 146:326–39

Harris ST, Watts NB, Genant HK, McKeever CD, Hangartner T, Keller M, Chesnut CH III, Brown J, Eriksen EF, Hoseyni MS, Axelrod DW, Miller PD (1999) Effects of risedronate treatment on vertebral and nonvertebral fractures in women with postmenopausal osteoporosis: a randomized controlled trial. Vertebral Efficacy With Risedronate Therapy (VERT) Study Group. JAMA 282:1344–1352

Heinonen A, Kannus P, Sievanen H, Oja P, Pasanen M, Rinne M, Uusi-Rasi K, Vuori I (1996) Randomised controlled trial of effect of high-impact exercise on selected risk factors for osteoporotic fractures. Lancet 348:1343–1347

Hesch RD, Busch U, Prokop M, Delling G, Rittinghaus EF (1989) Increase of vertebral density by combination therapy with pulsatile 1–38hPTH and sequential addition of calcitonin nasal spray in osteoporotic patients. Calcif Tissue Int 44:176–180

Hesch RD, Busch U, Prokop M, Delling G, Rittinghaus EF (1989) Increase of vertebral density by combination therapy with pulsatile 1–38hPTH and sequential addition of calcitonin nasal spray in osteoporotic patients. Calcif Tissue Int 44:176–180

Hodsman AB, Steer BM (1993) Early histomorphometric changes in response to parathyroid hormone therapy in osteoporosis: evidence for de novo bone formation on quiescent cancellous surfaces. Bone 14:523–527

Hodsman AB, Fraher LJ, Watson PH, Ostbye T, Stitt LW, Adachi JD, Taves DH, Drost D (1997) A randomized controlled trial to compare the efficacy of cyclical parathyroid hormone versus cyclical parathyroid hormone and sequential calcitonin to improve bone mass in postmenopausal women with osteoporosis. J Clin Endocrinol Metab 82:620–628

Holm K, Hedricks C (1989) Immobility and bone loss in the aging adult. Crit Care Nurs Q 12:46–51

Hosking D, Chilvers CE, Christiansen C, Ravn P, Wasnich R, Ross P, McClung M, Balske A, Thompson D, Daley M, Yates AJ (1998) Prevention of bone loss with alendronate in postmenopausal women under 60 years of age. Early Postmenopausal Intervention Cohort Study Group. N Engl J Med 338:485–492

Hughes-Fulford M, Tjandrawinata R, Fitzgerald J, Gasuad K, Gilbertson V (1998) Effects of microgravity on osteoblast growth. Gravit Space Biol Bull 11:51–60

Ireland P, Fordtran JS (1973) Effect of dietary calcium and age on jejunal calcium absorption in humans studied by intestinal perfusion. J Clin Invest 52:2672–2678

Jowsey J, Riggs BL, Kelly PJ, Hoffman DL (1978) Calcium and salmon calcitonin in treatment of osteoporosis. J Clin Endocrinol Metab 47:633–639

Kasting GB, Francis MD (1992) Retention of etidronate in human, dog and rat. J Bone Miner Res 7:513–522

Krolner B, Toft B (1983) Vertebral bone loss: an unheeded side effect of therapeutic bed rest. Clin Sci (Lond) 64:537–540

Kronhed AC, Moller M (1998) Effects of physical exercise on bone mass, balance skill and aerobic capacity in women and men with low bone mineral density, after one year of training – a prospective study. Scand J Med Sci Sports 8:290–298

Lane NE, Sanchez S, Modin GW, Genant HK, Pierini E, Arnaud CD (1998) Parathyroid hormone treatment can reverse corticosteroid-induced osteoporosis. Results of a randomized controlled clinical trial. J Clin Invest 102:1627–1633

Laurian L, Oberman Z, Graf E, Gilad S, Hoerer E, Simantov R (1986) Calcitonin induced increase in ACTH, beta-endorphin and cortisol secretion. Horm Metab Res 18:268–271

Liberman UA, Weiss SR, Broll J, Minne HW, Quan H, Bell NH, Rodriguez-Portales J, Downs RW Jr, Dequeker J, Favus M (1995) Effect of oral alendronate on bone mineral density and the incidence of fractures in postmenopausal osteoporosis. The Alendronate Phase III Osteoporosis Treatment Study Group. N Engl J Med 333:1437–1443

Lindsay R, Tohme JF (1990) Estrogen treatment of patients with established postmenopausal osteoporosis. Obstet Gynecol 76:290–295

Lindsay R, Hart DM, MacLean A, Clark AC, Kraszewski A, Garwood J (1978) Bone response to termination of oestrogen treatment. Lancet 1:1325–1327

Lindsay R, Hart DM, Forrest C, Baird C (1980) Prevention of spinal osteoporosis in oophorectomised women. Lancet 2:1151–1154

Lowik CW, Boonekamp PM, van de Pluym G, van de Wee-Pals L, Bloys van Treslong-de Groot H, Bijvoet OL (1986) Bisphosphonates can reduce osteoclastic bone resorption by two different mechanisms. Adv Exp Med Biol 208:275–281

Luengo M, Pons F, Martinez de Osaba MJ, Picado C (1994) Prevention of further bone mass loss by nasal calcitonin in patients on long term glucocorticoid therapy for asthma: a two year follow up study. Thorax 49:1099–1102

Lufkin EG, Wahner HW, O'Fallon WM, Hodgson SF, Kotowicz MA, Lane AW, Judd HL, Caplan RH, Riggs BL (1992) Treatment of postmenopausal osteoporosis with transdermal estrogen. Ann Intern Med 117:1–9

MacIntyre I, Craig RK (1982) Molecular evolution of the calcitonins. In: Fink G, Whalley LJ (eds) Neuropeptides: basic and clinical aspects. Proceedings of the eleventh Pfizer international symposium, September 1981. Churchill Livingstone, Edinburgh, pp 255–258

Marie PJ, Hott M, Modrowski D, De Pollak C, Guillemain J, Deloffre P, Tsouderos Y (1993) An uncoupling agent containing strontium prevents bone loss by depressing bone resorption and maintaining bone formation in estrogen-deficient rats. J Bone Miner Res 8:607–615

Marie PJ, Amman P, Boivin G, Rey C (2001) Mechanisms of action and therapeutic potentialof strontium in bone. Calcif Tissue Int 69:121–129

Mayoux-Benhamou MA, Bagheri F, Roux C, Auleley GR, Rabourdin JP, Revel M (1997) Effect of psoas training on postmenopausal lumbar bone loss: a 3-year follow-up study. Calcif Tissue Int 60:348–353

Mazzuoli GF, Passeri M, Gennari C, Minisola S, Antonelli R, Valtorta C, Palummeri E, Cervellin GF, Gonnelli S, Francini G (1986) Effects of salmon calcitonin in postmenopausal osteoporosis: a controlled double-blind clinical study. Calcif Tissue Int 38:3–8

McClung MR, Geusens P, Miller PD, Zippel H, Bensen WG, Roux C, Adami S, Fogelman I, Diamond T, Eastell R, Meunier PJ, Reginster JY (2001) Hip Intervention Program Study Group: effect of risedronate on the risk of hip fracture in elderly women. Hip Intervention Program Study Group. N Engl J Med 344:333–340

Meschia M, Brincat M, Barbacini P, Crossignani PG, Albiseti W (1993) A clinical trial on the effects of a combination of elcatonin (carbocalcitonin) and conjugated estrogens on vertebral bone mass in early postmenopausal women. Calcif Tissue Int 53:17–20

Meunier PJ, Roux C, Seeman E, Ortolani S, Badurski JE, Spector TD, Cannata J, Balogh A, Lemmel EM, Pors-Nielsen S, Rizzoli R, Genant HK, Reginster JY (2004) The effects of strontium ranelate on the risk of vertebral fracture in women with postmenopausal osteoporosis. N Engl J Med 350:459–68

Mezquita-Raya P, Munoz-Torres M, Luna JD, Luna V, Lopez-Rodriguez F, Torres-Vela E, Escobar-Jimenez F (2001) Relation between vitamin D insufficiency, bone density, and bone metabolism in healthy postmenopausal women. J Bone Miner Res 16:1408–1415

Miller PD, Watts NB, Licata AA, Harris ST, Genant HK, Wasnich RD, Ross PD, Jackson RD, Hoseyni MS, Schoenfeld SL, Valent DJ, Chesnut CH III (1997) Cyclical etidronate in the treatment of postmenopausal osteoporosis: efficacy and safety after seven years of treatment. Am J Med 103:468–476

Mortensen L, Charles P, Bekker PJ, Digennaro J, Johnston CC Jr (1998) Risedronate increases bone mass in an early postmenopausal population: two years of treatment plus one year of follow-up. J Clin Endocrinol Metab 83:396–402

Mosca L, Harper K, Sarkar S, O'Gorman J, Anderson PW, Cox DA, Barrett-Connor E (2001) Effect of raloxifene on serum triglycerides in postmenopausal women: influence of predisposing factors for hypertriglyceridemia. Clin Ther 23:1552–1565

Nachtigall LE, Nachtigall RH, Nachtigall RD, Beckman EM (1979) Estrogen replacement therapy I: a 10-year prospective study in the relationship to osteoporosis. Obstet Gynecol 53:277–281

Neer RM, Arnaud CD, Zanchetta JR, Prince R, Gaich GA, Reginster JY, Hodsman AB, Eriksen EF, Ish-Shalom S, Genant HK, Wang O, Mitlak BH (2001) Effect of parathyroid hormone (1–34) on fractures and bone mineral density in postmenopausal women with osteoporosis. N Engl J Med 344:1434–1441

Newsome FE, O'Dor RK, Parkes CO, Copp DH (1973) A study of the stability of calcitonin biological activity. Endocrinology 92:1102–1106

Nieves JW, Komar L, Cosman F, Lindsay R (1998) Calcium potentiates the effect of estrogen and calcitonin on bone mass: review and analysis. Am J Clin Nutr 67:18–24

O'Duffy JD, Wahner HW, O'Fallon WM, Johnson KA, Muhs JM, Beabout JW, Hodgson SF, Riggs BL (1986) Mechanism of acute lower extremity pain syndrome in fluoride-treated osteoporotic patients. Am J Med 80:561–566

Oganov VS, Rakhmanov AS, Novikov VE, Zatsepin ST, Rodionova SS, Cann C (1991) The state of human bone tissue during space flight. Acta Astronaut 23:129–133

Orimo H, Shiraki M, Hayashi T, Nakamura T (1987) Reduced occurrence of vertebral crush fractures in senile osteoporosis treated with 1 alpha (OH)-vitamin D3. Bone Miner 3:47–52

Orimo H, Shiraki M, Hayashi Y, Hoshino T, Onaya T, Miyazaki S, Kurosawa H, Nakamura T, Ogawa N (1994) Effects of 1 alpha-hydroxyvitamin D3 on lumbar bone mineral density and vertebral fractures in patients with postmenopausal osteoporosis. Calcif Tissue Int 54:370–376

Ormazabal MJ, Goicoechea C, Alfaro MJ, Sanchez E, Martin MI (1999) Study of mechanisms of calcitonin analgesia in mice. Involvement of 5-HT3 receptors. Brain Res 845:130–138

Ormazabal MJ, Goicoechea C, Sanchez E, Martin MI (2001) Salmon calcitonin potentiates the analgesia induced by antidepressants. Pharmacol Biochem Behav 68:125–133

Orwoll E, Ettinger M, Weiss S, Miller P, Kendler D, Graham J, Adami S, Weber K, Lorenc R, Pietschmann P, Vandormael K, Lombardi A (2000) Alendronate for the treatment of osteoporosis in men. N Engl J Med 343:604–610

Ott SM, Chesnut CH III (1989) Calcitriol treatment is not effective in postmenopausal osteoporosis. Ann Intern Med 110:267–274

Pak CY, Adams-Huet B, Sakhaee K, Bell NH, Licata A, Johnston C, Rubin B, Bonnick S, Piziak V, Graham H, Ballard J, Berger R, Fears W, Breslau N, Rubin C (1996) Comparison of nonrandomized trials with slow-release sodium fluoride with a randomized placebo-controlled trial in postmenopausal osteoporosis. J Bone Miner Res 11:160–168

Palmieri GM, Pitcock JA, Brown P, Karas JG, Roen LJ (1989) Effect of calcitonin and vitamin D in osteoporosis. Calcif Tissue Int 45:137–141

PEPI Trial Writing Group (1996) Effects of hormone therapy on bone mineral density: results from the postmenopausal estrogen/progestin interventions (PEPI) trial. The Writing Group for the PEPI. JAMA 276:1389–1396

Pfeifer M, Begerow B, Minne HW, Abrams C, Nachtigall D, Hansen C (2000) Effects of a short-term vitamin D and calcium supplementation on body sway and secondary hyperparathyroidism in elderly women. J Bone Miner Res 15:1113–1118

Preisinger E, Kerschan-Schindl K, Wober C, Kollmitzer J, Ebenbichler G, Hamwi A, Bieglmayer C, Kaider A (2001) The effect of calisthenic home exercises on postmenopausal fractures – a long-term observational study. Maturitas 40:61–67

Prestwood KM, Gunness M, Muchmore DB, Lu Y, Wong M, Raisz LG (2000) A comparison of the effects of raloxifene and estrogen on bone in postmenopausal women. J Clin Endocrinol Metab 85:2197–2202

Prince R (1994) Counterpoint: estrogen effects on calcitropic hormones and calcium homeostasis. Endocr Rev 15:301–309

Reginster JY, de Froidmont C, Lecart MP, Sarlet N, Defraigne JO (1999) Alphacalcidol in prevention of glucocorticoid-induced osteoporosis. Calcif Tissue Int 65:328–331

Reginster JY, Seeman E, De Vernejoul MC, Adami S, Compston J, Phenekos C, Devogelaer JP, Curiel MD, Sawicki A, Goemaere S, Sorensen OH, Felsenberg D, Meunier PJ (2005) Strontium ranelate reduces the risk of nonvertebral fractures in postmenopausal women with osteoporosis: Treatment of Peripheral Osteoporosis (TROPOS) study. J Clin Endocrinol Metab 90:2816–22

Reid DM, Hughes RA, Laan RF, Sacco-Gibson NA, Wenderoth DH, Adami S, Eusebio RA, Devogelaer JP (2000) Efficacy and safety of daily risedronate in the treatment of corticosteroid-induced osteoporosis in men and women: a randomized trial. European Corticosteroid-Induced Osteoporosis Treatment Study. J Bone Miner Res 15:1006–1013

Reid DM, Adami S, Devogelaer JP, Chines AA (2001) Risedronate increases bone density and reduces vertebral fracture risk within one year in men on corticosteroid therapy. Calcif Tissue Int 69:242–247

Riggs BL, Hodgson SF, O'Fallon WM, Chao EY, Wahner HW, Muhs JM, Cedel SL, Melton LJ III (1990) Effect of fluoride treatment on the fracture rate in postmenopausal women with osteoporosis. N Engl J Med 322:802–809

Riggs BL, O'Fallon WM, Lane A, Hodgson SF, Wahner HW, Muhs J, Chao E, Melton LJ III (1994) Clinical trial of fluoride therapy in postmenopausal osteoporotic women: extended observations and additional analysis. J Bone Miner Res 9:265–275

Rodan GA; Fleisch H (1996) Bisphosphonates: mechanisms of action. J Clin Invest 97:2692–2696

Rubin CD, Pak CY, Adams-Huet B, Genant HK, Li J, Rao DS (2001) Sustained-release sodium fluoride in the treatment of the elderly with established osteoporosis. Arch Intern Med 161:2325–2333

Sambrook P, Henderson NK, Keogh A, MacDonald P, Glanville A, Spratt P, Bergin P, Ebeling P, Eisman J (2000) Effect of calcitriol on bone loss after cardiac or lung transplantation. J Bone Miner Res 15:1818–1824

Schiessl H, Frost HM, Jee WS (1998) Estrogen and bone-muscle strength and mass relationships. Bone 22:1–6

Schmidt IU, Dobnig H, Turner RT (1995) Intermittent parathyroid hormone treatment increases osteoblast number, steadystate messenger ribonucleic acid levels for osteocalcin, and bone formation in tibial metaphysis of hypophysectomized female rats. Endocrinology 136:5127–5134

Schoutens A, Laurent E, Poortmans JR (1989) Effects of inactivity and exercise on bone. Sports Med 7:71–81

Selye H (1932) On the stimulation of new bone formation with parathyroid extract and irradiated ergosterol. Endocrinology 16:547

Shikari M, Kushida K, Yamazaki K, Nagai T, Inoue T, Orimo H (1996) Effects of 2 years' treatment of osteoporosis with 1 alpha-hydroxy vitamin D3 on bone mineral density and incidence of fracture: a placebo-controlled, double-blind prospective study. Endocr J 43:211–220

Simoncini T, Genazzani AR (2000) Raloxifene acutely stimulates nitric oxide release from human endothelial cells via an activation of endothelial nitric oxide synthase. J Clin Endocrinol Metab 85:2966–2969

Sogaard CH, Mosekilde L, Richards A, Mosekilde L (1994) Marked decrease in trabecular bone quality after five years of sodium fluoride therapy – assessed by biomechanical testing of iliac crest bone biopsies in osteoporotic patients. Bone 15:393–399

Stein MS, Wark JD, Scherer SC, Walton SL, Chick P, Di Carlantonio M, Zajac JD, Flicker L (1999) Falls relate to vitamin D and parathyroid hormone in an Australian nursing home and hostel. J Am Geriatr Soc 47:1195–1201

Strettle RJ, Bates RF, Buckley GA (1980) Evidence for a direct anti-inflammatory action of calcitonin: inhibition of histamine-induced mouse pinnal oedema by porcine calcitonin. J Pharm Pharmacol 32:192–195

Tilyard MW, Spears GF, Thomson J, Dovey S (1992) Treatment of postmenopausal osteoporosis with calcitriol or calcium. N Engl J Med 326:357–362

Toverud SU, Cooper CW, Munson PL (1978) Calcium metabolism during during lactation: elevated blood levels of calcitonin. Endocrinology 103:472–479

Turner RT, Riggs BL, Spelsberg TC (1994) Skeletal effects of estrogen. Endocr Rev 15:275–300

Uebelhart D, Demiaux-Domenech B, Roth M, Chantraine A (1995) Bone metabolism in spinal cord injured individuals and in others who have prolonged immobilisation. A review. Paraplegia 33:669–673

Ushiroyama T, Ikeda A, Sakai M, Higashiyama T, Ueki M (2001) Effects of the combined use of calcitonin and 1 alpha-hydroxycholecalciferol on vertebral bone loss and bone turnover in women with postmenopausal osteopenia and osteoporosis: a prospective study of long-term and continuous administration with low dose calcitonin. Maturitas 40:229–238

Van Beek ER, Lowik CW, Papapoulos SE (2002) Bisphosphonates suppress bone resorption by a direct effect on early osteoclast precursors without affecting the osteoclastogenic capacity of osteogenic cells: the role of protein geranylgeranylation in the action of nitrogencontaining bisphosphonates on osteoclast precursors. Bone 30:64–70

Vico L, Collet P, Guignandon A, Lafage-Proust MH, Thomas T, Rehaillia M, Alexandre C (2000) Effects of long-term microgravity exposure on cancellous and cortical weight-bearing bones of cosmonauts. Lancet 355:1607–1611

Vitte C, Fleisch H, Guenther HL (1996) Bisphosphonates induce osteoblasts to secrete an inhibitor of osteoclast-mediated resorption. Endocrinology 137:2324–2333

Wallach S, Cohen S, Reid DM, Hughes RA, Hosking DJ, Laan RF, Doherty SM, Maricic M, Rosen C, Brown J, Barton I, Chines AA (2000) Effects of risedronate treatment on bone density and vertebral fracture in patients on corticosteroid therapy. Calcif Tissue Int 67:277–285

Wener JA, Gorton SJ, Raisz LG (1972) Escape from inhibition or resorption in cultures of fetal bone treated with calcitonin and parathyroid hormone. Endocrinology 90:752–759

Whitehead M, Lane G, Young O, Campbell S, Abeyasekera G, Hillyard CJ, MacIntyre I, Phang KG, Stevenson JC (1981) Interrelations of calcium-regulating hormones during normal pregnancy. Br Med J (Clin Res Ed) 283:10–12

Writing Group for the Women's Health Initiative Investigators (2002) Risks and Benefits of Estrogen Plus Progestin in Healthy Postmenopausal Women. Principal Results from the Women's Health Initiative Randomized Controlled Trial. JAMA 288:321–333

Orthopedic Surgery

GEROLD HOLZER

CONTENTS

5.1
Introduction

The orthopedist accompanies human beings throughout their life span. Starting with the inspection of the newborn baby shortly after birth, orthopedic care continues with checks for malpositioning and provision of orthopedic shoe inlays during adolescence and conservative and surgical treatment of degenerative diseases in advanced age.

The lifelong care provided by the orthopedist carries an enormous responsibility since the con-

G. HOLZER, MD
Department of Orthopedics, Medical University of Vienna, Vienna General Hospital, Waehringer Guertel 18–20, 1090 Vienna, Austria

sequences of decisions taken reach far beyond the amelioration of the moment. However, this long-term care represents a great opportunity for the patient in that changes can be observed and diagnostic and – if necessary – therapeutic measures may be started early.

The medical history of the family and of the patient allows the specialist to identify risk factors for osteoporosis. Sometimes additional indications may derive from the patient's work or sports activities. Every suspicion will be followed up.

The orthopedic surgeon's responsibility in the diagnosis and treatment of osteoporosis covers all age groups and both genders (OBRANT 1998; NIH CONSENSUS DEVELOPMENT PANEL ON OSTEOPOROSIS PREVENTION, DIAGNOSIS, AND THERAPY 2001). The possibilities of orthopedic surgical treatment in osteoporosis mainly relate to complications and conditions resulting from osteoporosis (DOBBS et al. 1999; FITHIAN and PAGE 1999; FREEDMAN 1999; LANE and NYDICK 1999; TOSI and LANE 1998).

5.1.1
Definition of Osteoporosis

Osteoporosis (NIH CONSENSUS DEVELOPMENT PANEL ON OSTEOPOROSIS PREVENTION, DIAGNOSIS, AND THERAPY 2001) is the most common human metabolic bone disorder. It was defined as "a skeletal disorder characterized by compromised bone strength predisposing a person to an increased risk of fracture. Bone strength primarily reflects the integration of bone density and bone quality" (NIH CONSENSUS DEVELOPMENT PANEL ON OSTEOPOROSIS PREVENTION, DIAGNOSIS, AND THERAPY 2001). These changes can be assessed indirectly through noninvasive measurements of bone mineral density (BMD). Bone density accounts for 75%–85% of the variance in ultimate strength of bone tissue (MELTON et al. 1988) and correlates closely with the load-bearing capacity of the skeleton in vitro.

In practice, the disease is defined by an intermediate outcome (BMD) and not by a health outcome (fracture). This definition takes into account the strong correlation between BMD and the likelihood of fracture. However, other factors also influence the fracture risk.

The most common fractures observed by the orthopedic surgeon in patients with osteoporosis are fractures of the vertebrae, hip, and forearm (Colles' fracture). While spinal fractures lead to deformity and Colles' fracture produces dysfunction, hip fractures severely affect the patient's ultimate quality of life and threaten survival. Proximal femoral fractures account for only about 20% of osteoporotic fractures, but they are the most devastating and cause the highest costs for the health system.

Mortality during the first postoperative year in patients with a fracture of the proximal femur is about 20%. Two-thirds of the patients are unable to achieve their preoperative level of activity. Early surgical intervention in these cases is associated with a lower rate of perioperative morbidity and better long-term results.

5.1.2
Prevention of Osteoporosis

On the various occasions when the orthopedic surgeon deals with children and adolescents – whether in an orthopedic clinic or outpatients department or when caring for individual athletes or groups of athletes – there is an opportunity to discover disturbances of bone metabolism and to institute diagnostic and therapeutic measures.

Every practitioner with athletes under their care, especially female athletes, must be aware of the "athlete's triad" (DRINKWATER et al. 1984), in which extreme sports activity is associated with amenorrhea, anorexia nervosa, and reduced bone density. In young girls the regularity of the menstrual cycle should be given special attention, and if irregularities are noted, a gynecologic endocrinologist should be consulted (BALOGH and BETTEMBUK 1997). Furthermore, a certain percentage of fat of the total body weight is required for menarche to occur.

Conditions of the spine resulting from osteoporosis are a huge medical problem. The literature shows that by the age of 60 years one-quarter of the total population suffer from spinal pain and report a decrease in body height. Every year, 20% of the population aged over 70 years suffer a fracture of the spine, and 90% of all X-rays of the spine in patients older than 75 years show changes pointing to osteoporosis.

5.1.3
Pathology of Osteoporosis

Bone remodeling is a lifetime process comprised of bone resorption and bone formation. While bone formation predominates in adolescents and adults until peak bone mass is achieved, in old age bone resorption prevails.

Changes in the quantity and quality of the trabecular microstructures of the vertebral body are observed histologically with advancing age. This causes a reduction in the number of trabeculae except along the lines of tension and their replacement by tabular structures. These tabular structures in turn are later perforated by osteoclasts ultimately and rarefied, leading to the formation of rod-shaped trabeculae (RECKER 1993).

Microfractures occur beyond the age of 45 years, predominantly at the vertical trabeculae, especially in the immediate vicinity of the end-plates of the vertebral bodies. Histologic investigations in accordance with radiologic findings of osteolytic spots also point to the fact that the end-plates of the vertebral bodies might be the trouble spots of the spine.

It was shown that the percentage of body weight above the vertebral bodies L1, L2, L3, and L4 amounts to 50%, 53%, 56%, and 58%, respectively, of the total body weight, and that the mineral content of the bone increases with increasing cranial pressure on the vertebral body. This at least partially explains the increased incidence of fractures in the caudal parts of the thoracic and cranial parts of the lumbar spine. In animal experiments, fractures of wedge-shaped vertebrae predominantly occur in those with low mineral content. An increased number of more centrally located fractures was observed experimentally in bone with a higher mineral content. The degree of degeneration of the intervertebral bodies probably does not affect the ability of the bone to resist pressure.

Studies in the literature indicate that osteoporotic fractures may have a multifactorial origin. In general, the results achieved so far indicate that a close correlation between bone mineral content and the incidence of fractures in vertebral bodies is highly probably (MIRSKY and EINHORN 1998).

5.1.4
Diagnosis of Osteoporosis

Whereas fractures of the distal radius and the proximal femur cause immediate heavy pain and inability to bear weight on the fractured extremity, leading to immediate admission to a hospital, spinal fractures lead to equally severe pain but in most cases are not so devastating as to require hospital admission. Therefore, an extensive description of osteoporotic fractures of the vertebral bodies is given here.

The medical history of patients with compression fractures of vertebral bodies often shows a fall or minor trauma, often caused by lifting a heavy object, followed by acute severe back pain. The typical radiologic picture shows a ventral fracture of the vertebral body, resulting in a wedge-shaped vertebral body. When a single vertebral body is affected and the patient reacts to pressure or knocking against the spinous process with locally well defined pain and this correlates well with the radiologic finding, the diagnosis of a recent fracture is confirmed.

However, in the majority of cases the X-ray shows several wedge-shaped vertebral bodies and a kyphotic deformation of the spine, and the patient reports a loss of body height and pain in more than one segment. If the treating physician has known the patient for a long time and may therefore be certain of the diagnosis of osteoporosis, the clinical picture requires no further investigation.

If this is not the case, inflammatory, metabolic, and neoplastic diseases must be excluded by differential diagnosis. In addition to radiologic methods like computed tomography (CT) and magnetic resonance imaging (MRI), bone scintigraphy can prove helpful for determining the age of the fracture and ruling out the presence of metastases. Since merely osteolytic processes cannot be detected by technetium scintigraphy, serum protein electrophoresis should be included in the differential diagnostic investigations to exclude a plasmocytoma.

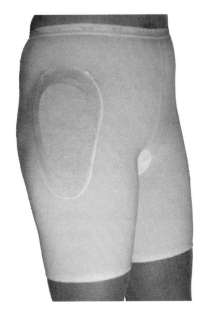

Fig. 5.1. Patient wearing an AHIP-Protector including a high-tech protection pad over the greater trochanter. Lateral view

avoided if all people at risk would wear a hip protector (wearing quota 100%). In clinical studies it was shown that hip protectors reduce the fracture rates (KANNUS et al. 2000).

The main disadvantage of hip protectors currently available lies in the material and shape. Either they consist of rigid, bulky structures or large elements covered with sweat producing fabrics. This is why most peoples refrain from wearing hip protectors long-term.

But new developments utilizing high-tech material in combination with new designs to implement medical considerations (AHIP-Protector, Astromed, Vienna) without reducing mechanical properties (HOLZER and HOLZER 2006). This leads to an increase in the wearing comfort and consequently to long-term use of the hip protector.

5.1.5
Mechanical Prevention of Osteoporotic Fractures

In principle hip-protectors exert mechanical protection of the hip region. By placing protection pads on the hip a force directed to the proximal femur during a fall will be absorbed. If worn they have an immediate effect. Half of hip fractures could be

5.2
Orthopedic Treatment of Osteoporosis

5.2.1
Conservative Treatment

For the majority of patients suffering from radial and vertebral body fractures, conservative management is the safest and most effective treatment. Only a brief indication of medical treatment of osteoporosis will be mentioned here: basically, calcium and vitamin D are given, and in the case of diagnosed osteoporosis, calcitonin, estrogen replacement therapy, and additionally bisphosphonates, depending on the severity of the disease.

High-risk patients without fractures, especially those with significantly low alimentary calcium uptake, should be advised to maintain a diet with sufficient calcium content. Vitamin D is recommended for patients who rarely expose themselves to the sun. Following diagnostic investigation with dual-energy X-ray absorptiometry (DEXA), quantitative CT, and possibly iliac crest puncture, additional therapy can be started.

Calcitonin administered as a nasal spray has proven an effective therapeutic modality in cases of osteoporosis, having an analgetic component, few side effects, and the potential for excellent patient compliance. Recently, selective estrogen receptor modulators (SERMs) have become available for women, and bisphosphonates for patients of both genders, besides estrogen replacement therapy. These medications have considerably enlarged the spectrum of therapy. Annual bone density checks are mandatory to monitor the treatment.

Therapy always starts with analgesia, which should allow continuous mobilization of the patient. It is important to select analgesics and psychophar-

maceuticals according to their side effects on neuromuscular coordination, as these drugs have been shown to considerably increase the danger of a fall and thus the risk of fracture in the elderly (NORDELL et al. 2000).

From an orthopedic point of view, treatment with braces is the method of choice to quickly achieve freedom from pain. A suitable orthosis supports the function of the abdominal muscles and thereby leads to raising of the spine. Stabilization of the spine prevents worsening of the existing spinal deformation. Orthoses remind patients to avoid certain movements, e.g., bending forward, and to adopt a kyphotic posture. Together with physiotherapeutic exercises, they induce a reduction of pain.

On the other hand, there are investigations (SNYDER et al. 1995) which show that fixation with braces and orthoses leads to increased osteopenia. Myoelectric studies in patients showed that orthoses – at least those acting like braces – do not contribute to a reduction in axial pressure on the spine. Despite these undesired side effects, however, there is still – at least at present – no alternative to treatment with orthoses. A full-contact brace such as the Boston brace, which passes the axial load to the iliac crest, might possibly produce the effects shown in the experiment. However, the main result of the limitation in motion brought about by the

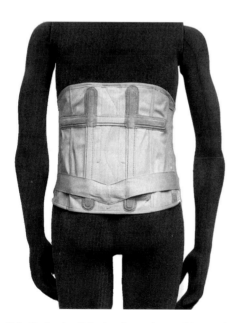

Fig. 5.2. Orthosis of the lumbar spine and lower thoracic spine as demonstrated on a dummy. Posterior view

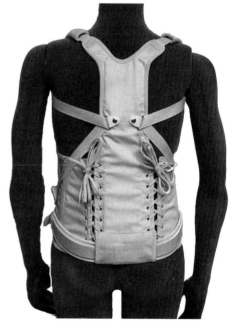

Fig. 5.3. Orthosis of the lumbar and thoracic region as demonstrated on a dummy. Posterior view

brace is reduction in pain, which is the aim of the treatment.

The orthosis of choice should be light and the patient should be able to put it on him- or herself. When a three-point fixation is aimed at, as is desirable in fractures of the upper and middle parts of the thoracic spine, a high brace must be prescribed (Figs. 5.2, 5.3). However, every specialist experienced in the treatment of osteoporosis well knows that elderly patients reject this sort of brace and will not wear it. As already pointed out, these orthoses should be worn for as short a time as possible after freedom from pain is achieved.

5.2.2
Acute Pain

Acute pain in patients suffering from osteoporosis mainly occurs with osteoporotic fractures. Depending on the location of the fracture, immediate surgery may be indicated (KOROVESSIS et al. 1994) or, in the case of compression fractures of vertebral bodies, immediate bed rest in the so-called K-position combined with infusion of analgesics. When bed rest alone is not sufficient, reduction of pain in the affected parts of the spine can be achieved by transient immobilization in a plaster jacket or a short plaster cast.

A determining factor is physiotherapeutic exercise. There is known to be a positive correlation between bone density and muscle mass (SINAKI et al. 1989). Physical loading influences activation of the muscle by induction of electric potentials stimulating new bone formation by osteoblasts. In addition, muscular activity strengthens the atrophic muscles, which are thereby enabled to hold the spine in a favorable position.

Once the patient is pain-free or at least the pain has been reduced, cautious mobilization with plastic braces should be started. In younger patients especially, but also in older ones, particular attention should be given to removing the brace when a considerable reduction in pain has been achieved. Patients should be recommended to use the brace only when they expect extended strain on the back or when leaving the house. Continuous use of the brace leads to atrophy of back muscles which are already weak. Ill-considered long-term use of a brace after osteoporotic fractures have healed makes it impossible to mobilize the patient without the brace.

5.2.3
Chronic Pain

When the acute pain has abated, chronic pain may develop despite prior medical and physiotherapeutic treatment of the cause. Often the patient has to be referred to the pain clinic for the pain to be successfully reduced. As pointed out earlier, providing the patient with a brace – watched with a critical eye – can be helpful.

5.3
Orthopedic Surgery of Osteoporosis

Most fractures are uncomplicated. A period of pain and partial disability is followed by restoration of function to the level before the fracture. However, in some cases fractures may lead to deformity, disability, dependence, the need for admission to a home for the aged, psychosocial problems, and even death (PAL et al. 1998; PERLAKY et al. 1994; SHEEHAN et al. 2000).

In general, treatment of fractures in older patients should follow these principles (LANE et al. 1988):
- Patients of advanced age are best served by a quick, definitive fixation of the fracture with immediate restoration of load and mobility. In most cases these patients are best suited for surgery on the day of the accident, although they may be suffering from other diseases which should be clarified precisely. The orthopedic surgical procedure should be as simple as possible in order to reduce the duration of surgery, blood loss, and psychological stress to a minimum.
- Orthopedic surgery should provide stable fixation of the fracture to enable normal function, which in the case of the lower extremity means weight bearing. In intra-articular fractures, anatomic reconstruction is important, whereas in metaphyseal and diaphyseal fractures stability is more important than anatomic reconstruction.
- Failure of internal fixation primarily means failure of the bone; only in rare cases does it mean failure of the fixation. The strength of bone is directly related to its mineral density (CARTER and HAYES 1977). Osteoporotic bone lacks the strength needed for screws and plates to be held securely. Moreover, comminution is generally more extensive in osteoporotic patients. The

internal fixation devices should be selected with a view to avoiding stress on bone–impact interfaces and stress shielding, and for this reason sliding nail plate devices and intramedullary nails are best suited for these cases.

The most common sites of fracture in osteoporotic patients are the distal radius, proximal femur, and vertebral bodies. The following review focuses on the principles of treatment for these fracture sites.

5.3.1
Fractures of the Distal Radius

Fractures of the distal radius (Colles' fractures) are very frequently observed in postmenopausal women, especially in winter. Sometimes minimal traumas such as those caused by supporting themselves with their hand while sitting down may cause a fracture in these subjects. In most cases the fractures are treated conservatively, typically with a plaster cast. The patients remain mobile and need not be admitted to hospital as long as they are still able to care for themselves and do not live alone.

5.3.2
Hip Fractures

Fractures in the hip region are more serious for patients with osteoporosis and are associated with the largest number of complications. An analysis of the US Congress Office of Technology Assessment (US CONGRESS OFFICE OF TECHNOLOGY ASSESSMENT 1995) showed proximal femur fracture impair most.

In the majority of cases a fall on the greater trochanter is an adequate trauma for hip fracture. Surgical treatment may be done by closed reduction and fixation with nails or screws or by hemiarthroplasty (VAHL et al. 1994). The biggest problem in the surgical treatment of a fracture of the greater trochanter is the high incidence of pseudarthrosis and avascular necrosis of the femoral head.

The Garden classification of fractures of the greater trochanter also recommends the surgical procedures: for Garden I and II, screw fixation of the fracture; for Garden III and IV, hemiarthroplasty. Despite the longer duration of the surgery and higher costs, hemiarthroplasty or total hip replacement (Fig. 5.4) are chosen in an increas-

ing number of cases, especially for pathologic and unstable fractures.

For intertrochanteric fractures the method of choice is implantation of a sliding screw plate (Fig. 5.5). Screws with large heads are available for use in osteoporotic bone.

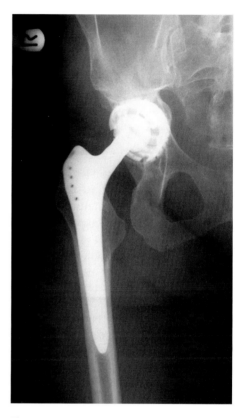

Fig. 5.4. Total hip replacement of the right side demonstrated on an anteroposterior conventional radiograph

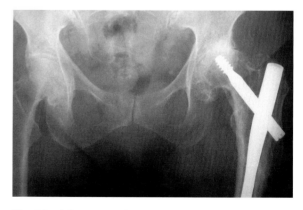

Fig. 5.5. Sliding screw plate in the left proximal femur demonstrated on an anteroposterior conventional radiograph

5.3.3
Fractures of the Vertebral Bodies

In general, the adverse effects of fractures of the vertebral bodies on health, function, and quality of life are underestimated. These fractures are associated with an increased rate of mortality. The occurrence of a single fracture increases the risk of future fractures and progressive kyphotic deformity. Owing to the challenges of reconstruction of an osteoporotic bone, open surgery is limited to those rare cases with neurologic deficits or unstable spines (Baba et al. 1995).

Nevertheless, most vertebral body fractures in osteoporotic patients do not require surgery, except for the described indications, and surgical treatment is limited to departments that specialize in this field. Such procedures only seem justified by the development of new instruments and implants for internal fixation and stabilization and by progress in the fields of intra- and perioperative anesthesia and intensive care.

Indications for surgical procedures such as decompression of the spinal cord (Shikata et al. 1990), reconstruction of vertebral bodies, and stabilization are neurologic complications such as paraplegia, typically developing slowly in cases of osteopenic fractures of vertebral bodies, or persistent pain despite treatment. Decompressing minimal surgical procedures without stabilization, such as laminectomy or costotransversectomy, are recommended to break the vicious circle of pain, inactivity, and increasing osteopenia (Ray 1987). If additional stabilization is needed, Cotrel-Dubousset, Kostuik-Harrington, Zielke, Kaneda, or Steffee instruments are recommended in addition to decompression.

Recently there has been increased interest in two "minimally invasive" procedures for acute vertebral fractures: i.e., vertebroplasty (Belkoff et al. 2000; Wenger and Markwalder 1999) and kyphoplasty, in which polymethylmethacrylate bone cement is injected into the fractured vertebral body. Single reports of both techniques claim prompt reduction of pain. However, controlled trials of these surgical methods to prove the advantages and disadvantages in comparison to the established methods are still lacking. Furthermore, the long-term effects of one or more vertebral bodies reinforced by bone cement on the neighboring vertebral bodies are unknown.

Some problems are of special importance for the orthopedic management of an acute osteoporotic fracture. Above all, the impression should be avoided that surgery is the only possible treatment for an acute osteoporotic fracture. Management of the perioperative period for long-term hospitalized patients must include thrombosis prophylaxis, avoidance of substances that inhibit bone healing (nicotine, corticosteroids), and, frequently, an additional high-calorie diet. Finally, the occurrence of the acute fracture should be used as an opportunity for additional diagnostic and therapeutic procedures in order to avoid further surgical operations. The orthopedic surgeon should initiate outpatient evaluation of the patient for osteoporosis and a treatment program.

Whether treated surgically or conservatively, patients should be confined to bed for as short a time as possible, and pharmacologic treatment for osteoporosis should be started immediately a fracture of osteopenic vertebral bodies is diagnosed.

5.4
Osteoporosis as a Complication

Osteoporosis is mainly a disease of age. Socioeconomic change and the greater life expectancy of the general population mean that the number of people suffering from osteoporosis will increase dramatically in the next few decades.

There is a long list of risk factors which increase the chance of developing osteoporosis. Different diseases and their treatment regimens were neglected until recently: glucocorticoid induced osteoporosis (GIOP) and chemotherapy induced osteoporosis (CIOP), as it was shown in patients with breast cancer and osteosacoma (Holzer et al. 2003), just to name the most important.

Moreover, many old patients also suffer from degenerative diseases such as osteoarthritis (Healey et al. 1985). Progress in orthopedic endoprosthetic devices may help a large number of these people. Elective total hip and knee replacements render these joints painfree, enabling longer mobility. However, osteoporosis is a complication during implantation of an endoprosthesis, because the rarified and softer bone offers a poorer bed for the implantation (Levitz et al. 1995) and therefore parts of the prosthesis must be implanted with cement. The information given above for the implantation of hip or knee endoprostheses also hold for surgery of other parts of the locomotive apparatus, e.g., feet or spine (Hirano et al. 1998; Lim et al. 1995).

References

Anonymous (2001) Osteoporosis prevention, diagnosis and therapy. JAMA 285:785–795)

Baba H, Maezawa Y, Kamitani K, Furusawa N, Imura S, Tomita K (1995) Osteoporotic vertebral collapse with late neurological complications. Paraplegia 33:281–289

Balogh A, Bettembuk P (1997) Hormone replacement therapy and prevention of osteoporosis: risk assessment and practical advice. Eur J Obstet Gynecol Reprod Biol 71:189–191

Belkoff SM, Mathis JM, Erbe EM, Fenton DC (2000) Biomechanical evaluation of a new bone cement for use in vertebroplasty. Spine 25:1061–1064

Carter DR, Hayes WC (1977) The compressive behavior of bone as a two-phase porous structure. J Bone Joint Surg 59:954–962

Dobbs MB, Buckwalter J, Saltzman C (1999) Osteoporosis: the increasing role of the orthopaedist. Iowa Orthop J 19:43–52

Drinkwater BL, Nilson K, Chesnut CH III, Bremner WJ, Shainholtz S, Southworth MB (1984) Bone mineral content of amenorrheic and eumenorrheic athletes. N Engl J Med 311:277–281

Fithian DC, Page AE (1999) Osteoporosis prevention and the orthopaedic surgeon: when fracture care is not enough. J Bone Joint Surg [Am] 81:1653–1654

Freedman KB (1999) Osteoporosis prevention and the orthopaedic surgeon: when fracture care is not enough. J Bone Joint Surg [Am] 81:1652–1653

Healey JH, Vigorita VJ, Lane JM (1985) The coexistence and characteristics of osteoarthritis and osteoporosis. J Bone Joint Surg [Am] 67:586–592

Hirano T, Hasegawa K, Washio T, Hara T, Takahashi H (1998) Fracture risk during pedicle screw insertion in osteoporotic spine. J Spinal Disord 11:493–497

Holzer L, Holzer G (2006) Mechanical protection of hip fractures by the use of hip protectors – review and mechanical comparison Wien Med Wschr (in press)

Holzer G, Krepler P, Koschat MA, Grampp S, Dominkus M, Kotz R (2003) Bone mineral density in long-term survivors of highly malignant osteosarcoma. J Bone Joint Surg Br 85:231–237

Kannus kP, Parkkari J, Niemi S, Pasanen M, Palvanen M, Jarvinen M, Vuori I (2000) Prevention of hip fracture in elderly people with use of a hip protector. N Engl J Med 343:1506–13

Korovessis P, Maraziotis T, Piperos G, Spyropoulos P (1994) Spontaneous burst fracture of the thoracolumbar spine in osteoporosis associated with neurological impairment: a report of seven cases and review of the literature. Eur Spine J 3:286–288

Lane JM, Nydick M (1999) Osteoporosis: current modes of prevention and treatment. J Am Acad Orthop Surg 7:19–31

Lane JM, Cornell CN, Healey JH (1988) Orthopaedic consequences of osteoporosis. In: Riggs BL, Melton LJ III (eds) Osteoporosis: etiology, diagnosis, and management. Raven, New York, pp 443–455

Levitz CL, Lotke PA, Karp JS (1995) Long-term changes in bone mineral density following total knee replacement. Clin Orthop 321:68–72

Lim TH, An HS, Evanich C, Hasanoglu KY, McGrady L, Wilson CR (1995) Strength of anterior vertebral screw fixation in relationship to bone mineral density. J Spinal Disord 8:121–125

Melton LJ, Chao EYS, Lane J (1988) Biochemical aspects of fractures. In: Riggs BL, Melton LJ (eds) Osteoporosis: etiology, diagnosis, and management. Raven, New York, p 111–131

Mirsky EC, Einhorn TA (1998) Bone densitometry in orthopaedic practice. J Bone Joint Surg [Am] 80:1687–1698

Nordell E, Jarnlo GB, Jetsen C, Nordstrom L, Thorngren KG (2000) Accidental falls and related fractures in 65–74 year olds: a retrospective study of 332 patients. Acta Orthop Scand 71:175–179

Obrant KJ (1998) Prevention of osteoporotic fractures – should orthopedic surgeons care? Acta Orthop Scand 69:333–338

Pal B, Morris J, Muddu B (1998) The management of osteoporosis-related fractures: a survey of orthopaedic surgeons' practice. Clin Exp Rheumatol 16:61–62

Perlaky G, Szendroi M, Varga PP (1994) Osteoporosis – a modifying factor of surgical treatment. Acta Med Hung 50:245–256

Ray CD (1987) Extensive lumbar decompression. In: White A, Rothman R, Ray C (eds) Lumbar spine surgery. Mosby, St Louis, p 165–184

Recker RR (1993) Architecture and vertebral fracture. Calcif Tissue Int 53 [Suppl 1]:S139–S142

Sheehan J, Mohamed F, Reilly M, Perry IJ (2000) Secondary prevention following fractured neck of femur: a survey of orthopaedic surgeons practice. Ir Med J 93:105–107

Shikata J, Yamamuro T, Iida H, Shimizu K, Yoshikawa J (1990) Surgical treatment for paraplegia resulting from vertebral fractures in senile osteoporosis. Spine 15:485–489

Sinaki M, Wahner HW, Offord KP, Hodgson SF (1989) Efficacy of nonloading exercises in prevention of vertebral bone loss in postmenopausal women. Mayo Clin Proc 64:762–769

Snyder BD, Zaltz I, Breitenbach MA, Kido TH, Myers ER, Emans JB (1995) Does bracing affect bone density in adolescent scoliosis? Spine 20:1554–1560

Tosi LL, Lane JM (1998) Osteoporosis prevention and the orthopaedic surgeon: when fracture care is not enough. J Bone Joint Surg [Am] 80:1567–1569

US Congress Office of Technology Assessment (1995) Effectiveness and costs of osteoporosis screening and hormone replacement therapy, vol 2. Evidence on benefits, risks and costs, OTA-BP-H-144. US Government Printing Office, Washington DC

Vahl AC, Dunki-Jacobs PB, Patka P, Haarman HJ (1994) Hemiarthroplasty in elderly, debilitated patients with an unstable femoral fracture in the trochanteric region. Acta Orthop Belg 60:274–279

Wenger M, Markwalder TM (1999) Surgically controlled, transpedicular methyl methacrylate vertebroplasty with fluoroscopic guidance. Acta Neurochir (Wien) 141:625–631

Radiology of Osteoporosis

MICHAEL JERGAS

CONTENTS

MICHAEL JERGAS, MD
Priv.-Doz., Department of Radiology and Nuclear Medicine,
St. Elisabeth-Krankenhaus, Werthmannstrasse 1, 50935
Cologne, Germany

The term osteoporosis is widely used clinically to mean generalized loss of bone, or osteopenia, accompanied by relatively atraumatic fractures of the spine, wrist, hips or ribs. Because of uncertainties of specific radiologic interpretation, the term osteopenia ("poverty of bone") has been used as a generic designation for radiographic signs of decreased bone density. Radiographic findings suggestive of osteopenia and osteoporosis are frequently encountered in everyday medical practice and can result from a wide spectrum of diseases ranging from highly prevalent causes such as postmenopausal and involutional osteoporosis to rare endocrinologic and hereditary or acquired disorders (Table 6.1). Histologically, in each of these disorders there is a deficient amount of osseous tissue, although different pathogenic mechanisms may be involved. Conventional radiography is widely available, and alone, or in conjunction with other imaging techniques it is widely used for the detection of complications of osteopenia, for the differential diagnosis of osteopenia, or for follow-up examinations in specific clinical settings. Bone scintigraphy, computed tomography and magnetic resonance imaging are additional diagnostic methods that are applied almost routinely to aid in the differential diagnosis of osteoporosis and its sequelae.

6.1
Radiographic Findings in Osteopenia and Osteoporosis

Knowledge of both the physical nature of X-ray absorption by biologic tissues as well as the histopathologic changes leading to osteopenia and osteoporosis is required to understand the radiographic findings. The absorption of X-rays by a tissue depends on the quality of the X-ray beam, the character of the atoms composing the tissue, the physical density

Table 6.1. Disorders associated with radiographic osteoporosis (osteopenia).

I. Primary osteoporosis

1. Involutional osteoporosis (postmenopausal and senile)
2. Juvenile osteoporosis

II. Secondary osteoporosis

A. Endocrine
   1. Adrenal cortex (Cushing's disease)
   2. Gonadal disorders (hypogonadism)
   3. Pituitary (hypopituitarism)
   4. Pancreas (diabetes)
   5. Thyroid (hyperthyroidism)
   6. Parathyroid (hyperparathyroidism)

B. Marrow replacement and expansion
   1. Myeloma
   2. Leukemia
   3. Metastatic disease
   4. Gaucher's disease
   5. Anemias (sickle cell disease, thalassemia)

C. Drugs and substances
   1. Corticosteroids
   2. Heparin
   3. Anticonvulsants
   4. Immunosuppressants
   5. Alcohol (in combination with malnutrition)

D. Chronic disease
   1. Chronic renal disease
   2. Hepatic insufficiency
   3. Gastrointestinal malabsorption
   4. Chronic inflammatory polyarthropathies
   5. Chronic immobilization

E. Deficiency states
   1. Vitamin D
   2. Vitamin C (scurvy)
   3. Calcium
   4. Malnutrition

F. Inborn errors of metabolism
   1. Osteogenesis imperfecta
   2. Homocystinuria

of the tissue, and the thickness of the penetrated structure. The amount of X-ray absorption defines the density of X-ray shadow that a tissue casts on the film. Because absorption rises with the third power of the atomic number, and because calcium has a high atomic number, it is primarily the amount of calcium that affects the X-ray absorption of bone. The amount of calcium per unit mineralized bone volume in osteoporosis remains constant at about 35% (ALBRIGHT et al. 1941; LeGEROS 1994). There-

fore, a decrease in the mineralized bone volume results in a decrease of the total bone calcium and consequently a decreased absorption of the X-ray beam. On the X-ray film this phenomenon is referred to as increased radiolucency.

As bone mass is lost, changes in bone structure occur, and these can be observed radiographically (Fig. 6.1). Bone is composed of two compartments, cortical bone and trabecular bone. The structural changes seen in cortical bone represent bone resorption at different sites (e.g., the inner and outer surfaces of the cortex, or within the cortex in the Haversian and Volkmann channels). These three sites (endosteal, intracortical and periosteal) may react differently to distinct metabolic stimuli, and careful investigation of the cortices may be of value in the differential diagnosis of metabolic disease affecting the skeleton.

Cortical bone remodeling typically occurs in the endosteal "envelope", and the interpretation of subtle changes in this layer may be difficult at times. With increasing age, there is a widening of the marrow canal due to an imbalance of endosteal bone formation and resorption that leads to a "trabeculization" of the inner surface of the cortex. Endosteal scalloping due to resorption of the inner bone surface can be seen in high bone turnover states such as reflex sympathetic dystrophy.

Intracortical bone resorption may cause longitudinal striation or tunneling, predominantly in the subendosteal zone. These changes are seen in various high turnover metabolic diseases affecting the bone such as hyperparathyroidism, osteomalacia, renal osteodystrophy, and acute osteoporosis from disuse or the reflex sympathetic dystrophy syndrome but also postmenopausal osteoporosis. Intracortical tunneling is a hallmark of rapid bone turnover. It is usually not apparent in disease states with relatively low bone turnover such as senile osteoporosis. Accelerated endosteal and intracortical resorption with intracortical tunneling and indistinct border of the inner cortical surface, is best depicted with high resolution radiographic techniques. Intracortical tunneling must be distinguished from nutritional foramina, which are isolated and present with an oblique orientation. Intracortical resorption is also a sign of bone viability and is not seen in necrotic or allograft bone.

Subperiosteal bone resorption is associated with an irregular definition of the outer bone surface. This finding is pronounced in diseases with a high bone turnover, principally primary and secondary

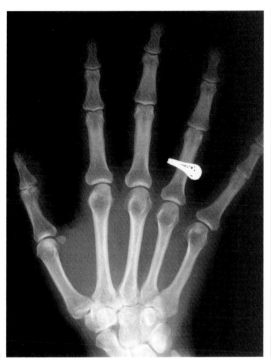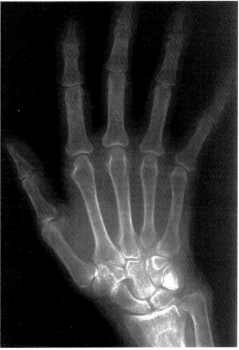

a

b

Fig. 6.1a,b. Conventional radiographs of the hand in a healthy woman (**a**) and in a patient suffering from osteoporosis (**b**). Aside from a general increase in radiolucency of the bone there is also a diminution of cortical bone and widening of the marrow space

hyperparathyroidism. However, rarely it may also be present in other diseases. Cortical thinning with expansion of the medullary cavity occurs as endosteal bone resorption exceeds periosteal bone apposition in most adults. In the late stages of osteoporosis, the cortices appear paper-thin with the endosteal surface usually being smooth.

Trabecular bone has a greater surface and responds faster to metabolic changes than does cortical (FROST 1964). These changes are most prominent in the axial skeleton and in the ends of the long and tubular bones of the appendicular skeleton (juxtaarticular), e.g., proximal femur, distal radius. These are sites with a relatively great amount of trabecular bone. Loss of trabecular bone (in cases with low rates of loss) occurs in a predictable pattern. Nonweight bearing trabeculae are resorbed first. This leads to a relative prominence of the weight bearing trabeculae. The remaining trabeculae may become thicker, which may result in a distinct radiographic trabecular pattern. For example, early changes of osteopenia in the lumbar spine typically include a rarefication of the horizontal trabeculae accompanied by a relative accentuation of the vertical trabeculae, radiographically appearing as vertical

striation of the bone. With decreasing density of the trabecular bone the cortical rim of the vertebrae is accentuated, and the vertebrae may have a "picture-frame" appearance (Fig. 6.2). In addition to changes in the trabecular bone, thinning of the cortical bone occurs. Changes of the bone structure at distinct skeletal sites are assessed for the differential diagnosis of various skeletal conditions. For the evaluation of very subtle changes, such as different forms of bone resorption, high resolution radiographic techniques with optical or geometric magnification may be required (GENANT et al. 1977).

The anatomic distribution of the osteopenia or osteoporosis depends on the underlying cause. Osteopenia can be generalized affecting the whole skeleton, or regional, affecting only a part of the skeleton, usually in the appendicular skeleton. Typical examples of generalized osteopenias are involutional and postmenopausal osteoporosis and osteoporosis caused by endocrine disorders such as hyperparathyroidism, hyperthyroidism, osteomalacia and hypogonadism. Regional forms of osteoporosis result from factors affecting only parts of the appendicular skeleton such as disuse, reflex sympathetic syndrome and transient osteoporosis of large

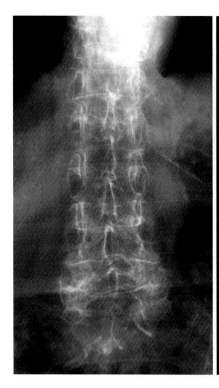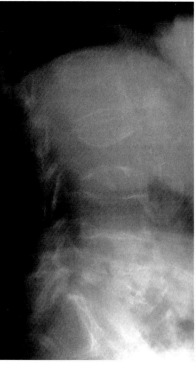

Fig. 6.2. Severe osteopenia. The transparency of the vertebral bodies matches that of the intervertebral disc space. There are multiple fractures of the vertebral endplates leading to biconcave deformities of the vertebrae as well as a severe fracture of L5

joints. The distribution of osteopenia may vary considerably between different diseases and may be suggestive of a specific diagnosis. Focal osteopenia primarily reflects the underlying cause such as inflammation, fracture or tumor.

Thus, it seems that a number of characteristic features by conventional radiography make the diagnosis of osteopenia or osteoporosis possible. However, the detection of osteopenia by conventional radiography is inaccurate since it is influenced by many technical factors such as radiographic exposure factors, film development, soft tissue thickness of the patient, etc. (Table 6.2). It has been estimated that as much as 20%–40% of bone mass must be lost before a decrease in bone density can be seen in lateral radiographs of the thoracic and lumbar spine (LACHMANN and WHELAN 1936). Finally, the diagnosis of osteopenia from conventional radiographs is dependent on the experience of the reader and his/her subjective interpretation (JERGAS et al. 1994a).

In summary, a radiograph may reflect the amount of bone mass, histology and gross morphology of the skeletal part examined. The principal findings of osteopenia are increased radiolucency, changes in bone microstructure, e.g. rarefication of trabeculae, thinning of the cortices, eventually resulting in changes of the gross bone morphology, i.e., changes in the shape of the bone and fractures.

Table 6.2. Factors influencing the radiographic appearance of objects (HEUCK and SCHMIDT 1960)

Radiation source
Exposure time
Film-focus distance
Anode characteristics
Voltage
Beam filtration
Object
Thickness of bone
Bone mineral content
Soft tissue composition
Scattering
Film and screen
Film granularity
Emulsion of film
Film speed
Screen properties
Film processing
Developing time
Temperature of developer
Type of developer
Type of fixer
Type of processing (automated vs. manual)

6.2
Diseases Characterized by Generalized Osteopenia

6.2.1
Involutional Osteoporosis

Involutional osteoporosis is the most common generalized skeletal disease. It has been classified as a type I or postmenopausal osteoporosis and a type II or senile osteoporosis (ALBRIGHT 1947; RIGGS and MELTON 1983). GALLAGHER (1990) added a third type meaning secondary osteoporosis (Table 6.3). Even though the importance of estrogen deficiency for postmenopausal osteoporosis has been established, the distinction between the first two types of osteoporosis is not generally accepted. Distinctions between postmenopausal and senile osteoporosis may sometimes be arbitrary, and the assignment of fracture sites to the different types of osteoporosis is uncertain. Postmenopausal osteoporosis is believed to represent that process occurring in a subset of postmenopausal women, typically between the ages of 50 and 65 years. There is accelerated trabecular bone resorption related to estrogen deficiency, and the fracture pattern in this group of women primarily involves the spine and the wrist. In senile osteoporosis, there is a proportionate loss of cortical and trabecular bone. The characteristic fractures of senile osteoporosis include fractures of the hip, the proximal humerus, the tibia and the pelvis in elderly women and men, usually 75 years or older. Major factors in the etiology of senile osteoporosis include the age-related decrease in bone formation, diminished adrenal function, reduced intestinal calcium absorption and secondary hyperparathyroidism.

The radiographic appearance of the skeleton in involutional osteoporosis may include all of the aforementioned characteristics for generalized osteoporosis. The high prevalence of involutional osteoporosis with its typical radiographic manifestations has lead to numerous attempts to diagnose and quantify osteoporosis based on its radiographic characteristics.

6.2.1.1
Osteopenia and Osteoporosis of the Axial Skeleton

The radiographic manifestation of osteopenia of the axial skeleton includes increased radiolucency of the vertebrae. The vertebral body's radiographic density may assume the density of the intervertebral disk space. Further findings include vertical striation of the vertebrae due to reinforcement of vertical trabeculae in the osteopenic vertebra, framed appearance of the vertebrae ("picture framing" or "empty box") due to an accentuation of the cortical outline, and increased biconcavity of the vertebral endplates (Fig. 6.3). Biconcavity of the vertebrae results from protrusion of the intervertebral disk into the weakened vertebral body. A classification of these characteristics can be found with the Saville index (Table 6.4) (SAVILLE 1967). This index, however, has never gained widespread acceptance, being prone to great subjectivity and experience of the reader. DOYLE and colleagues (1967) found that neither of aforementioned signs of osteopenia reflect the bone mineral status of an individual reliably and cannot be used for follow-up of osteopenic patients. Thus, bone density measurements using dedicated densitometric methods have widely replaced the subjective analysis of bone density from conventional radiographs. Densitometric results may suggest osteopenia even if the bone loss is not detectable on a spine radiograph. Nevertheless, the aforementioned radiographic signs of osteoporosis have been found to be significantly related to measured bone density, and normal bone densitometry measurements may

Table 6.3. Classification of osteoporosis acording to Albright, Riggs and Melton, and Gallagher (Table adapted from GALLAGHER 1992)

Type	I Postmeno- pausal	II Senile	III Secondary
Age	55-70	75-90	Any age
Years past menopause	5-15	25-40	-
Sex ratio (female:male)	20:1	2:1	1:1
Fracture site	Spine	Hip, spine, pelvis, humerus	Spine, hip, peripheral skeleton
Bone loss			
– Trabecular	+++	++	+++
– Cortical	+	++	+++
Contributing factor			
– Menopause	+++	++	++
– Age	+	+++	++

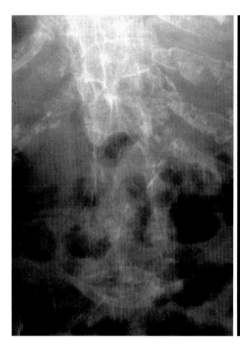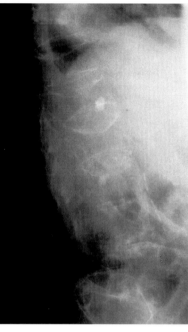

Fig. 6.3. Severe osteopenia in a patient with long-standing osteoporosis. There are multiple vertebral deformities. Due to the decreased bone density bone tissue can hardly be differentiated from soft tissue

Table 6.4. Osteopenia score for vertebrae by SAVILLE (1967)

Grade	Radiographic appearance of vertebra
0	Normal bone density
1	Minimal loss of density; endplates begin to stand out giving a stenciled effect
2	Vertical striation is more obvious; endplates are thinner
3	More severe loss of bone density than grade 2; endplates becoming less visible
4	Ghost-like vertebral bodies; density is no greater than soft tissue; no trabecular pattern is visible

sometimes have to be considered false if the radiograph displays characteristic changes of osteopenia (JERGAS et al. 1994b; AHMED et al. 1998).

6.2.2
Vertebral Fractures and Their Diagnosis

Vertebral fractures are the hallmarks of osteoporosis, and even though one may argue that osteopenia per se may not be diagnosed reliably from spinal radiographs, spinal radiography continues to be a substantial aid in diagnosing and following vertebral fractures (GENANT et al. 1993). Furthermore, along with a low bone density the vertebral

fracture has been recognized as the strongest risk factor for future osteoporotic fractures (ROSS et al. 1991, 1993; KOTOWICZ et al. 1994). Thus, the presence of vertebral fracture has become a key factor in patient evaluation as expressed in the NOF guidelines (NATIONAL OSTEOPOROSIS FOUNDATION 2000; LENCHIK et al. 2004). Educational efforts, such as the Vertebral Fracture Initiative by the IOF, aim at raising the awareness of physicians to recognize the importance of vertebral fracture as a trigger for therapeutic decisions to prevent future fractures (DELMAS et al. 2005).

Changes in the gross morphology of the vertebral body have a wide range of appearances from increased concavity of the end plates to a complete destruction of the vertebral anatomy in vertebral crush fractures. In clinical practice conventional radiographs of the thoracolumbar region in lateral projection are analyzed qualitatively by radiologists or experienced clinicians to identify vertebral deformities or fractures. For an experienced radiologist, this assessment generally is uncomplicated, and it can be aided by additional radiographic projections such as anteroposterior and oblique views, or by complimentary examinations such as bone scintigraphy, computed tomography (Fig. 6.4) and magnetic resonance imaging (Fig. 6.5) (McAFEE et al. 1983; BALLOCK et al. 1992; CAMPBELL et al. 1995; TEHRANZADEH and TAO 2004).

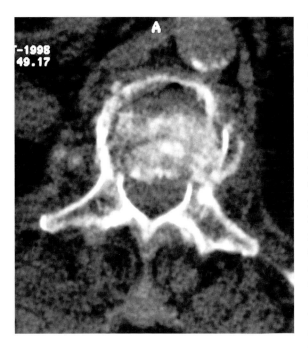

Fig. 6.4. Computed tomography of the osteoporotic fracture may reveal involvement of the posterior border as well as narrowing of the spinal canal

In the context of conducting epidemiologic studies or clinical drug trials in osteoporosis research, where vertebral fractures are an important end point, the requirements and expectations differ considerably from the clinical environment (KLEEREKOPER

et al. 1992). The examinations are frequently performed without specific clinical indications and without specific therapeutic ramifications. The evaluation for fractures is generally limited to lateral conventional thoracolumbar radiographs, and the number of subjects to be reviewed is often quite large, requiring high efficiency. The assessment may be performed by a variety of observers with different levels of experience. The detection of vertebral fractures certainly depends on the reader's expertise. Early experience with qualitative readings indicated that considerable variability in fracture identification exists when radiologists or clinicians interpreted radiographs without specific training, standardization, reference to an atlas or prior consensus readings (JENSEN et al. 1984; DEYO et al. 1985; GENANT et al. 1995).

Therefore, several approaches to standardizing visual qualitative readings have been proposed and applied in clinical studies. An early approach for a standardized description of vertebral fractures was made by SMITH and colleagues (1960). These authors assigned one of three grades (normal, indeterminate or osteoporotic) to a patient depending on the most severe deformity (SMITH et al. 1960). The spinal radiographs were evaluated on a per patient and not on a per vertebra basis, a serious limitation for the follow-up of vertebral fractures and also for the assessment of the severity of osteoporosis. Other standardized visual approaches allow for an assess-

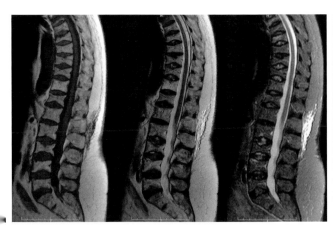
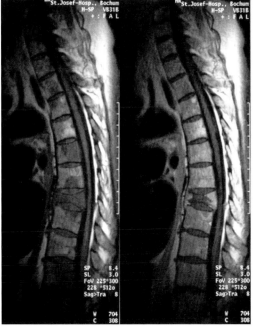

Fig. 6.5a,b. Magnetic resonance imaging of benign vertebral collapse (**a**) and metastatic disease of the spine in breast cancer (**b**). Abnormal signal that parallels the fracture, the absence of abnormal signal in non-fractured vertebrae, other vertebral deformities with normal signal and the absence of paravertebral soft tissue mass usually indicates benign vertebral collapse. Diffusion weighted images may also help differentiate between benign (low signal) and malignant (high signal) vertebral collapse

ment of vertebral deformities on a per vertebra rather than on a per patient basis and thus make a more accurate assessment of the fracture status of a person and the follow-up of individual fractures possible. Meunier et al. (1978) proposed an approach in which each vertebra is graded depending on its shape or deformity. Grade 1 is assigned to a normal vertebra without any deformity, grade 2 is assigned to a biconcave vertebra, and grade 4 is assigned to an end plate fracture or a wedged or crushed vertebra. The sum of all grades of the vertebrae T7 to L4 is the radiological vertebral index (RVI). This approach is limited since it considers only the type of the vertebral deformity, i.e., biconcavity versus fracture, without assessing fracture severity. For prevalent fractures, each fracture, whether it is diminutive or severe, would have the same weight in the RVI, and for the application of this approach to follow-up examinations this means that refractures of pre-existing fractures may not be detected at all. With the distinction between biconcavity and fracture in this approach, the concept of «vertebral deformity» versus vertebral fracture was introduced. However, it was not expressively attempted to distinguish non-fracture deformities, such as degenerative remodeling, from actual fracture appearances.

Kleerekoper and colleagues (1984) modified Meunier's radiological vertebral index and introduced the "vertebra deformity score" VDS (Nielsen et al. 1991; Olmez et al. 2005), by which each vertebra from T4 to L5 is assigned an individual score from 0 to 3 depending on the type of vertebral deformity. This grading scheme is based on the reduction of the anterior, middle, and posterior vertebral heights, H_a, H_m and H_p, respectively. A vertebral deformity (to be graded 1 to 3) is present when any vertebral height, H_a, H_m, or H_p, is reduced by at least 4 mm or 15%. A vertebral deformity score 0 is assigned to a normal vertebra without any vertebral height reduction. A VDS 1 deformity corresponds to a vertebral end plate deformity with the heights H_a and H_p being normal. A wedge deformity with a reduction of H_a and – to a lesser extent H_m – is assigned a VDS of 2. A compression deformity, which is assigned a VDS of 3, is characterized by a reduction of all vertebral heights H_a, H_m and H_p. Grading all vertebrae T4 to L5 using this score, the minimum VDS for the whole spine would thus be zero with all vertebrae intact and the maximum score would be 42 with compression fractures of all vertebrae. The vertebral deformity score still relies on the type of deformity, i.e., the vertebral shape, and changes of the vertebral shape

would be required to account for incident vertebral fractures on follow-up radiographs. A quantitative extension of the VDS with measurements of the vertebral heights accounts for the continuous character of vertebral fractures.

The radiologist's perspective of vertebral fracture diagnosis, i.e., considering the differential diagnosis as well as the severity of a fracture, is probably best reflected in the semiquantitative fracture assessment used in several studies (Genant 1990; Genant et al. 1993). The severity of a fracture is assessed solely by visual determination of the extent of a vertebral height reduction and morphological change, and vertebral fractures are differentiated from other nonfracture deformities. With this approach the type of the deformity (wedge, biconcavity, or compression) is no longer linked to the grading of a fracture as is done with the other standardized visual approaches. Thoracic and lumbar vertebrae from T4 to L4 are graded on visual inspection and without direct vertebral measurement as normal (grade 0), mildly deformed (grade 1, approximately 20%–25% reduction in anterior, middle and/or posterior height and a reduction of 10%–20% of the projected vertebral area), moderately deformed (grade 2, approximately 25%–40% reduction in anterior, middle and/or posterior height and a reduction of 20%–40% of the projected vertebral area), and severely deformed (grade 3, approximately 40% or greater reduction in anterior, middle and/or posterior height and in the projected vertebral area) (Fig. 6.6). From this semiquantitative assessment a "spinal fracture index", SFI, can be calculated as the sum of all grades assigned to the vertebrae divided by the number of the evaluated vertebrae. In addition to height reductions, careful attention is given to alterations in the shape and configuration of the vertebrae relative to adjacent vertebrae and expected normal appearances. These features add a strong qualitative aspect to the interpretation and also render this method less readily definable. Several studies, however, have demonstrated that semiquantitative interpretation, after careful training and standardization, can produce results with excellent intra- and interobserver reproducibility within the same school of training (Genant et al. 1993; Wu et al. 1995).

In a further effort to provide definable, reproducible, and objective methods to detect vertebral fractures and in order to accommodate the assessment of large numbers of radiographs by technicians (in the absence of radiologists or experienced clinicians), various quantitative morphometric approaches

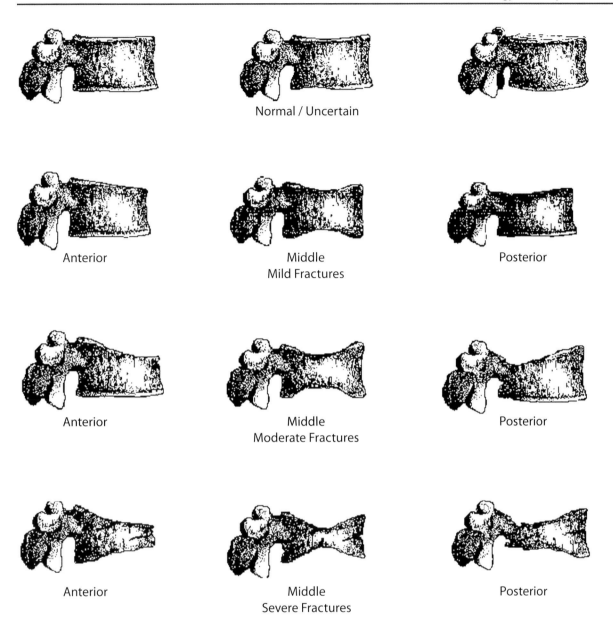

Normal / Uncertain

Anterior   Middle   Posterior
Mild Fractures

Anterior   Middle   Posterior
Moderate Fractures

Anterior   Middle   Posterior
Severe Fractures

Fig. 6.6. Grading scheme for a semiquantitative assessment of vertebral deformities after Genant. The drawing illustrates the reductions of vertebral height that correspond to the grade of deformity. (Drawing courtesy of Dr. C.Y. Wu)

have been explored and employed. Early studies using direct measurements of vertebral dimensions on lateral radiographs were described by FLETCHER in 1946, HURXTHAL in 1968, JENSEN and TOUGAARD in 1981, and KLEEREKOPER et al. in 1984, with the rationale being a reduction in the subjectivity considered intrinsic to the qualitative assessment of spinal radiographs.

Increasingly sophisticated morphometric approaches have been derived for the definition of vertebral dimensions, most of them making 4 to 10 points on a vertebral body to define vertebral heights (NELSON et al. 1990; SPENCER et al. 1990; JERGAS and SAN VALENTIN 1995) (Fig. 6.7). Typically, H_a, H_m and H_p are measured, as is the projected vertebral area. Newer techniques are based on digitally captured conventional radiographs to assess the vertebral dimensions (KALIDIS et al. 1992; EVANS et al. 1993; WU et al. 2000). These techniques then rely on either marking points manually to define vertebral heights or finding those points and measuring in an automated or semiautomated fashion.

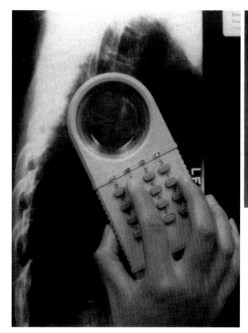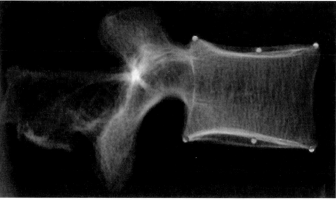

Fig. 6.7. In six-point digitization for quantitative morphometric assessment of vertebral fractures the endpoints of the vertebral height are marked directly on the vertebra. Point placement is fairly easy when the vertebra is ideally projected with perfect superposition of the vertebral contours. When the vertebra is rotated and oblique, point placement is more difficult

HEDLUND and GALLAGHER (1988) used criteria such as percent reduction of vertebral height, wedge angles, and areas in various combinations. DAVIES and co-workers (1993) employed two distinct morphometric cut-off thresholds for the detection of either vertebral compression or wedge fractures using vertebral height ratios that were defined by a radiologist's assessment of vertebral deformities. SMITH-BINDMAN et al. (1991) initially reported the use of vertebral level specific reductions in anterior, middle, or posterior height ratios expressed as a percentage relative to normal data. MELTON et al. (1989) used this level-specific approach, and subsequently EASTELL et al. (1991) modified it by applying height ratio reductions in terms of standard deviations rather than percentage. With this approach, each vertebral level has its own specific mean and standard deviation. MINNE et al. (1988) developed a method by which vertebral height measures are adjusted according to the height of T4 as a means of standardization, and the resulting values are compared to a normal population. BLACK et al. (1991) derived a statistical method for establishing normative data from morphometric measures of vertebral heights based upon deletion of the tails of the Gaussian distribution of an unselected population. McCLOSKEY et al. (1993) used vertebral height ratios and introduced an additional parameter defined as a predicted posterior height in addition to the measured posterior height. Ross et al. (1993) further

refined morphometric criteria for fracture by utilizing height reductions in standard deviations based on the overall patient specific vertebral dimensions combined with population based level-specific vertebral dimensions.

Several comprehensive studies have compared the various methods or cut-off criteria in the same populations to examine the impact of methodology on estimates of vertebral prevalence and on identification of individual patients or individual vertebrae as fractured. In these studies the expected trade-offs between sensitivity and specificity were observed. Two- to fourfold differences in estimates of fracture prevalence and generally poor or modest kappa scores between the different algorithms for defining fractures were reported (SMITH-BINDMAN et al. 1991; SAUER et al. 1991; HANSEN et al. 1992; ADAMI et al. 1992). Therefore, despite having developed sophisticated, describable, and objective methods, the application and interpretation of the results have been complicated by the large differences observed from one technique to the next. Unfortunately, no true gold standard for defining fractures exists, by which one can judge the methods or their variable cut-off criteria. However, as a first approximation, there is some rationale for comparing visual assessment and morphometric data on a per vertebra basis in order to develop a consensus interpretation based upon the expertise of experienced radiologists and highly trained research assistants (GENANT et al.

1996). This may help to understand the reasons for concordant and discordant results and to utilize the strengths of the respective methods. When relying solely on quantitative morphometry one has to consider that no real distinction between osteoporotic fractures and other nonfracture deformities can be made. Besides the uncertainties that are introduced by vertebral projection, differences in the applied technique and intra- and interobserver precision of quantitative morphometry, this may have a substantial impact on the prevalence and to a lesser extent on the incidence of vertebral fractures in a population.

When comparing a standardized visual approach with quantitative morphometry substantial differences between both techniques have been reported, while the agreement between different, centrally trained readers for the semiquantitative approach is reportedly very good (GENANT et al. 1993; WU et al. 1995; HANSEN et al. 1992; LEIDIG-BRUCKNER et al. 1994). This applies to the diagnosis of both prevalent and incident fractures. Drawing on the strength of each of the approaches both a quantitative approach as well as a standardized visual approach may be applied in combination to reliably diagnose vertebral fractures in clinical drug trials (GENANT et al. 1996; CUMMINGS et al. 1995; GRADOS et al. 2001).

Since dual X-ray absorptiometry is applied in almost all patients suffering from osteoporosis it has been proposed to use this technique to depict the thoracolumbar spine. Initially this technique has been termed morphometric X-ray analysis or MXA (STEIGER et al. 1993, 1994). Especially the effect of different projections and magnification effects between two films of the spine will be minimized due to the technical specifications of this technique, and radiation dose may be reduced to a minimum allowing for serial assessment of the fracture status. Since its inception improvements in image quality and the application of refined diagnostic approaches have overcome some of the inherent limitations of the technique such as poor image resolution and relatively high noise levels (FERRAR et al. 2001, 2005) (Fig. 6.8). Since its inception vertebral fracture assessment has been adopted by the major manufacturers of DXA devices, and improvements in image acquisition and vertebral fracture detection have been applied. Depending on the manufacturer, the technique has been termed vertebral fracture assessment (VFA), computer aided fracture assessment (CADfx) or dual energy

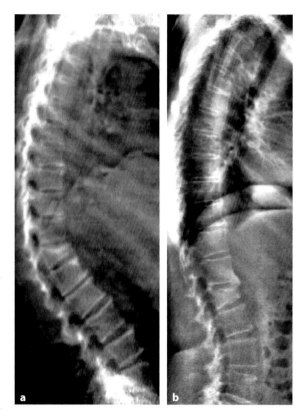

Fig. 6.8a,b. The lateral assessment of vertebral deformities using a dual energy X-ray absorptiometry scanner is termed vertebral fracture assessment (VFA). The resulting image of the spine allows for a morphometric analysis of vertebral deformities as well as an identification of vertebral fractures using a semiquantitative technique

vertebral assessment (DVA). Several quantitative or semiquantitative techniques may be applied to the acquired scans. The restrictions that are inherent to quantitative morphometry also apply to those scans, potentially even more since image quality does not always warrant a thorough diagnostic evaluation of a vertebral deformity. While vertebral fracture detection may be helpful in the serial assessment of vertebral deformities and it is now widely applied, its diagnostic validity still requires thorough evaluation by the experienced technologist and physician (CHAPPARD et al. 1998; FERRAR et al. 2000; REA et al. 2000; GUERMAZI et al. 2002; JACOBS-KOSMIN et al. 2005). Vertebral fracture assessment in its present form is an effective tool to identify moderate and severe vertebral deformities (SCHWARTZ and STEINBERG 2005). Thus, VFA may serve as a valuable tool for the identification of high-risk patients and as a screening tool for clinical trials.

6.2.2.1
Osteopenia and Osteoporosis at Other Skeletal Sites

The axial skeleton is not the only site where characteristic changes of osteopenia and osteoporosis can be depicted radiographically. Changes in the trabecular and cortical bone can also be seen in the appendicular skeleton. It is first apparent at the ends of long and tubular bones due to the predominance of cancellous bone in these regions. Endosteal resorption has a prominent role particularly in senile osteoporosis. The net result of this chronic process is widening of the medullary canal and thinning of the cortices. In late stages of senile osteoporosis, the cortices are paper-thin and the endosteal surfaces are smooth. In rapidly evolving postmenopausal osteoporosis accelerated endosteal and intracortical bone resorption may be seen and can be directly assessed by high-resolution radiographic techniques. Methods to quantitate the changes at the peripheral skeleton have been proposed and also clinically applied (e.g., Singh index, radiogrammetry) (SINGH et al. 1970; BARNETT and NORDIN 1961; MEEMA and MEEMA 1981). Conventional radiography is the basis for a number of recent studies exploring new aspects of assessing bone structure using sophisticated image analysis procedures such as fractal analysis or fast Fourier transforms (BENHAMOU et al. 1994; GERAETS et al. 1998; LINK et al. 1997; LESPESSAILLES et al. 1998). These techniques have also been applied to the study of bone structure using high resolution images acquired with magnetic resonance imaging or computed tomography in a research setting (MAJUMDAR et al. 1998, 1999; MILLARD et al. 1998; LINK et al. 1998; LAIB and RUEGSEGGER 1999; CORTET et al. 1999).

6.2.3
Differential Diagnosis of Reduced Bone Mass

Aside from senile and postmenopausal states there are various other conditions that may be accompanied by generalized osteoporosis. While most of the previously mentioned radiographic characteristics are shared by a variety of conditions, there may be some apparent differences in the appearance of osteoporosis as compared to involutional osteoporosis.

6.2.3.1
Endocrine Disorders Associated with Osteoporosis

Increased serum concentrations of parathyroid hormone in hyperparathyroidism may result from autonomous hypersecretion by a parathyroid adenoma or diffuse hyperplasia of the parathyroid glands (primary hyperparathyroidism). A long sustained hypocalcaemic stimulus may result in hyperplasia of all parathyroid glands and secondary hyperparathyroidism (Fig. 6.9). The cause of hypocalcaemia usually is chronic renal failure or rarely malabsorption states. Patients with long-standing hyperparathyroidism may develop autonomous function and hypercalcaemia (tertiary hyperparathyroidism). While it is the increase in serum parathyroid hormone and calcium that establishes the diagnosis, radiographs document the severity and course of the disease. Hyperparathyroidism leads to both increased bone resorption and bone formation. Changes induced by hyperparathyroidism may affect all bone surfaces resulting in subperiosteal, intracortical, endosteal, subchondral, subepiphyseal, subligamentous, subtendinous and trabecular bone resorption (GENANT et al. 1973, 1974; RICHARDSON et al. 1986).

Subperiosteal bone resorption is the most characteristic radiographic feature of hyperparathyroidism (CAMP and OCHSNER 1931). It is especially prominent in the hand, wrist and foot but may also be seen other sites. Radiographically, the outer margin of the bone becomes indistinct. Scalloping and spiculations of the cortex may occur in later stages.

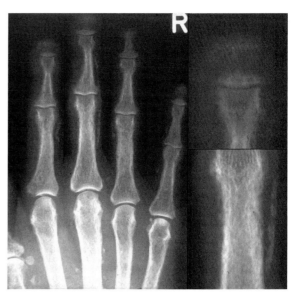

Fig. 6.9. Conventional radiograph of the hand in secondary hyperparathyroidism. The magnification illustrates periosteal bone resorption with indistinct delineation of the outer cortical border. There is also osteolytic appearance of the distal phalanges due to undermineralization of the osseous substance

Undermineralization of the tela ossea leads to the distinctive radiographic appearance of acro-osteolyses (RESNICK and NIWAYAMA 1995). Intracortical resorption results in longitudinally oriented linear striations within the cortex (cortical tunneling), and endosteal bone resorption leads to scalloping of the inner cortex, cortical thinning and widening of the medullary canal (MEEMA and MEEMA 1972). Cortical tunneling is nonspecific and may be seen in other diseases of rapid bone turnover, including hyperthyroidism, reflex sympathetic dystrophy, acute disuse osteoporosis and Paget's disease.

Subchondral bone resorption frequently also affects the joints of the axial skeleton causing undermineralization of the Tela ossea. For example, it may mimic widening of the sacroiliac joint space leading to 'pseudo-widening' of the joint (HAYES and CONWAY 1991). The osseous surface may collapse, and thus may simulate subchondral lesions of inflammatory disease. Osteopenia occurs frequently in hyperparathyroidism and may be observed throughout the skeleton. Other radiographic signs of hyperparathyroidism include focal bone lesions ("brown tumors"), cartilage calcification resulting from the deposition of of calcium pyrophosphate dehydrate crystals (CPPD) and also bone sclerosis (STEINBACH et al. 1961). Increased amounts of trabecular bone leading to bone sclerosis may occur especially in patients with renal osteodystrophy and secondary hyperparathyroidism. Increased bone density may occur preferably in the axial skeleton, sometimes leading to deposition of bone in subchondral areas of the vertebral body resulting in an appearance of radiodense bands across the superior and inferior border and normal or decreased density of the center ("rugger-jersey spine") (RESNICK 1981).

While osteoporosis is defined by a reduction of regularly mineralized osteoid, findings in osteomalacia include an abnormally high amount of non-mineralized osteoid, and a reduction in mineralized bone volume. Thus, radiographic abnormalities in osteomalacia include osteopenia (reduction of mineralized bone), coarsened, indistinct trabeculae and unsharp delineation of cortical bone (excessive apposition of non-mineralized osteoid), deformities, insufficiency fractures and true fractures (bone softening and weakening) (REGINATO et al. 1999). Deformations include bowing and bending of the long bones, and biconcave deformities of the vertebrae (KIENBÖCK 1940). Pseudofractures, or Looser's zones (focal accumulations of osteoid in compact

bone at right angles of the long axis), are diagnostic of osteomalacia and often occur bilateral and symmetrical. There are more than 50 different diseases that may cause osteomalacia of which chronic renal insufficiency, hemodialysis and renal transplantation are the most common causes (PITT 1991; KAINBERGER et al. 1992). Modern patient management has resulted in typical radiographic features of osteomalacia being present in only a minority of these patients (ADAMS 1999). A decrease of vitamin D and reduced responsiveness in chronic renal insufficiency leads to osteomalacia and rickets. The additional secondary hyperparathyroidism leads to a superimposition of radiographic changes from both osteomalacia and secondary hyperparathyroidism (SUNDARAM 1989). This radiographic appearance is termed renal osteodystrophy. A common finding in secondary hyperparathyroidism associated with renal osteodystrophy is the osteosclerosis resulting in typical appearance of the vertebral bodies as seen in the rugger-jersey spine (PITT 1991). Several other radiographic abnormalities may be frequently seen in renal osteodystrophy (Fig. 6.10) including amyloid deposits, destructive spondyloarthropathy, inflammatory changes, and avascular necrosis, soft tissue calcification and arteriosclerosis (KRIEGSHAUSER et al. 1987; MURPHEY et al. 1993).

Hyperthyroidism is a high-turnover disease, and it is associated with an increase in both bone resorption and bone formation (MOSEKILDE et al. 1990). Since bone resorption exceeds bone formation rapid bone loss may occur and result in generalized osteoporosis with the largest effect on cortical bone (GREENSPAN and GREENSPAN 1999). This effect is especially pronounced in patients with thyrotoxicosis, or with a history of thyrotoxicosis (TOH et al. 1985). TSH-suppressive doses of thyroid hormone have been reported to decrease, or have no effect on bone density (NUZZO et al. 1998). Radiological findings of hyperthyroidism-induced osteoporosis are those that are commonly seen in involutional or senile osteoporosis including generalized osteopenia and cortical thinning and tunneling. The fractures associated with this condition affect the spine, the hip, as well as the distal radius (CHEW 1991; SOLOMON et al. 1993).

6.2.3.2
Medication-Induced Osteoporosis

Hypercortisolism is probably the most common cause of medication induced generalized osteoporo-

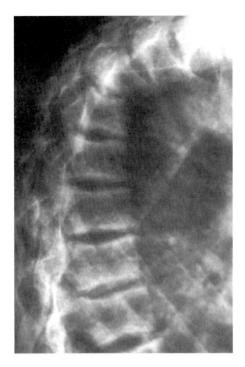

Fig. 6.10. Renal osteodystrophy presenting with increased sclerosis of the vertebral endplates. There is a vertebral fracture in the upper thoracic spine leading to increased kyphosis

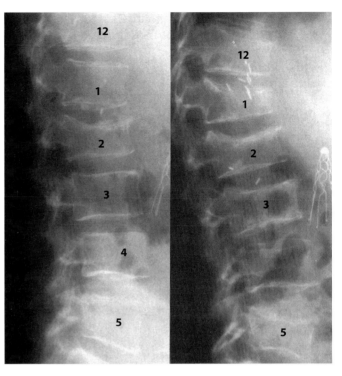

Fig. 6.11. Serial radiographs in heparin-induced osteoporosis. The follow-up radiograph (*right*) reveals newly developed fractures of the 1st, 3rd and 5th lumbar vertebrae

sis while the endogenous form of hypercortisolism, Cushing's disease, is relatively rare (Laan et al. 1993; Saito et al. 1995; Adachi et al. 1993). That is why this form of osteoporosis is listed in this section on medication-induced osteoporosis. Decreased bone formation and increased bone resorption have been observed in hypercortisolism. This has attributed to inhibition of osteoblast formation, either direct stimulation of osteoclast activity or increased secretion of parathyroid hormone. The typical radiographic appearance of steroid-induced osteoporosis comprises generalized osteoporosis, at predominantly trabecular sites, with decreased bone density and fractures of the axial but also of the appendicular skeleton. A characteristic finding in steroid-induced osteoporosis is the marginal condensation of the vertebral bodies resulting from exuberant callus formation. Avascular osteonecrosis is another complication of hypercortisolism, most frequently involving the femoral head, and to a lesser extent the humeral head and the femoral condyles (Heimann and Freiberger 1969; Hurel and Kendall-Taylor 1997). Unlike the avascular osteonecrosis of joints, these bone marrow infarcts are clinically silent and insignificant.

Generalized osteoporosis has been observed in patients receiving high dose heparin therapy (Griffith et al. 1965; Rupp et al. 1982; Nelson-Piercy 1998) (Fig. 6.11). The radiological features of heparin-induced osteoporosis include generalized osteopenia and vertebral compression fractures (Sackler and Liu 1973). The pathomechanism of heparin-induced osteoporosis is not completely clear, and there may be a prolonged effect on bone even after cessation of therapy (Walenga and Bick 1998; Shaughnessy et al. 1999).

6.2.3.3
Other Causes of Generalized Osteoporosis

Other causes of generalized osteoporosis include malnutrition, chronic alcoholism (if associated with malnutrition), smoking and caffein intake, Marfan syndrome and, somewhat infrequently, pregnancy (Seeman et al. 1992; Kohlmeyer et al. 1993; Smith et al. 1985; Hopper and Seeman 1994; Diez et al. 1994). Marrow abnormalities associated with osteoporosis are anemias (sickle cell anemia, thalassemia), plasma cell myeloma, leukemia, Gaucher's disease and glycogen storage disease (Resnick

Fig. 6.12a,b. Multiple myeloma often cannot be distinguished from osteoporosis on conventional radiographs. Magnetic resonance imaging often reveals the bone marrow involvement and makes it possible to distinguish multiple myeloma from osteoporosis. In this patient with multiple myeloma, extensive inhomogeneities ("salt and pepper") of the bone marrow signal can be seen on T1-weighted images suggesting the nature of the disease as well as the extent of bone marrow involvement. There is a fracture of L1

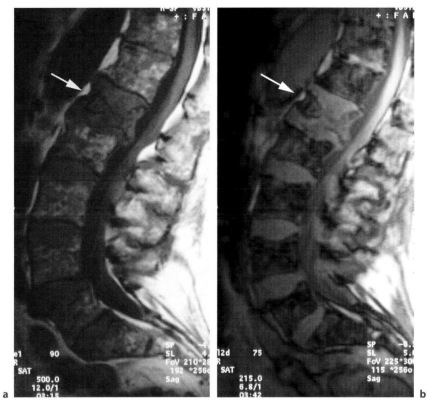

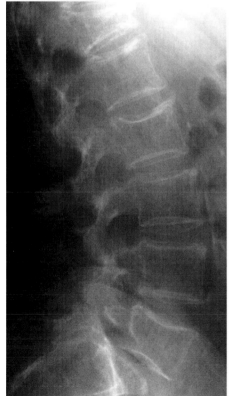

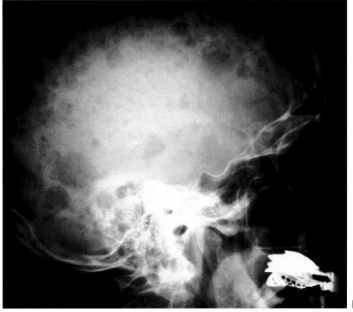

Fig. 6.13a,b. Conventional radiography of the long bones and the skull may reveal extensive lytic lesions in multiple myeloma

1995a,b) (Fig. 6.12, Fig. 6.13). This list is certainly far from being complete but it represents some of the major causes of osteoporosis. Additional imaging techniques such as computed tomography, magnetic resonance tomography and bone scintigraphy, as well as clinical information, may be helpful in the differential diagnosis of the various conditions associated with osteoporosis (Stäbler et al. 1996; Baur et al. 1998; Moulopoulos and Dimopoulos 1997; Lecouvet et al. 1997a,b).

There are some conditions of the juvenile skeleton that result in generalized osteoporosis. Rickets is characterized by inadequate mineralization of the bone matrix, and some of its radiographic appearance may resemble that of osteomalacia (Molpus et al. 1991). Widening of the growth plates, cupping of the metaphysis, and decreased density and irregularities of the metaphyseal margins may be present (Pitt 1995). Epiphyseal ossification centers may show delayed ossification and unsharp borders (Steinbach et al. 1954). Overgrowth of the hyaline cartilage may lead to prominence of costochondral junctions of the ribs (rachitic rosary). The child's age at the onset of the disease determines the pattern of bone deformity, with bowing of the long bone being more pronounced in infancy and early childhood, and vertebral deformities and scoliosis in older children (Rosenberg 1991). Further deformities that may be observed in rickets include pseudofractures, basilar invagination and triradiate configuration of the pelvis.

Idiopathic juvenile osteoporosis is a self-limited disease of childhood with recovery occurring as puberty progresses (Smith 1995). A typical feature of this condition is the increased vulnerability of the metaphyses, often resulting in metaphyseal injuries of the knees and ankles. Idiopathic juvenile osteoporosis must be distinguished from osteogenesis imperfecta, another disease often presenting with radiographic signs of generalized osteoporosis (Smith 1995). The pathogenesis of osteogenesis imperfecta is quantitative or qualitative abnormalities of type I collagen. There are four major types of osteogenesis imperfecta, and the degree of osteoporosis in osteogenesis imperfecta depends strongly on the type of disease (Minch and Kruse 1998). The clinical features of each type usually correspond to the type of mutation. The abnormal maturation of collagen seen in this disorder results in a primary defect in bone matrix. This, combined with a defective mineralization, result in overall loss of bone density involving both the axial and peripheral skeleton. Patients with type III disease have a significantly decreased bone density presenting with generalized osteopenia, thinned cortices, fractures of long bones and ribs, exuberant callus formation and bone deformation (Hanscom et al. 1992). The degree of osteopenia is highly variable, however, and at the mildest end of the spectrum some patients do not have any radiographic signs of osteopenia (Zionts et al. 1995).

6.3
Regional Osteoporosis

Osteoporosis may also be confined to only a segment of the body. This type of osteoporosis is called regional osteoporosis, and it is commonly caused by some disorder of the appendicular skeleton. Osteoporosis due to immobilization or disuse characteristically occurs in the immobilized regions of patients with fractures, motor paralysis due to central nervous system disease or trauma and bone and joint inflammation (Kiratli 1996). Chronic and acute disease may vary in their radiographic appearance somewhat, showing diffuse osteopenia, linear radiolucent bands, speckled radiolucent areas and cortical bone resorption.

Reflex sympathetic dystrophy, sometimes also termed Sudeck's atrophy or algodystrophy, has the radiographic appearance of a high turnover process. It most often occurs in patients with trauma, such as Colles' fracture but also in patients with any neurally related musculoskeletal, neurologic, or vascular condition such as hemiplegia or myocardial infarction (Sudeck 1901; Oyen et al. 1993; Sarangi et al. 1993). This condition is probably related to overactivity of the sympathetic nervous system with increased blood flow and increased intravenous oxygen saturation in the affected extremity (Gellman et al. 1992; Schwartzman and McLellan 1987). Its radiographic appearance includes soft tissue swelling as well as regional osteoporosis showing with bandlike, patchy, or periarticular osteoporosis. Additional radiographic features include subperiosteal bone resorption, intracortical tunneling, endosteal bone resorption with initial excavation and scalloping of the endosteal surface and subsequent remodeling and widening of the medullary canal, as well as subchondral and juxtaarticular erosions (Resnick and Niwayama 1995). Especially in the early stages of reflex sympathetic dystrophy, bone scintigraphy may be helpful to establish the diagnosis (Todorovic Tirnanic et al. 1995; Leitha et al. 1996).

Transient regional osteoporosis includes conditions that have in common the development of self-limited pain and radiographic osteopenia affecting one or several joints, most commonly the hip. Transient osteoporosis typically occurs in middle-aged men and women in the third trimester of pregnancy. At the onset of clinical symptoms, there may be normal radiographic findings, and within several weeks, patients develop variable osteopenia of the hip, sometimes involving the acetabulum. Some patients later develop similar changes in the opposite hip or in other joints, in which case the term regional migratory osteoporosis may be used. The cause of transient regional osteoporosis is not known, and it appears that it may be related to reflex sympathetic dystrophy. In some patients with clinically similar or identical manifestations, magnetic resonance imaging presents with transient regional bone marrow edema (Hayes et al. 1993; Boos et al. 1993). Since not all patients with identical clinical symptoms and transient bone marrow edema develop regional osteoporosis, the sensitivity as to the detection of regional osteoporosis has to be questioned as well as the interrelationship between transient regional osteoporosis and transient bone marrow edema (Palit et al. 2006). There also seems to be a relationship of transient bone marrow edema to ischemic necrosis of bone, and there is a need to define criteria for allowing differentiation of transient bone marrow edema and the edema pattern associated with osteonecrosis (Trepman and King 1992; Froberg et al. 1996; Guerra and Steinberg 1995; Gil et al. 2006).

6.4
Quantifying Bone Mineral in Conventional Radiography

6.4.1
Standardized Evaluation of Conventional Radiographs

The lack of methods to objectively assess bone density in the past made some researchers use the characteristic radiographic appearance of bone in

osteoporosis to grade or classify osteoporosis, e.g., Saville's score (Saville 1967). Doyle and coworkers (1967) studied radiological criteria of osteoporosis and found, with the exception of biconcavity, none of the other criteria to be valid criteria for the diagnosis of osteoporosis. For follow-up even increased biconcavity was not a useful criterion. 'Can Radiologists Detect Osteopenia on Plain Radiographs?' Garton and colleagues (1994) asked and concluded that even though the reproducibility of Saville's score was only moderate, bone density was significantly correlated with this score. Potentially, aside from single criteria, the radiographic impression of the spine as a whole may hint to a reduced bone density (Ahmed et al. 1998). Therefore, and because it is essential for differential diagnosis of osteoporosis and for the diagnosis and follow-up of vertebral deformities, conventional radiography will remain an important asset to the diagnosis of osteoporosis.

In an attempt to quantitate the degree of osteoporosis, Barnett and Nordin (1960, 1961), and in a similar form Dent and colleagues (1953), proposed that the increased biconcavity of a vertebra could be used to diagnose and follow osteoporosis. The quotient of middle and anterior vertebral height today is associated with the names of Barnett and Nordin. However, the authors only used one vertebra to calculate their score (usually L3) which may not represent the bone mineral status of the whole spine (Jergas et al. 1994). Furthermore, following the course of osteoporosis using only one vertebra may also be regarded as problematic.

Urist (1960) reported that in women with hip fracture the principal compressive trabeculae in the proximal femur become more prominent while other groups of trabeculae are resorbed. Based on this observation in women with advanced osteoporosis Singh et al. (1970) proposed a femoral index for the diagnosis of osteoporosis based on the assumption that the trabeculae in the proximal femur disappear in a predictable sequence depending on their original thickness (Fig. 6.14). The authors considered that the thickness and spacing of trabeculae in the various trajectorial groups (principal compressive, secondary compressive, greater trochanter, principal tensile, and secondary tensile group) depend on the intensity of stresses normally carried by these trabeculae. With advancing bone loss trabeculae that are thinner become invisible first on the radiograph. Singh and coworkers (1970) introduced a classification rang-

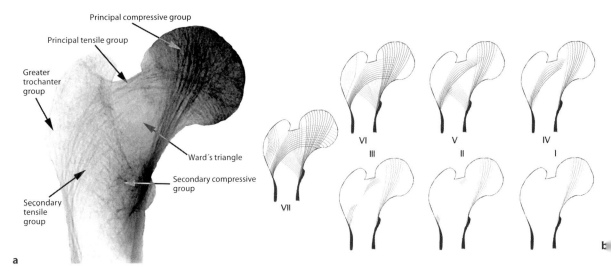

Fig. 6.14a,b. The Singh index is based on the assumption that the trabeculae in the proximal femur (**a**) disappear in a predictable sequence depending on their original thickness. The classification ranges from grade VII (normal, all trabecular groups visible) to grade I (marked reduction of even the principal compressive trabeculae) according to the degree of bone loss (**b**)

ing from grade VI (normal, all trabecular groups visible) to grade I (marked reduction of even the principal compressive trabeculae) according to the degree of bone loss. Singh et al. (1972) later added a grade VII to their scale for individuals with dense bone, meaning that the Ward's triangle (an area on radiographs of the proximal femur enclosed by the principle and secondary compressive, and the tensile groups) contained trabeculae that were as dense as the other surrounding trabeculae. The authors reported a relatively good discrimination of individuals with and without vertebral fractures. Interobserver variation for the Singh index is highly variable being influenced strongly by the quality of the radiographs, the degree of osteoporosis (moderate changes being harder to agree on than on the extremes), and the experience of the observer. Right-left comparisons of the Singh index show a concordance on the order of 80%. The Singh index has been applied in a number of studies in which varying results in the relationship to bone mass and vertebral appearance have been shown (Griffiths and Virtama 1990; Peacock et al. 1995; Koot et al. 1996). More recent observations indicate that the underlying assumption of the Singh index, the organized sequential loss of trabeculae, may be false and a generalized loss of bone mineral in both the tensile and compressive occurs. A similar grading scheme for estimating bone loss exists for the calcaneus (Jhamaria et al. 1983).

6.4.2
Radiogrammetry

Radiogrammetry, a simple measurement of cortical thickness in virtually any tubular bone, is easy to perform with a caliper or with a graduated magnifying glass. Simple cortical measurements may be represented in several ways (Fig. 6.15): One method involves summing the thickness of both cortices as an index of bone mass; another method uses the combined cortical thickness divided by the total bone width as a measure of density; finally, a circular cross-section of bone can be assumed with the measurements of bone width and cortical thickness converted to cortical areas that more closely parallel actual physical mass. Radiogrammetry is applied most often to the metacarpal bones (Kalla et al. 1989). The use of a caliper, the combination of a number of metacarpals or repeated measurements of one metacarpal and the use of digitization techniques or automated edge detection on digitally acquired radiographs may improve the precision error (Horsman and Simpson 1975; Bloom et al. 1983; Rico and Hernandez 1989). Variations in soft tissue thickness and in radiographic geometry cause systematic errors. As a consequence of these inaccuracies and the imprecision of the measurements, the values for compact bone area derived from radiogrammetry at different skeletal locations are correlated only moderately. The correlation between right-

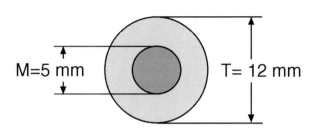

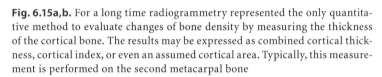

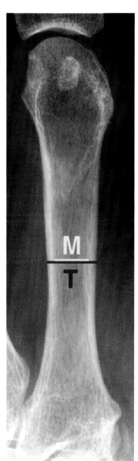

a

Combined Cortical Thickness (CCT)   T-M
Cortical Index   (T-M)/T
Cortical Area $0.785 * (T^2-M^2)$

Fig. 6.15a,b. For a long time radiogrammetry represented the only quantitative method to evaluate changes of bone density by measuring the thickness of the cortical bone. The results may be expressed as combined cortical thickness, cortical index, or even an assumed cortical area. Typically, this measurement is performed on the second metacarpal bone

b

and left-sided bones is higher (HELELA and VIRTAMA 1970; BLOOM 1980; PLATO and PURIFOY 1982). While MEEMA and MEINDOK (1992) reported a good correlation between radiogrammetric measurements and dual photon absorptiometry of the spine, other studies suggest only a poor to moderate correlation with other methods of bone mineral measurements (GUESENS et al. 1986; ROSENTHAL et al. 1987).

Simple cortical measurements, particularly when obtained at several anatomic sites, provide information that is more useful in clinical research than in individual patient management. For example, extensive data on metacarpal changes in populations show a loss with aging in men and women (GEUSENS et al. 1986; DEQUEKER 1976; EVANS et al. 1978; GARN et al. 1967; FALCH and SANDVIK 1990; MAGGIO et al. 1997). Studies of patients with primary hyperparathyroidism, rheumatoid arthritis and systemic lupus erythematosus have revealed substantial reductions of the combined cortical thickness compared to normal controls (GENANT et al. 1973; KALLA et al.

1992). MEEMA (1991) and MEEMA and MEEMA (1987) found radiogrammetry to be a good discriminator between postmenopausal women with and without vertebral fractures. While the aforementioned studies all used radiogrammetry on plain films, CRESPO and colleagues (1998) reported on the use of computed tomography for the determination of cortical area. The authors found that cortical bone loss was associated with prevalent Colles' fractures in postmenopausal women.

A variation of radiogrammetry was introduced a few years ago and is called digital X-ray radiogrammetry, or DXR. In this technique a radiogram of the hand or forearm is scanned with a commercial high-resolution scanner, and the digital image of the forearm is analyzed using various regions of interest in three metacarpals II to IV. A BMD equivalent DXR bone density is calculated from cortical thickness of these bones and image procession algorithms are applied to calculate additional parameters, striation and porosity (MALICH et al. 2004). Initial results showed the method provided adequate precision as well as a good association with age and with the history of fracture (JORGENSEN et al. 2000; TOLEDO and JERGAS 2006). In the context of the large epidemiological 'Study of Osteoporotic Fractures' digital radiogrammetry proved to be predictive of incident fractures of the wrist, hip and spine (BOUXSEIN et al. 2002).

One major limitation of radiogrammetry is its failure to measure intracortical resorption or porosity and irregular endosteal scalloping or erosion. As intracortical and trabecular bone resorptions are important indicators of high bone turnover states, the fact that they are not measured by this technique is significant. Despite its shortcomings when applied to individual patients, radiogrammetry remains an important research tool, especially for studying changes in cortical bone (VAN RIJN et al. 2004, 2006; GOERRES et al. 2007; BOTTCHER et al. 2005).

6.4.3
Photodensitometry or
Radiographic Absorptiometry (RA)

It has been known for many years that the photographic density on a film is roughly proportional to the mass of bone located in the X-ray beam. A relatively large change in bone mineral content (25%–50%) must occur, however, before it can be detected with visual observation of radiographs (LACHMANN and WHELAN 1936; VIRTAMA 1960). Some investigator proposed to include a standard bone on an the X-ray of the hand, or even with a spine radiograph (STEVEN 1947; NORDIN et al. 1962). In an effort to quantitate bone mass, a number of investigators have measured the optical density of bone contained in radiographs, in which both the anatomic part to be studied and a reference wedge are included in the exposure area (HODGE et al. 1935; STEIN 1937; MACK et al. 1939; COSMAN et al. 1991; TROUERBACH et al. 1987) (Fig. 6.16). The simultaneous exposure of a reference system (usually a wedge or step wedge consisting of aluminum or hydroxyapatite) allows for a reproducible determination of bone density with an appropriate exposure technique. Following film processing, bone and reference wedge are evaluated using a photo densitometer. In its long history, many names have been assigned to this technique like radiographic photodensitometry, radiographic absorptiometry, quantitative Röntgen microdensitometry, and even digital image processing. They

are all basically the same technique using more or less sophisticated approaches.

Photodensitometry is a low dose and low cost technique, which measures integral bone (trabecular and cortical). Moreover, photodensitometry is easy to perform. Multiple technical problems arise, however, such as nonuniformity of X-ray intensity beam hardening due to the polychromatic radiation source, and variation in film sensitivity related to processing. Photodensitometry is limited to the peripheral skeleton because of soft tissue inhomogeneities. Various measurement sites in the upper and lower extremities are reported in the literature. Metacarpal or phalangeal bones are preferred sites. HEUCK and SCHMIDT (1960) reported an accuracy of 5%–10% for photodensitometry of the femoral neck and the calcaneus. Some results using more advanced photodensitometric techniques suggest that precision on the order of 1%–3.5% for photodensitometry of the phalangeal or metacarpal bones is possible (TROUERBACH et al. 1987; HAYASHI et al. 1990; MEEMA and MEEMA 1969).

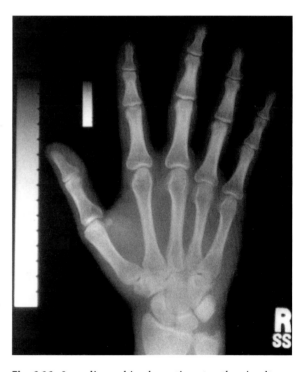

Fig. 6.16. In radiographic absorptiometry the simultaneous exposure of a reference system (usually a wedge or step wedge consisting of aluminum or hydroxyapatite) enables the reproducible determination of bone density with an appropriate exposure technique. By comparing the attenuation values of the reference with known density values one determines corresponding density of a region of interest in the bone

Hagiwara et al. (1993) found the correlation coefficient between photodensitometry of the metacarpal bones and their ash density to be r = 0.95 (CV% = 3.4%). Results derived from photodensitometry of the hand compared significantly with other bone density measurements in vivo. Moderate correlation coefficients between spinal BMD using a dual photon absorptiometry technique and photodensitometry of the hand were reported. The correlation with other measurement sites was found to be in the same order (Cosman et al. 1991).

The early investigations of Meema and Meema (1976) showed that, at all ages, women have less cortical bone than men and that age-related bone loss starts earlier, proceeds more rapidly, and results in a much greater depletion of the skeleton in women than in men (Trouerbach et al. 1987, 1993). Several investigators have studied the association between BMD of the phalanges assessed by radiographic absorptiometry and fracture risk in cross-sectional studies. Here the significant relationship with prevalent vertebral fractures could be confirmed (Ross et al. 1995; Takada et al. 1997; Hagiwara et al. 1998; Versluis et al. 2000). Mussolino et al. (1997) examined the relationship between phalangeal bone density in women and future hip fracture risk using prospective fracture data with a maximum follow-up of 16 years from the NHANES I study. They found a significant association between phalangeal bone density at baseline and future hip fractures with an age-adjusted relative risk of approximately 1.8 per 1 standard deviation decrease in bone mass. These results for the female study cohort could also be confirmed in the male NHANES study cohort (Mussolino et al. 1998). However, in a cross-sectional study Ekman and colleagues (2001) found that neither quantitative ultrasound nor densitometry of the phalanges could discriminate between women with and without hip fracture. As a plus, cost effectiveness, ease of use and its theoretically ubiquitous availability make this technique an interesting option for the assessment of bone mass. Nevertheless, the value of peripheral measurements for the diagnosis of osteoporosis and the prediction of the significant hip fractures and vertebral fractures have to be studied further.

Even some of the methods used to study bone density at the axial skeleton are derived from radiographic absorptiometry. Classic photodensitometry cannot be applied to the axial skeleton due to the greater amount and inhomogeneity of the surrounding soft tissue. Krokowski and Schlungbaum already reported on a photodensitometric method for determining the bone mineral content at the lumbar spine in 1959. The authors used two lateral radiographs of the lumbar spine taken at two distinct energies (62 and 250 kV) to calculated bone density in a region of interest (Krokowski and Schlungbaum 1959). This method described the basic principles of what was to become the most widespread technique to assess bone density at the axial skeleton, dual photon or X-ray absorptiometry (DPA, DXA).

References

Adachi JD, Bensen WG, Hodsman AB (1993) Corticosteroid-induced osteoporosis. Semin Arthr Rheum 22:375–384

Adami S, Gatti D, Rossini M, Adamoli A, James G, Girardello S, Zamberlan N (1992) The radiological assessment of vertebral osteoporosis. Bone 13[Suppl]:S33–S6

Adams JE (1999) Renal bone disease: radiological investigation. Kidney Int Suppl 73:S38–S41

Ahmed AIH, Ilic D, Blake GM, Rymer JM, Fogelman I (1998) Review of 3530 referrals for bone density measurements of spine and femur: evidence that radiographic osteopenia predicts low bone mass. Radiology 207:619–624

Albright F(1947) Osteoporosis. Annals of internal medicine. 27:861–882

Albright F, Smith PH, Richardson AM (1941) Postmenopausal osteoporosis. Its clinical features. JAMA 116:2465–2474

Ballock RT, Mackersie R, Abitbol JJ, Cervilla V, Resnick D, Garfin SR (1992) Can burst fractures be predicted from plain radiographs? J Bone Joint Surg [Br] 74:147–150

Barnett E, Nordin BEC (1960) The radiological diagnosis of osteoporosis: a new approach. Clin Radiol 11:166–174

Barnett E, Nordin BEC (1961) Radiological assessment of bone density. I. The clinical and radiological problem of thin bones. Br J Radiol 34:683–692

Baur A, Stäbler A, Steinborn M, Schnarkowski P, Pistitsch C, Lamerz R, Bartl R, Reiser M (1998) Magnetresonanztomographie beim Plasmozytom: Wertigkeit verschiedener Sequenzen bei diffuser und lokaler Infiltrationsform. RöFo Fortschr Röntgenstr 168:323–329

Benhamou CL, Lespessailles E, Jacquet G, Harba R, Jennane R, Loussot T, Tourliere D, Ohley W (1994) Fractal organization of trabecular bone images on calcaneus radiographs. J Bone Miner Res 9:1909–1918

Black DM, Cummings SR, Stone K, Hudes E, Palermo L, Steiger P (1991) A new approach to defining normal vertebral dimensions. J Bone Miner Res 6:883–892

Bloom RA (1980) A comparative estimation of the combined cortical thickness of various bone sites. Skeletal Radiol 5:167–170

Bloom RA, Pogrund H, Libson E (1983) Radiogrammetry of the metacarpal: a critical reappraisal. Skeletal Radiol 10:5–9

Boos S, Sigmund G, Huhle P, Nurbakhsch I (1993) Magnetresonanztomographie der sogenannten transitorischen Osteoporose. Primärdiagnostik und Verlaufskontrolle nach Therapie. Röfo Fortschr Geb Rontgenstr Neuen Bildgeb Verfahr 158:201–206

Böttcher J, Pfeil A, Rosholm A, Petrovitch A, Seidl BE, Malich A, Schäfer ML, Kramer A, Mentzel HJ, Lehmann G, Hein G, Kaiser WA (2005) Digital X-ray radiogrammetry combined with semiautomated analysis of joint space widths as a new diagnostic approach in rheumatoid arthritis: a cross-sectional and longitudinal study. Arthritis Rheum 52:3850–3859

Bouxsein ML, Palermo L, Yeung C, Black DM (2002) Digital X-ray radiogrammetry predicts hip, wrist and vertebral fracture risk in elderly women: a prospective analysis from the study of osteoporotic fractures. Osteoporos Int 13:358–365

Camp JD, Ochsner HC (1931) The osseous changes in hyperparathyroidism associated with parathyroid tumor: a roentgenologic study. Radiology 17:63

Campbell SE, Phillips CD, Dubovsky E, Cail WS, Omary RA (1995) The value of CT in determining potential instability of simple wedge-compression fractures of the lumbar spine. AJNR Am J Neuroradiol 16:1385–1392

Chappard C, Kolta S, Fechtenbaum J, Dougados M, Roux C (1998) Clinical evaluation of spine morphometric X-ray absorptiometry. Br J Rheumatol 37:496–501

Chew FS (1991) Radiologic manifestations in the musculoskeletal system of miscellaneous endocrine disorders. Radiol Clin North Am 29:135–147

Cortet B, Dubois P, Boutry N, Bourel P, Cotten A, Marchandise X (1999) Image analysis of the distal radius trabecular network using computed tomography. Osteoporos Int 9:410–419

Cosman F, Herrington B, Himmelstein S, Lindsay R (1991) Radiographic absorptiometry: a simple method for determination of bone mass. Osteoporosis Int 2:34–38

Crespo R, Revilla M, Usabiago J, Crespo E, Garcia-Arino J, Villa LF, Rico H (1998) Metacarpal radiogrammetry by computed radiography in postmenopausal women with Colles' fracture and vertebral crush fracture syndrome. Calcif Tissue Int 62:470–473

Cummings SR, Melton III LJ, Felsenberg D (1995) National Osteoporosis Foundation Working Group on Vertebral Fracture. Report: Assessing vertebral fractures. J Bone Miner Res 10:518–523

Davies KM, Recker RR, Heaney RP (1993) Revisable criteria for vertebral deformity. Osteoporosis Int 3:265–270

Delmas PD, Genant HK, Adams JE (2005) Vertebral fracture initiative. [cited 2007; Available from: http://www.iof-bonehealth.org/vfi/index-flash.html

Dent RV, Milne MD, Roussak NJ, Steiner G (1953) Abdominal topography in relation to senile osteoporosis of the spine. Br Med J 2:1082–1084

Dequeker J (1976) Quantitative radiology: radiogrammetry of cortical bone. Br J Radiol 49:912–920

Deyo RA, McNiesh LM, Cone III RO (1985) Observer variability in the interpretation of lumbar spine radiographs. Arthritis Rheum 28:1066–1070

Diez A, Puig J, Serrano S, Marinoso M-L, Bosch J, Marrugat J (1994) Alcohol-induced bone disease in the absence of severe chronic liver damage. J Bone Miner Res 9:825–831

Doyle FH, Gutteridge DH, Joplin GF, Fraser R (1967) An assessment of radiological criteria used in the study of spinal osteoporosis. Brit J Radiol 40:241–250

Eastell R, Cedel SL, Wahner HW, Riggs BL, Melton LJ III (1991) Classification of vertebral fractures. J Bone Miner Res 6:207–215

Ekman A, Michaelsson K, Petren-Mallmin M, Ljunghall S, Mallmin H (2001) DXA of the hip and heel ultrasound but not densitometry of the fingers can discriminate female hip fracture patients from controls: a comparison between four different methods. Osteoporos Int 12:185–191

Evans RA, MdDonnell GD, Schieb M (1978) Metacarpal cortical area as an index of bone mass. Br J Radiol 51:428–431

Evans SF, Nicholson PHF, Haddaway MJ, Davie MWJ (1993) Vertebral morphometry in women aged 50–81 years. Bone Mineral 21:29–40

Falch JA, Sandvik L (1990) Perimenopausal appendicular bone loss: a 10-year prospective study. Bone 11:425–428

Ferrar L, Jiang G, Barrington NA, Eastell R (2000) Identification of vertebral deformities in women: comparison of radiological assessment and quantitative morphometry using morphometric radiography and morphometric X-ray absorptiometry. J Bone Miner Res 15:575–585

Ferrar L, Jiang G, Eastell R (2001) Short-term precision for morphometric X-ray absorptiometry. Osteoporos Int 12:710–715

Ferrar L, Jiang G, Adams J, Eastell R (2005) Identification of vertebral fractures: an update. Osteoporos Int 16:717–728

Fletcher H (1947) Anterior vertebral wedging – frequency and significance. AJR Am J Roentgenol 57:232–238

Froberg PK, Braunstein EM, Buckwalter KA (1996) Osteonecrosis, transient osteoporosis, and transient bone marrow edema: current concepts. Radiol Clin North Am 34:273–291

Frost HM (1964) Dynamics of bone remodelling. In: Frost HM (ed) Bone biodynamics. Little Brown, Boston, pp 315–334

Gallagher JC (1990) The pathogenesis of osteoporosis. Bone Miner 9:215–227

Garn SM, Rohmann CG, Wagner B (1967) Bone loss as a general phenomenon of man. Fed Proc 26:1729–1736

Garton MJ, Robertson EM, Gilbert FJ, Gomersall L, Reid DM (1994) Can radiologists detect osteopenia on plain radiographs? Clin Radiol 49:118–122

Gellman H, Keenan MA, Stone L, Hardy SE, Waters RL, Stewart C (1992) Reflex sympathetic dystrophy in brain-injured patients. Pain 51:307–311

Genant HK, Heck LL, Lanzl LH, Rossmann K, Vander Horst J, Paloyan E (1973) Primary hyperparathyroidism. A comprehensive study of clinical, biochemical and radiographic manifestations. Radiology 109:513–519

Genant HK, Vander Horst J, Lanzl LH, Mall JC, Doi K (1974) Skeletal demineralization in primary hyperparathyroidism. In: Mazess RB (ed) Proceedings of international conference on bone mineral measurement. National Institute of Arthritis, Metabolism and Digestive Diseases, Washington, DC, p 177

Genant HK, Doi K, Mall JC, Sickles EA (1977) Direct radiographic magnification for skeletal radiology. Radiology 123:47–55

Genant HK (1990) Radiographic assessment of the effects of intermittent cyclical treatment with etidronate. In:

Christiansen C, Overgaard K (eds) Third International Conference on Osteoporosis, Osteopress ApS, Copenhagen, p 2047–2054

Genant HK, Wu CY, van Kuijk C, Nevitt M (1993) Vertebral fracture assessment using a semi-quantitative technique. J Bone Miner Res 8:1137–1148

Genant HK, Jergas M, van Kuijk C (1995) Vertebral fracture in osteoporosis. Radiology Research and Education Foundation, San Francisco

Genant HK, Jergas M, Palermo L, Nevitt M, San Valentin R, Black D, Cummings SR (1996) Comparison of semiquantitative visual and quantitative morphometric assessment of prevalent and incident vertebral fractures in osteoporosis. J Bone Miner Res 11:984–996

Geraets W, Van der Stelt P, Lips P, Van Ginkel F (1998) The radiographic trabecular pattern of hips in patients with hip fractures and in elderly control subjects. Bone 22:165–173

Geusens P, Dequeker J, Verstraeten A, Nijs J (1986) Age-, sex-, and menopause-related changes of vertebral and peripheral bone: population study using dual and single photon absorptiometry and radiogrammetry. J Nucl Med 27:1540–1549

Gil HC, Levine SM, Zoga AC (2006) MRI findings in the subchondral bone marrow: a discussion of conditions including transient osteoporosis, transient bone marrow edema syndrome, SONK, and shifting bone marrow edema of the knee. Semin Musculoskelet Radiol 10:177–186

Goerres GW, Frey D, Hany TF, Seifert B, Hauselmann HJ, Studer A, Hauser D, Zilic N, Michel BA, Hans D, Uebelhart D (2007) Digital X-ray radiogrammetry better identifies osteoarthritis patients with a low bone mineral density than quantitative ultrasound. Eur Radiol 17:965–974

Grados F, Roux C, de Vernejoul MC, Utard G, Sebert JL, Fardellone P (2001) Comparison of four morphometric definitions and a semiquantitative consensus reading for assessing prevalent vertebral fractures. Osteoporos Int 12:716–722

Greenspan SL, Greenspan FS (1999) The effect of thyroid hormone on skeletal integrity. Ann Intern Med 130:750–758

Griffith GC, Nichols G, Ashey JD, Flannagan B (1965) Heparin osteoporosis. JAMA 193:85–88

Griffiths HJ, Virtama P (1990) Cortical thickness and trabecular pattern of the femoral neck as a measure of osteopenia. Invest Radiol 25:1116–1119

Guermazi A, Mohr A, Grigorian M, Taouli B, Genant HK (2002) Identification of vertebral fractures in osteoporosis. Semin Musculoskelet Radiol 6:241–252

Guerra JJ, Steinberg ME (1995) Distinguishing transient osteoporosis from avascular necrosis of the hip. J Bone Joint Surg 77:616–624

Hagiwara S, Yang S-O, Dhillon MS et al (1993) Precision and accuracy of photodensitometry of metacarpal bone (digital image processing). J Bone Miner Res 8[Suppl 1]:S 346

Hagiwara S, Engelke K, Takada M, Yang SO, Grampp S, Dhillon MS, Genant HK (1998) Accuracy and diagnostic sensitivity of radiographic absorptiometry of the second metacarpal. Calcif Tissue Int 62:95–98

Hanscom DA, Winter RB, Lutter L, Lonstein JE, Bloom BA, Bradford DS (1992) Osteogenesis imperfecta. Radiographic classification, natural history, and treatment of spinal deformities. J Bone Joint Surgery 74:598–616

Hansen M, Overgaard K, Nielsen V, Jensen G, Gotfredsen A, Christiansen C (1992) No secular increase in the prevalence of vertebral fractures due to postmenopausal osteoporosis. Osteoporosis Int 2:241–246

Hayashi Y, Yamamoto K, Fukunaga M, Ishibashi T, Takahashi K, Nishii Y (1990) Assessment of bone mass by image analysis of metacarpal bone roentgenograms: a quantitative digital image processing (DIP) method. Radiation medicine 8:173–178

Hayes CW, Conway WF (1991) Hyperparathyroidism. Radiol Clin North Am. 29:85–96

Hayes CW, Conway WF, Daniel WW (1993) MR imaging of bone marrow edema pattern: transient osteoporosis, transient bone marrow edema syndrome, or osteonecrosis. Radiographics 13:1001–1011

Hedlund LR, Gallagher JC (1988) Vertebral morphometry in diagnosis of spinal fractures. Bone Mineral 5:59–67

Heimann WG, Freiberger RH (1969) Avascular necrosis of the femoral and humeral heads after high-dosage corticosteroid therapy. N Engl J Med 263:672–674

Helela T, Virtama P (1970) Cortical thickness of long bones in different age groups. Symposium ossium. Livingstone, London, pp 238–240

Heuck F, Schmidt E (1960) Die quantitative Bestimmung des Mineralgehaltes des Knochens aus dem Röntgenbild. Fortschr Röntgenstr 93:523–554

Hodge HC, Bale WF, Warren SL, van Huysen G (1935) Factors influencing the quantitative measurement of the roentgen-ray absorption of tooth slabs. Am J Roentgenol 34:817–838

Hopper JL, Seeman E (1994) The bone density of twins discordant for tobacco use. N Engl J Med 330:387–392

Horsman A, Simpson M (1975) The measurement of sequential changes in cortical bone geometry. Br J Radiol 48:471–476

Hurel SJ, Kendall-Taylor P (1997) Avascular necrosis secondary to postoperative steroid therapy. Br J Neurosurg 11:356–358

Hurxthal L (1968) Measurement of anterior vertebral compressions and biconcave vertebrae. AJR Am J Roentgenol 103:635–644

Jacobs-Kosmin D, Sandorfi N, Murray H, Abruzzo JL (2005) Vertebral deformities identified by vertebral fracture assessment: associations with clinical characteristics and bone mineral density. J Clin Densitom 8:267–272

Jensen GF, McNair P, Boesen J, Hegedüs V (1984) Validity in diagnosing osteoporosis. Europ J Radiol 4:1–3

Jensen KK, Tougaard L (1981) A simple X-ray method for monitoring progress of osteoporosis. Lancet 2:19–20

Jergas M, San Valentin R (1995) Techniques for the assessment of vertebral dimensions in quantitative morphometry. In: Genant HK, Jergas M, van Kuijk C (eds) Vertebral fracture in osteoporosis. Radiology Research and Education Foundation, San Francisco, pp 163–88

Jergas M, Uffmann M, Escher H, Schaffstein J, Nitzschke E, Köster O (1994a) Visuelle Beurteilung konventioneller Röntgenaufnahmen und duale Röntgenabsorptiometrie in der Diagnostik der Osteoporose. Z Orthop Grenzgeb 132:91–98

Jergas M, Uffmann M, Escher H, Glüer CC, Young KC, Grampp S, Köster O, Genant HK (1994b) Interobserver variation in the detection of osteopenia by radiography and comparison with dual X-ray absorptiometry (DXA) of the lumbar spinc. Skclctal Radiol 23:195–199

Jhamaria NL, Lal KB, Udawat M, Banerji P, Kabra SG (1983) The trabecular pattern of the calcaneum as an index of osteoporosis. J Bone Joint Surg 65-B:195–198

Jorgensen JT, Andersen PB, Rosholm A, Bjarnason NH (2000) Digital X-ray radiogrammetry: a new appendicular bone densitometric method with high precision. Clin Physiol 20:330–335

Kainberger F, Traindl O, Baldt M, Helbich T, Breitenseher M, Seidl G, Kovarik J (1992) Renale Osteodytrophie: Spektrum der Röntgensymptomatik bei modernen Formen der Nierentransplantation und Dauerdialysetherapie. Fortschr Röntgenstr 157:501–505

Kalidis L, Felsenberg D, Kalender W, Eidloth H, Wieland E (1992) Morphometric analysis of digitized radiographs: description of automatic evaluation. In: Ring EFG (ed) Current research in osteoporosis and bone mineral measurement II: 1992. British Institute of Radiology, Bath, pp 14–16

Kalla AA, Meyers OL, Parkyn ND, Kotze TJvW (1989) Osteoporosis screening – radiogrammetry revisited. Br J Rheumatol 28:511–517

Kalla AA, Kotze TJvW, Meyers OL (1992) Metacarpal bone mass in systemic lupus erythematotus. Clin Rheumatol 11:475–482

Kienböck R (1940) Osteomalazie, Osteoporose, Osteopsathyrose, porotische Kyphose. Fortschr Röntgenstr 61:159

Kiratli BJ (1996) Immobilization osteopenia. In: Marcus R, Feldman D, Kelsey J (eds) Osteoporosis. Academic Press, San Diego, pp 833–853

Kleerekoper M, Parfitt AM, Ellis BI (1984) Measurement of vertebral fracture rates in osteoporosis. In: Christiansen C, Arnaud CD, Nordin BEC, Parfitt AM, Peck WA, Riggs BL (eds) Copenhagen International Symposium on Osteoporosis June 3–8, 1984; Department of Clinical Chemistry, Glostrup Hospital, Copenhagen, p 103–108

Kleerekoper M, Nelson DA, Peterson EL, Tilley BC (1992) Outcome variables in osteoporosis trials. Bone 13:S29–S34

Kohlmeyer L, Gasner C, Marcus R (1993) Bone mineral status of women with Marfan syndrome. Am J Med 95:568–572

Koot VC, Kesselaer SM, Clevers GJ, de Hooge P, Weits T, van der Werken C (1996) Evaluation of the Singh index for measuring osteoporosis. J Bone Joint Surg Br 78:831–834

Kotowicz MA, Melton III LJ, Cooper C, Atkinson EJ, O'Fallon WM, Riggs LB (1994) Risk of hip fracture in women with vertebral fracture. J Bone Miner Res 9:599–605

Kriegshauser JS, Swee RG, McCarthy JT, Hauser MF (1987) Aluminum toxicity in patients undergoing dialysis: radiographic findings and prediction of bone biopsy results. Radiology 164:399–403

Krokowski E, Schlungbaum W (1959) Die Objektivierung der röntgenologischen Diagnose "Osteoporose". Fortschr Röntgenstr 91:740–746

Laan RF, Buijs WC, van Erning LJ, Lemmens JA, Corstens FH, Ruijs SH, van de Putte LB, van Riel PL (1993) Differential effects of glucocorticoids on cortical appendicular and cortical vertebral bone mineral content. Calcif Tissue Int 52:5–9

Lachmann E, Whelan M (1936) The roentgen diagnosis of osteoporosis and its limitations. Radiology 26:165–177

Laib A, Ruegsegger P (1999) Comparison of structure extraction methods for in vivo trabecular bone measurements. Comput Med Imaging Graph 23:69–74

Lecouvet F, Vande Berg B, Maldague B, Michaux L, Laterre E, Michaux J, Ferrant A, Malghem J (1997a) Vertebral compression fractures in multiple myeloma. Part I. Distribution and appearance at MR imaging. Radiology 204:195–199

Lecouvet F, Malghem J, Michaux L, Michaux J, Lehmann F, Maldague B, Jamart J, Ferrant A, Vande Berg B (1997b) Vertebral compression fractures in multiple myeloma. Part II. Assessment of fracture risk with MR imaging of spinal bone marrow. Radiology 204:201–205

LeGeros RZ (1994) Biological and synthetic apatites. In: Brown PW, Constantz B (eds) Hydroxyapatite and related materials. CRC Press, Boca Raton, pp 3–28

Leidig-Bruckner G, Genant HK, Minne HW, Storm T, Thamsborg G, Bruckner T, Sauer P, Schilling T, Soerensen OH, Ziegler R (1994) Comparison of a semiquantitative and a quantitative method for assessing vertebral fractures in osteoporosis. Osteoporosis Int 4:154–161

Leitha T, Staudenherz A, Korpan M, Fialka V (1996) Pattern recognition in five-phase bone scintigraphy: diagnostic patterns of reflex sympathetic dystrophy in adults. Eur J Nucl Med 23:256–262

Lenchik L, Rogers LF, Delmas PD, Genant HK (2004) Diagnosis of osteoporotic vertebral fractures: importance of recognition and description by radiologists. AJR Am J Roentgenol 183:949–958

Lespessailles E, Roux JP, Benhamou CL, Arlot ME, Eynard E, Harba R, Padonou C, Meunier P (1998) Fractal analysis of bone texture on os calcis radiographs compared with trabecular microarchitecture analyzed by histomorphometry. Calcif Tissue Int 63:121–125

Link T, Majumdar S, Konermann W, Meier N, Lin J, Newitt D, Ouyang X, Peters PE, Genant HK (1997) Texture analysis of direct magnification radiographs of vertebral specimens: correlation with bone mineral density and biomechanical properties. Acad Radiol 4:167–176

Link TM, Lin JC, Newitt D, Meier N, Waldt S, Majumdar S (1998) [Computer-assisted structure analysis of trabecular bone in the diagnosis of osteoporosis]. Der Radiologe 38:853–859

Mack PB, O'Brian AT, Smith JM, Bauman AW (1939) A method for estimating degree of mineralization of bones from tracings of roentgenograms. Science 89:467

Maggio D, Pacifici R, Cherubini A, Simonelli G, Luchetti M, Aisa MC, Cucinotta D, Adami S, Senin U (1997) Age-related cortical bone loss at the metacarpal. Calcif Tissue Int 60:94–97

Majumdar S, Kothari M, Augat P, Newitt DC, Link TM, Lin JC, Lang T, Lu Y, Genant HK (1998) High-resolution magnetic resonance imaging: three-dimensional trabecular bone architecture and biomechanical properties. Bone 22:445–454

Majumdar S, Link TM, Augat P, Lin JC, Newitt D, Lane NE, Genant HK (1999) Trabecular bone architecture in the distal radius using magnetic resonance imaging in subjects with fractures of the proximal femur. Magnetic Resonance Science Center and Osteoporosis and Arthritis Research Group. Osteoporos Int 10:231–239

Malich A, Boettcher J, Pfeil A, Sauner D, Heyne JP, Petrovitch A, Hansch A, Linss W, Kaiser WA (2004) The impact of technical conditions of X-ray imaging on reproducibility and precision of digital computer-assisted X-ray radiogrammetry (DXR). Skeletal Radiol 33:698–703

McAfee PC, Yuan HA, Fredrickson BE, Lubicky JP (1983) The value of computed tomography in thoracolumbar fractures. An analysis of one hundred consecutive cases and a new classification. J Bone Joint Surg [Am] 65:461–473

McCloskey EV, Spector TD, Eyres KS, Fern ED, O'Rourke N, Vasikaran S, Kanis JA (1993) The assessment of vertebral deformity: a method for use in population studies and clinical trials. Osteoporosis Int 3:138–147

Meema HE (1991) Improved vertebral fracture threshold in postmenopausal osteoporosis by radiographic measurements: its usefulness in selection for preventative therapy. J Bone Miner Res 6:9–14

Meema HE, Meema S (1969) Cortical bone mineral density versus cortical thickness in the diagnosis of osteoporosis: a roentgenologic densitometric study. J Am Geriat Soc 17:120–141

Meema HE, Meema S (1972) Microradioscopic and morphometric findings in the hand bones with densitometric findings in the proximal radius in thyrotoxicosis and in renal osteodystrophy. Investigative Radiol 7:88

Meema S, Meema HE (1976) Menopausal bone loss and estrogen replacement. Isr J Med Sci 12:601–606

Meema HE, Meema S (1981) Radiogrammetry. In: Cohn SH (ed) Non-invasive measurements of bone mass. CRC Press, Boca Raton, pp 5–50

Meema HE, Meema S (1987) Postmenopausal osteoporosis: simple screening method for diagnosis before structural failure. Radiology 164:405–410

Meema HE, Meindok H (1992) Advantages of peripheral radiogrametry over dual-photon absorptiometry of the spine in the assessment of prevalence of osteoporotic vertebral fractures in women. J Bone Miner Res 7:897–903

Melton III LJ, Kan SH, Frye MA, Wahner HW, O'Fallon WM, Riggs BL (1989) Epidemiology of vertebral fractures in women. Am J Epidemiol 129:1000–1011

Meunier PJ, Bressot C, Vignon E et al (1978) Radiological and histological evolution of post-menopausal osteoporosis treated with sodium fluoride-vitamin D-calcium. Preliminary results. In: Courvoisier B, Donath A, Baud CA (eds) Fluoride and bone. Hans Huber Publishers, Bern, 263–276

Millard J, Augat P, Link TM, Kothari M, Newitt DC, Genant HK, Majumdar S (1998) Power spectral analysis of vertebral trabecular bone structure from radiographs: orientation dependence and correlation with bone mineral density and mechanical properties. Calcif Tissue Int 63:482–489

Minch CM, Kruse RW (1998) Osteogenesis imperfecta: a review of basic science and diagnosis. Orthopedics 21:558–567

Minne HW, Leidig G, Wüster C, Siromachkostov L, Baldauf G, Bickel R, Sauer P, Lojen M, Ziegler R (1988) A newly developed spine deformity index (SDI) to quantitate vertebral crush fractures in patients with osteoporosis. Bone Mineral 3:335–349

Molpus WM, Pritchard RS, Walker CW, Fitzrandolph RL (1991) The radiographic spectrum of renal osteodystrophy. Am Fam Physician 43:151–158

Mosekilde L, Eriksen EF, Charles P (1990) Effects of thyroid hormones on bone and mineral metabolism. Endocrinol Metab Clin North Am 19:35–63

Mouloopoulos LA, Dimopoulos MA (1997) Magnetic resonance imaging of the bone marrow in hematologic malignancies. Blood 90:2127–2147

Murphey MD, Sartoris DJ, Quale JL, Pathria MN, Martin NL (1993) Musculoskeletal manifestations of chronic renal insufficiency. Radiographics 13:357–379

Mussolino ME, Looker AC, Madans JH, Edelstein D, Walker RE, Lydick E, Epstein RS, Yates AJ (1997) Phalangeal bone density and hip fracture risk. Arch Intern Med 157:433–438

Mussolino ME, Looker AC, Madans JH, Langlois JA, Orwoll ES (1998) Risk factors for hip fracture in white men: the NHANES I epidemiologic follow-up study. J Bone Miner Res 13:918–924

National Osteoporosis Foundation (NOF) (2000) Physician's guide to prevention and treatment of osteoporosis. Washington DC

Nelson D, Peterson E, Tilley B, O'Fallon W, Chao E, Riggs BL, Kleerekoper M (1990) Measurement of vertebral area on spine X-rays in osteoporosis: reliability of digitizing techniques. J Bone Miner Res 5:707–716

Nelson-Piercy C (1998) Heparin-induced osteoporosis. Scand J Rheumatol Suppl 107:68–71

Nielsen VAH, Pødenphant J, Martens S, Gotfredsen A, Riis BJ (1991) Precision in assessment of osteoporosis from spine radiographs. Europ J Radiol 13:11–14

Nordin BEC, Barnett E, MacGregor J, Nisbet J (1962) Lumbar spine densitometry. Br Med J I:1793–1796

Norman ME (1996) Juvenile osteoporosis. In: Favus MJ (ed) Primer on the metabolic diseases and disorders of mineral metabolism, 3rd edn. Lippincott-Raven, Philadelphia, pp 275–278

Nuzzo V, Lupoli G, Esposito Del Puente A, Rampone E, Carpinelli A, Del Puente AE, Oriente P (1998) Bone mineral density in premenopausal women receiving levothyroxine suppressive therapy. Gynecol Endocrinol 12:333–337

Olmez N, Kaya T, Gunaydin R, Vidinli BD, Erdogan N, Memis A (2005) Intra- and interobserver variability of Kleerekoper's method in vertebral fracture assessment. Clin Rheumatol 24:215–218

Oyen WJ, Arntz IE, Claessens RM, Van der Meer JW, Corstens FH, Goris RJ (1993) Reflex sympathetic dystrophy of the hand: an excessive inflammatory response? Pain 55:151–157

Palit G, Kerremans M, Gorissen J, Jacquemyn Y (2006) Transient bone marrow oedema of the femoral head in pregnancy – case report. Clin Exp Obstet Gynecol 33:244–245

Peacock M, Turner CH, Liu G, Manatunga AK, Timmerman L, Johnston CC Jr (1995) Better discrimination of hip fracture using bone density, geometry and architecture. Osteoporos Int 5:167–173

Pitt MJ (1991) Rickets and osteomalacia are still around. Radiol Clin North Am 29:97–118

Pitt MJ (1995) Rickets and osteomalacia. In: Resnick D (ed) Diagnosis of bone and joint disorders, 3rd edn. W.B. Saunders Company, Philadelphia, pp 1885–1922

Plato CC, Purifoy FE (1982) Age, sex and bilateral variability in cortical bone loss and measurements of the second metacarpal. Growth 46:100–112

Rea JA, Chen MB, Li J, Blake GM, Steiger P, Genant HK, Fogelman I (2000) Morphometric X-ray absorptiometry and morphometric radiography of the spine: a comparison of prevalent vertebral deformity identification. J Bone Miner Res 15:564–574

Reginato AJ, Falasca GF, Pappu R, McKnight B, Agha A (1999) Musculoskeletal manifestations of osteomalacia: report of 26 cases and literature review. Semin Arthritis Rheum 28:287–304

Resnick D (1981) The "rugger jersey" vertebral body. Arthritis Rheum 24:1191–1194

Resnick D (1995a) Hemoglobinopathies and other anemias. In: Resnick D (ed) Diagnosis of bone and joint disorders, 3rd edn. WB Saunders Company, Philadelphia, pp 2107–2146

Resnick D (1995b) Plasma cell dyscrasias and dysgamma-globulinemias. In: Resnick D (ed) Diagnosis of bone and joint disorders, 3rd edn. WB Saunders Company, Philadelphia, pp 2147–2189

Resnick D, Niwayama G (1995a) Parathyroid disorders and renal osteodystrophy. In: Resnick D (ed) Diagnosis of bone and joint disorders, 3rd edn. WB Saunders, Philadelphia, pp 2012–2075

Resnick D, Niwayama G (1995b) Osteoporosis. In: Resnick D (ed) Diagnosis of bone and joint disorders, 3rd edn. WB Saunders Company, Philadelphia, pp 1783–1853

Richardson ML, Pozzi-Mucelli RS, Kanter AS, Kolb FO, Ettinger B, Genant HK (1986) Bone mineral changes in primary hyperparathyroidism. Skeletal Radiol 15:85–95

Rico H, Hernandez ER (1989) Bone radiogrametry: caliper versus magnifying glass. Calcif Tissue Int 45:285–287

Riggs BL, Melton LJ (1983) Evidence for two distinct syndromes of involutional osteoporosis. Am J Med 75:899–901

Rosenberg AE (1991) The pathology of metabolic bone disease. Radiol Clin North Am 29:19–35

Rosenthal DI, Gregg GA, Slovik DM, Neer RM (1987) A comparison of quantitative computed tomography to four techniques of upper extremity bone mass measurement. In: Genant HK (ed) Osteoporosis Update 1987. Radiology Research and Education Foundation, San Francisco, pp 87–93

Ross PD, Davis JW, Epstein RS, Wasnich RD (1991) Pre-existing fractures and bone mass predict vertebral fracture incidence in women. Ann Intern Med 114:919–923

Ross PD, Genant HK, Davis JW, Miller PD, Wasnich RD (1993a) Predicting vertebral fracture incidence from prevalent fractures and bone density among non-black, osteoporotic women. Osteoporosis Int 3:120–126

Ross PD, Yhee YK, He Y-F, Davis JW, Kamimoto C, Epstein RS, Wasnich RD (1993b) A new method for vertebral fracture diagnosis. J Bone Miner Res 8:167–174

Ross PD, Huang C, Davis JW, Imose K, Yates J, Vogel J, Wasnich RD (1995) Predicting vertebral deformity using bone densitometry at various skeletal sites and calcaneus ultrasound. Bone 16:325–332

Rupp WM, McCarthy HB, Rohde TD, Blackshear PJ, Goldenberg FJ, Buchwald H (1982) Risk of osteoporosis in patients treated with long-term intravenous heparin therapy. Curr Surg 39:419–422

Sackler JP, Liu L (1973) Heparin-induced osteoporosis. Br J Radiol 46:548–550

Saito JK, Davis JW, Wasnich RD, Ross PD (1995) Users of low-dose glucocorticoids have increased bone loss rates: a longitudinal study. Calcif Tissue Int 57:115–119

Sarangi PP, Ward AJ, Smith EJ, Staddon GE, Atkins RM (1993) Algodystrophy and osteoporosis after tibial fractures. J Bone Joint Surg Br 75:450–452

Sauer P, Leidig G, Minne HW, Duckeck G, Schwarz W, Siromachkostov L, Ziegler R (1991) Spine deformity index (SDI) versus other objective procedures of vertebral fracture identification in patients with osteoporosis. J Bone Miner Res 6:227–238

Saville PD (1967) A quantitative approach to simple radiographic diagnosis of osteoporosis: its application to the osteoporosis of rheumatoid arthritis. Arthritis Rheumatism 10:416–422

Schwartz EN, Steinberg D (2005) Detection of vertebral fractures. Curr Osteoporos Rep 3:126–135

Schwartzman RJ, McLellan TL (1987) Reflex sympathetic dystrophy: a review. Arch Neurol 44:555–561

Seeman E, Szmukler GI, Formica C, Tsalamandris C, Mestrovic R (1992) Osteoporosis in anorexia nervosa: the influence of peak bone density, bone loss, oral contraceptive use, and exercise. J Bone Miner Res 7:1467–1474

Shaughnessy SG, Hirsh J, Bhandari M, Muir JM, Young E, Weitz JI (1999) A histomorphometric evaluation of heparin-induced bone loss after discontinuation of heparin treatment in rats. Blood 93:1231–1236

Singh YM, Nagrath AR, Maini PS (1970) Changes in trabecular pattern of the upper end of the femur as an index of osteoporosis. J Bone Joint Surg 52-A:457–467

Singh YM, Riggs BL, Beabout JW, Jowsey J (1972) Femoral trabecular-pattern index for evaluation of spinal osteoporosis. Ann Int Med 77:63–67

Smith R (1995) Idiopathic juvenile osteoporosis: experience of twenty-one patients. Br J Rheumatol 34:68–77

Smith RW, Eyler WR, Mellinger RC (1960) On the incidence of senile osteoporosis. Ann Int Med 52:773–781

Smith R, Stevenson JC, Winearls CG, Woods CG, Wordsworth BP (1985) Osteoporosis of pregnancy. Lancet 1:1178–1180

Smith-Bindman R, Cummings SR, Steiger P, Genant HK (1991) A comparison of morphometric definitions of vertebral fracture. J Bone Miner Res 6:25–34

Solomon BL, Wartofsky L, Burman KD (1993) Prevalence of fractures in postmenopausal women with thyroid disease. Thyroid 3:17–23

Spencer NE, Steiger P, Cummings SR, Genant HK (1990) Placement for points for digitizing spine films. J Bone Miner Res 5[Suppl 2]:S247

Stäbler A, Baur A, Bartl R, Munker R, Lamerz R, Reiser MF (1996) Contrast enhancement and quantitative signal analysis in MR imaging of multiple myeloma: assessment of focal and diffuse growth patterns in marrow correlated with biopsies and survival rates. AJR Am J Roentgenol 167:1029–1036

Steiger P, Weiss H, Stein JA (1993) Morphometric X-ray absorptiometry of the spine: a new method to assess vertebral osteoporosis. In: Christiansen C, Riis B (eds) Proceedings of the 4th International Symposium on Osteoporosis and Consensus Development Conference, 1993, Hong Kong, p 292

Steiger P, Cummings SR, Genant HK, Weiss H (1994) Morphometric X-ray absorptiometry of the spine: correlation in vivo with morphometric radiography. Osteoporosis Int 4:238–244

Stein I (1937) The evaluation of bone density in the roentgenogram by the use of an ivory wedge. AJR Am J Roentgenol 37:678–682

Steinbach HL, Kolb FO, Gilfillan R (1954) A mechanism of the production of pseudofractures in osteomalacia (Milkman's syndrome). Radiology 62:388

Steinbach HL, Gordan GS, Eisenberg E, Carne JT, Silverman S, Goldman L (1961) Primary hyperparathyroidism: a correlation of roentgen, clinical, and pathologic features. Am J Roentgenol Radium Ther Nucl Med 86:239–243

Steven GD (1947) "Standard bone". A description of radiographic technique. Ann Rheum Dis 6:184–185

Sudeck P (1901) Über die akute (reflectorische) Knochenatrophie nach Entzündungen und Verletzungen an den Extremitäten und ihre klinischen Erscheinungen. RöFo 5:277

Sundaram M (1989) Renal osteodystrophy. Skeletal Radiol 18:415–426

Takada M, Engelke K, Hagiwara S, Grampp S, Jergas M, Glüer CC, Genant HK (1997) Assessment of osteoporosis: comparison of radiographic absorptiometry of the phalanges and dual X-ray absorptiometry of the radius and the lumbar spine. Radiology 202:759–763

Tehranzadeh J, Tao C (2004) Advances in MR imaging of vertebral collapse. Semin Ultrasound CT MR 25:440–460

Todorovic Tirnanic M, Obradovic V, Han R, Goldner B, Stankovic D, Sekulic D, Lazic T, Djordjevic B (1995) Diagnostic approach to reflex sympathetic dystrophy after fracture: radiography or bone scintigraphy? Eur J Nucl Med 22:1187–1193

Toh SH, Claunch BC, Brown PH (1985) Effect of hyperthyroidism and its treatment on bone mineral content. Arch Intern Med 145:883–886

Toledo VA, Jergas M (2006) Age-related changes in cortical bone mass: data from a German female cohort. Eur Radiol 16:811–817

Trepman E, King TV (1992) Transient osteoporosis of the hip misdiagnosed as osteonecrosis on magnetic resonance imaging. Orthop Rev 21:1089–1091, 1094–1098

Trouerbach WT, Birkenhäger JC, Collette BJA, Drogendijk AC, Schmitz PIM, Zwamborn AW (1987) A study on the phalanx bone mineral content in 273 normal pre- and post-menopausal females (transverse study of age-dependent bone loss). Bone Miner 3:53–62

Trouerbach WT, Vecht-Hart CM, Collette HJA, Slooter GD, Zwamborn AW, Schmitz PIM (1993) Cross-sectional and longitudinal study of age-related phalangeal bone loss in adult females. J Bone Miner Res 8:685–691

Urist MR (1960) Observations bearing on the problem of osteoporosis. In: Rodahl K, Nicholson JT, Brown EM Jr (eds) Bone as a tissue. McGraw-Hill, New York, pp 18–45

van Rijn RR, Grootfaam DS, Lequin MH, Boot AM, van Beek RD, Hop WC, van Kuijk C (2004) Digital radiogrammetry of the hand in a pediatric and adolescent Dutch Caucasian population: normative data and measurements in children with inflammatory bowel disease and juvenile chronic arthritis. Calcif Tissue Int 74:342–350

van Rijn RR, Boot A, Wittenberg R, van der Sluis IM, van den Heuvel-Eibrink MM, Lequin MH, de Muinck Keizer-Schrama SM, Van Kuijk C (2006) Direct X-ray radiogrammetry versus dual-energy X-ray absorptiometry: assessment of bone density in children treated for acute lymphoblastic leukaemia and growth hormone deficiency. Pediatr Radiol 36:227–232

Versluis RGJA, Petri H, Vismans FJFE, van de Ven CM, Springer MP, Papapoulos SE (2000) The relationship between phalangeal bone density and vertebral deformities. Calcif Tissue Int 66:1–4

Virtama P (1960) Uneven distribution of bone mineral and covering effect of non-mineralized tissue as reasons for impaired detectability of bone density from roentgenograms. Ann Med Int Fenn 49:57–65

Walenga JM, Bick RL (1998) Heparin-induced thrombocytopenia, paradoxical thromboembolism, and other side-effects of heparin therapy. Med Clin North Am 82:635–658

Wu CY, Li J, Jergas M, Genant HK (1995) Comparison of semiquantitative and quantitative techniques for the assessment of prevalent and incident vertebral fractures. Osteoporosis Int 5:354–370

Wu C, van Kuijk C, Li J, Jiang Y, Chan M, Countryman P, Genant HK (2000) Comparison of digitized images with original radiography for semiquantitative assessment of osteoporotic fractures. Osteoporos Int 11:25–30

Zionts LE, Nash JP, Rude R, Ross T, Stott NS (1995) Bone mineral density in children with mild osteogenesis imperfecta. J Bone Joint Surg Br 77:143–147

Dual-Energy X-Ray Absorptiometry

Judith E. Adams

CONTENTS

J. E. Adams, MBBS, FRCP, FRCP
Professor, Department of Clinical Radiology, Imaging Science and Biomedical Engineering, Stopford Medical School, University of Manchester, Oxford Road, Manchester, M13 9PT, UK

7.1
Introduction

Osteoporosis is the most common metabolic bone disease. It is characterised by reduced bone mass, altered bone architecture and the clinical consequence of fracture with little or no trauma (low-trauma fractures, insufficiency fractures). These fractures tend to occur most commonly in sites of the skeleton that are rich in trabecular bone: the wrist, spine and hip. It is the last of these which has the greatest morbidity and mortality, but all osteoporotic fractures result in pain and suffering for patients and have considerable socio-economic impact on health care systems and society generally (COOPER 1996). 1 in 2 women and 1 in 5 men over the age of 50 years will suffer a fracture in their lifetime in the Western world (VAN STAA et al. 2001). In the past 20 years there have been significant advances in knowledge of the epidemiology, patho-physiology, and treatment of osteoporosis (SAMBROOK and COOPER 2006). These therapies increase bone mineral density (BMD) by between 5–12% and, more importantly, reduce future fracture risk to a greater magnitude (decrements between 30–70%) (ROYAL COLLEGE OF PHYSICIANS 1999, 2000; MEUNIER 2001; COMPSTON 2005; POOLE and COMPSTON 2006; KEEN 2007). Such therapies include bisphosphonates (etidronate, alendronate, risedronate, ibandronate, zoledronate), selective oestrogen modulator regulators (SERMs), strontium ranelate and anabolic parathyroid hormone, together with ensuring adequate calcium and vitamin D intake (PRINCE 2007). These developments have made it even more relevant to identify accurately those patients at risk of osteoporosis, and to do so before they suffer a fracture.

The diagnosis of osteoporosis can be made from radiographs when multiple fractures are present, or if structural abnormalities characteristic of osteoporosis are present (reduction in bone density and the number of trabeculae, thinned cortices, promi-

nent vertical trabeculae in the vertebrae) (QUEK and PEH 2002; ADAMS 2008). However, judging bone density on a radiograph can be imprecise, as technical aspects such as patient size, exposure and processing factors influence how radio-dense the bones appear. Although whether a patient suffers a fracture depends on a number of factors (age, propensity to fall and the nature of, and the response to, a fall), about 60%–70% of bone strength and what determines whether a fracture occurs is related to BMD (BLAKE et al. 2006a; ENGELKE and GLUER 2006). These factors lead to the importance of having available accurate and reproducible methods to measure the BMD of the skeleton in order to:
- Diagnose osteoporosis
- Predict fracture risk
- Determine therapeutic intervention
- Monitor response to therapy, or change with time,

which are the diagnostic and management roles of bone densitometry.

Quantitative measurements of bone mineral content (BMC) of the skeleton first became available in 1963, with the introduction of single photon absorptiometry (SPA) for peripheral bone densitometry (CAMERON and SORENSON 1963). For application to central sites (lumbar spine and proximal femur), a dual photon source (DPA) was required to correct for the overlying soft tissues (DUNN et al. 1980). These techniques used radionuclide sources for the production of the photons; the sources decayed and needed regular replacement, and scanning took a considerable length of time (15–30 min) because the photon flux was low. Thus, the patient might move during the scan, and the image quality was relatively poor; both these factors limited reproducibility (precision).

However, much useful clinical data were collected using these methods. In the mid-1980s the radionuclide sources of these scanners were replaced with low-dose X-ray tubes. These had a higher photon flux and so allowed faster scanning (10–15 min) and improved spatial resolution (better image quality) (KELLY et al. 1988; CULLUM et al. 1989). This heralded the introduction of single- and dual-energy X-ray absorptiometry (SXA, DXA), with improved precision, which could be applied to peripheral and central skeletal sites respectively.

7.2
Technical Aspects

The first DXA scanners were introduce in the late 1980s, and DXA is now the most widely used and available method amongst the techniques applied to bone densitometry (FAULKNER et al. 1991; GRAMPP et al. 1993; PEEL and EASTELL 1993; BLAKE and FOGELMAN 2007a), although its availability varies greatly in different countries (EUROPEAN COMMUNITIES/EUROPEAN FOUNDATION FOR OSTEOPOROSIS 1998). The dual-energy X-ray beams are required to correct bone density measurements for overlying soft tissue, and are produced by a variety of techniques by different manufacturers (energy switching; k-edge filtration) (BLAKE and FOGELMAN 1997; ADAMS 1998). The energies used are selected to optimise the separation of the mineralised and soft tissue components of the skeletal site analysed. Scanners manufactured by Hologic (Bedford, Mass., USA) use an energy-switching system in which the X-ray tube potential is switched rapidly from 70 to 140 kVp, alternating 60 times per second. The problems (in quantitative applications) of beam hardening that are usually associated with the polychromatic beam produced by an X-ray tube are overcome by simultaneous calibration and correction using a disc of reference bone and soft tissue equivalents which rotates synchronously with the X-ray pulses. The scanners manufactured by General Electric/Lunar (Madison, Wis., USA), Norland Medical Systems (Fort Atkinson, Wis., USA) and Sopha (Buc, France) use a constant potential X-ray source, combined with a rare-earth filter with energy-specific absorption characteristics due to the k-edge of the atomic structure of the element (k-edge filtration). The k-edge filter separates the X-ray distribution into two separate components of "high-energy" and "low-energy" photons (70 keV and 40 keV using cerium; 45 keV and 80 keV using a samarium filter) (BLAKE et al. 1999). If a single-energy photon beam is used (only applicable to peripheral skeletal sites), then the site has to be placed in a water bath, to allow correction for the overlying soft tissues.

7.2.1
Technical Developments

The original DXA scanners used a pencil X-ray beam and a single detector, and scanned in a rectilinear fashion across the anatomical site being examined. Scanning time was approximately 10–15 min per single site, and up to 30–40 min for whole body scanning in a large patient. Technical developments in DXA have taken place over recent years (Genant et al. 1996; Blake et al. 1999; Fogelman and Blake 2005; Engelke and Gluer 2006). These include fan-beam X-ray sources and a bank of detectors (Fig. 7.1). This allows faster scanning (approximately 1 min per site; similar times for whole body scans) with improved image quality and spatial resolution (Eiken et al. 1994). The spatial resolution of DPA was 3 mm; for the original DXA scanners the resolution was approximately 1mm and that of third-generation DXA scanners is approximately 0.5 mm (Kastl et al. 2002). With fan-beam scanners there is some magnification (approximately 7%) in the horizontal plane, but not in the cranio-caudal plane. This magnification does not affect BMD, but there are significant difference in BMC, bone area and parameters of hip geometry. This can be corrected by performing two scans at different distances from the X-ray tube (Griffiths et al. 1997). Some scanners have a "C" arm which allows lateral BMD scanning with the patient remaining in the supine position, rather than having to be repositioned into the lateral decubitus position. The latter is not often performed in clinical practice, because of the additional time required for repositioning. Lateral scanning enables views to be obtained of the vertebrae in the thoracic and lumbar spine. From these, assessments for vertebral fracture can be made (Rea et al. 1998, 2000, 2001; Genant et al. 2000; Ferrar et al. 2003, 2005, Link et al 2005; Vokes et al 2006).

7.2.2
Sites of Application and Measures Provided by DXA

DXA can be applied to sites of the skeleton where osteoporotic fractures occur; in the central skeleton this includes the lumbar spine (L1–4) (Fig. 7.1) and proximal femur (total hip, femoral neck, trochanter, and Ward's area) (Fig. 7.2). DXA can also be applied to peripheral skeletal sites (forearm and calcaneus), using either full-sized, or dedicated peripheral, DXA scanners (Fig. 7.3). Central DXA measures of lumbar spine, femoral neck and total hip are currently used as the "gold standard" for the clinical diagnosis of osteoporosis by bone densitometry (Figs. 7.1, 7.2).

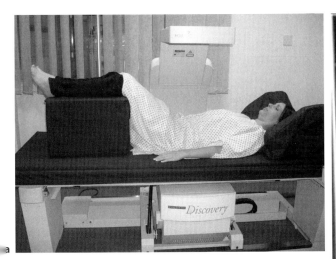
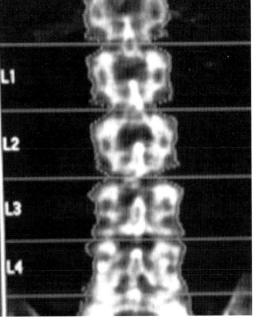

Fig. 7.1a,b. DXA of lumbar spine. **a** Patient positioned on fan-beam DXA scanner (with 'C' arm) for postero-anterior (PA – the X-ray source is below the table and the detectors in the scanning arm) scanning of the lumbar spine (L1–4). The legs are flexed at the hip and knee, and rest on a foam pad, to eliminate the natural lumbar lordosis; **b** DXA of normal lumbar spine L1–4. Measurements of BMC (g) and area (cm²) are provided for each vertebra. Results are generally expressed as a mean "areal" density (BMD$_a$; g/cm²) for all four vertebrae. For interpretation an appropriate ethnic- and gender-matched reference database must be available (usually provided by the manufacturer of the scanner) and expressed as a standard deviation score (SD) from the mean of either peak bone mass (T-score) or age-matched BMD$_a$ (Z-score)

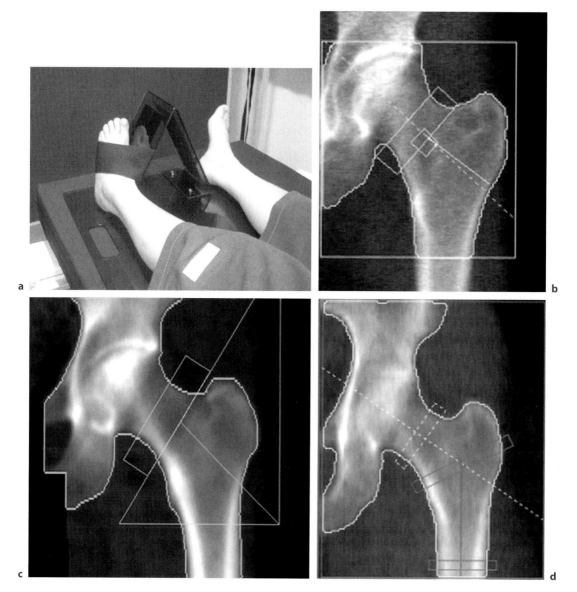

Fig. 7.2a–d. DXA of left hip. **a** with the leg well positioned - a little abducted and internally rotated with foot secured to positioner provided by scanner manufacturer. This brings the anteverted femoral neck parallel to the table, to avoid foreshortening of the neck (the lesser trochanter should not be seen prominently); DXA image of well positioned hip obtained on (**b**) Hologic and (**c**) General Electric Lunar scanners; note that the regions analysed are not identical between scanners. Although "areal" bone mineral density (g/cm²) is provided in a number of different sites (femoral neck, *oblong box*; Ward's area, *small box*; trochanter and total hip), for clinical diagnosis of osteoporosis (WHO T-Score below –2.5) femoral neck and total hip are used. For change in BMD$_a$ total hip is optimum as this measure is the most precise (CV=1%) in this site. The morphometric measure of the hip (hip axis length [HAL]) is the length of a line drawn parallel and between the margins of the femoral neck and extending from the inner margin of the bony pelvis to the lateral margin of the femur. An increase in this length has been found to be predictive of hip fracture. This measurement may be magnified on some fan-beam DXA. **d** Hip Strength Analysis (HSA) is calculated making mathematical assumptions of mineral distribution at the neck, trochanter and proximal shaft (*oblong boxes*) (Beck TJ (2007) Curr Osteoporos Rep 5:49–55)

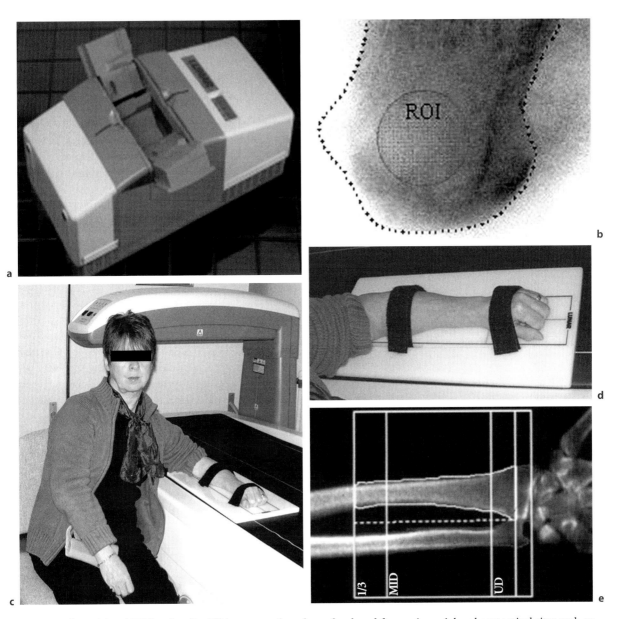

Fig. 7.3a–d. Peripheral DXA. **a** Smaller DXA scanners have been developed for use in peripheral anatomical sites such as the calcaneus (and forearm); these are less expensive than central DXA scanners and portable, so have the potential for use in a community, rather than a hospital, setting. **b** DXA of the calcaneus with the region of interest (ROI) in which the measurements are made indicated. The calcaneus is predominantly (95%) trabecular bone and is a better predictor of hip fracture than spinal DXA in the elderly, in whom artefacts (degenerative and hyperostotic spinal disease) confound central DXA. The WHO definition of osteoporosis (T-score less than –2.5) does not apply to this site. **c** Peripheral measures can be performed on central DXA scanners (**d**) the non-dominant forearm is positioned on the board provided by the scanner manufacturer. **e** The anatomical sites measured and their names vary between scanner manufacturers, but are generally the distal (designated as 'MID' in figure – predominantly cortical bone, and the most precise measure, CV = 1%), and the ultra-distal sites (predominantly trabecular bone, but less precise, CV = 2.5%). This peripheral cortical measure is particularly pertinent in patients with hyperparathyroidism (primary or secondary), and can be used if the patient's excessive size and weight preclude central DXA. The WHO definition of osteoporosis (T-Score below –2.5) is only applicable to the 'MID' (distal) site

The measurements provided by DXA are BMC in grams and projected area (BA) of the measured site in square centimetres. X-ray attenuation values are converted to bone mineral content (BMC in g); bone area (BA in cm) is calculated by summing the pixels within the bone edges; software algorithms detect the bone edges. 'Areal' bone mineral density (BMD_a in g/cm^2) is then calculated by dividing BMC/BA (BLAKE et al. 1999; ENGELKE and GLUER 2006). As the DXA image is a two-dimensional image of a three-dimensional object, this is an "areal", rather than a true volumetric, density; there is the depth of the bones which cannot be taken into account with a single postero-anterior (PA) projection. This results in one of the limitations of DXA, as the measurement is size-dependent. This is a particular problem in children, in whom the bones change markedly in size and shape during growth, especially during puberty, and in patients whose disease might result in them being small in stature or having slender, small bones.

With appropriate software whole-body scanning can also be performed, from which can be extracted whole-body and regional bone mineral content (BMC in grams) and whole-body and regional body composition [lean (muscle) and fat mass] (Fig. 7.4) (PIETROBELLI et al. 1996; TOTHILL and HANNAN 2000; KIM et al. 2006).

7.2.3
Precision and Accuracy

Precision measures the reproducibility of a bone densitometry technique, and is usually expressed as a coefficient of variation (CV) or standardised CV, which takes into account the range of measurements of the particular method (GLUER et al. 1995). To be clinically useful the precision needs ideally to be in the region of CV = 1%, and certainly better that 3%. The precision for total hip and lumbar spine is approximately 1%; for femoral neck and trochanter CV is 2.5% and for Ward's area it is 2.5%–5%. In peripheral sites precision is 1% in the distal forearm, 2.5% in the ultra-distal forearm and 1.4% in the calcaneus (SIEVANEN et al 1992; GRAMPP et al. 1993; PACHECO et al. 2002). The measurement sites generally used in clinical diagnosis (in contrast to research) are therefore lumbar spine (L1–4), femoral neck and total hip (KANIS and GLUER 2000); if hyperparathyroidism (primary or secondary) is suspected a forearm measurement is relevant, since cortical bone can be lost preferentially from this site (WISHART et al. 1990). Precision can be measured in either phantoms, normal individuals or in patients with osteoporosis. Precision is optimum in phantoms, and will be less good in patients with osteoporosis than in normal people, because positioning is more problematic in the former. Precision can be calculated by making repeat BMD measurements in the same individual after repositioning (usually a minimum of 10, but preferably 30 individuals or patients). Departments performing bone densitometry should calculate their own precision. Precision is optimised by using the minimum number of expert, highly motivated and well trained technical staff; it is not ideal to

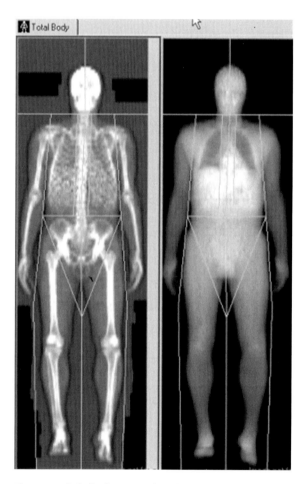

Fig. 7.4. Whole-body DXA takes about 1 min to obtain on fan beam scanners and provides total and regional information about the skeleton (*left image*) (BMC in g; BMD_a in g/cm^2) and body composition (lean muscle and fat mass (*right image*)

have a large number of staff who rotate through different departments and perform bone density scanning only infrequently.

Accuracy is how close the BMD measured by densitometry is to the actual calcium content of the bone (ash weight). The accuracy of DXA lies between 3% and 8%. The inaccuracies are related to marrow fat and DXA taking soft tissue as a reference (Blake et al. 1999).

Sensitivity is the ability of the measurement to discriminate between patients with and without fractures, and to measure small changes with time and/or treatment. A statistically significant change in BMD is calculated as 2.77 multiplied by precision of the measurement technique at the site of measurement. Changes in bone density are generally small; even in the early post-menopausal period in women, when bone loss is greatest, bone density decrements may only be in the region of 1–2% per annum. Therefore, when performing follow-up BMD measures in an individual patient it is essential to leave an adequate time interval between measures, usually 18–24 months (Gluer 1999).

Since whether a patient develops a fracture depends on factors in addition to BMD (age, whether the patient falls, the nature of the fall and the patient's response to the fall), it is impossible for BMD techniques to completely discriminate between those with and without fractures. However, the lower the DXA BMD, the more at risk the patient is of suffering a fracture (Melton et al. 1993; Kroger et al. 1995; Marshall et al. 1996; de Laet et al. 1998; Schott et al. 1998).

7.2.4
Correlations

DXA provides an "areal" density (g/cm^2) of integral (cortical and trabecular) bone. The cortical/trabecular ratios vary in different sites (Eastell et al. 1989; Faulkner et al. 1991), being approximately:
- 50/50 in the PA lumbar spine
- 10/90 in the lateral lumbar spine scan
- 60/40 in total hip
- 80/20 in total body
- 5/95 in calcaneus
- 95/5 in distal radius
- 40/60 in ultra-distal radius (depending on site of region of interest)

As a result of the different composition of bones and rates of change in these various skeletal sites, it is not surprising that measurements in different sites in the same individual will not give the same results (Eastell et al. 1989). The correlations between the BMD measurements made in the same patient vary between $r=0.4$ and $r=0.9$; it is not possible to predict from a DXA BMD measurement made in one site, what the BMD will be in another site using DXA or other bone densitometry methods (Grampp et al. 1997). In research studies, BMD measurements in different anatomical sites and by various bone density methods (DXA, QCT, QUS) may be complementary.

7.2.5
Radiation Dose

These quantitative photon absorptiometric techniques involve very low radiation doses, which are similar to those of natural background radiation (2,400 μSv per annum; about 7 μSv per day) (Kalender 1992; Huda and Morin 1996; Blake et al. 2006b) (Table 7.1). For the first-generation pencil-beam scanners the dose per site scanned is about 1 μSv, but it may be up to 6 μSv for the hip scan in pre-menopausal women, as the ovary may be included in the scan field (Lewis et al. 1994). The doses are a little higher for the fan-beam scanners (generally 3–6 μSv), but may be up to 62 μSv with some scanners (Lunar Expert – no longer manufactured) (Eiken et al. 1994; Njeh et al. 1996). Radiation doses for forearm and calcaneus scans are extremely low (0.5 and 0.03 μSv respectively). These DXA doses are generally less than one-tenth of a chest radiograph (20 μSv), and considerably lower than doses involved in other radiographic examinations carried out to confirm the diagnosis of osteoporosis in patients at risk (e.g. lateral spinal radiographs involve doses in the region of 700–2000 μSv per projection, depending on patient size and exposure factors). Assessment of the spine for vertebral fracture using DXA equipment by Lateral Vertebral Assessment (LVA[TM]) or Instant Vertebral Assessment (LVA[TM]) has the advantage over conventional spinal radiography of a lower radiation dose (1/100th; 12 μSv PA and lateral single energy image; 42 μSv for dual energy image [personal communication Dr Glen Blake, London]).

7.3
Indications

There has been much debate concerning the appropriate use of bone densitometry, particularly in population screening in women at the menopause (Melton et al. 1990), and the cost-effectiveness of such a programme has not been established (Tostestan et al. 1990). However, there is consensus that central DXA bone densitometry is the 'gold standard' measurement to make in appropriate individuals to assess fracture risk and make the diagnosis of osteoporosis in terms of bone densitometry (Peel and Eastell 1993; Compston et al. 1995; Kanis et al. 1997; Blake and Fogelman 2007a). Bone densitometry has high specificity but low sensitivity. Selection of patients who would most appropriately be referred for DXA bone densitometry is based on a case-finding strategy in those who have had a fragility (low-trauma) fracture or have other strong risk factors (Table 7.2) (Royal College of Physicians 1999). There may be national differences in such referral guidelines.

7.4
Positioning, Artefacts, and Errors

7.4.1
Patient Positioning

For measurement of the lumbar spine the patient is positioned supine on the scanner table with the legs flexed at the hips and knees and the calves resting on a square pad (Fig. 7.1). This removes the natural lumbar lordosis, so that the lumbar spine lies flat on the scanner table. For scanning of the proximal femur the leg is slightly abducted and internally rotated and fixed to a shaped block provided by the scanner manufacturer (Fig. 7.2). This ensures that the femoral neck is parallel to the table to avoid foreshortening which will result in false elevation of BMD (same amount of calcium in reduced area), and poor positioning of the femur can result in errors in BMD of the femoral neck of 0.95%–4.5% (Wilson et al. 1991; Goh et al. 1995). For whole-body DXA, the technician must ensure that all parts of the body, including arms and hands, are positioned inside the marker line on the scanner table.

For scanning of the forearm the hand is pronated and the arm and hand are positioned flat on the scanner table (Fig. 7.3). In some dedicated peripheral scanners the forearm is scanned in a horizontal position with the hand gripping a short vertical pole to ensure reproducible positioning. It is usual to scan the non-dominant forearm unless there are contraindications to this (e.g. previous fracture, etc.), when the dominant forearm is scanned. For measurements of the calcaneus the foot is positioned in a foot well, as prescribed by the manufacturer of the equipment.

7.4.2
Artefacts

Imaging artefacts can cause inaccuracies in DXA measurements. They are most common in the lumbar spine, particularly in the more elderly population. All the calcium in the path of the X-ray beam will contribute to the BMD measured. If there are degenerative disc disease with osteophytes, osteoarthritis with hyperostosis of the facet joints or a vertebral fracture (same amount of calcium before fracture contained in vertebra which is reduced in area) present, then the BMD will be falsely elevated (Orwoll et al. 1990; Frohn et al. 1991; Laskey et al. 1993; Franck et al. 1995; Jaovisidha et al. 1997; Adams 1998). Other aetiologies can also cause false elevation or underestimation of BMD measured by DXA (Table 7.3) (Fig. 7.5). It is therefore essential that all DXA images be scrutinised for such artefacts. The vertebra affected significantly by artefact should be excluded from analysis. Anomalies in spinal segmentation may be quite frequent (16.5%), and may cause the vertebral bodies to be misidentified (Peel et al. 1993). Strontium ranelate is a relatively new oral therapy for osteoporosis which results in large increases in bone mineral density compared to other treatments, such as bisphosphonates. However, some of this apparent increase is artefactual and related to the high atomic number strontium accumulating in the bone and contributing to the attenuation of X-rays. Methods to correct for this artefact have been proposed (Blake and Fogelman 2007b).

To overcome the problems of degenerative disc disease and hyperostosis in PA DXA of the spine, lateral DXA has been developed (Fig. 7.6). On scanners with "C" arms lateral scanning can be performed with the patient remaining in the supine position;

Table 7.1. Radiation doses of DXA and some comparable investigations

Examination	Site	EDE (µSv)	NBR	FC
DXA	Spine	2.4–4	13 hours	< 1 in few million
	Femur	2.4–5.4	20 hours	< 1 in few million
	Total body	0.01–3.4	11 hours	< 1 in few million
Vertebral assessment	Spine: Single energy Dual energy	12 42	2 days 6 days	1 in 1 million 1 in 1 million
Radiograph	Hand	< 1	< 1 hour	< 1 in few million
	Chest Lumbar spine	20 700–1000	3 days 7 months	1 in 1 million 1 in 200,000
Return flight UK/USA		80	12 days	
Background radiation		7–20 per day (2400–7300 per year)		

EDE = effective dose equivalent; NBR = natural background radiation; FC = fatal cancer risk

Table 7.2. Factors used to indicate appropriate referral for bone densitometry

Presence of strong risk factors:

Oestrogen (testosterone) deficiency

Premature menopause – age < 45 years

Prolonged secondary amenorrhoea (> 1 year)

Primary hypogonadism

Glucocorticoid therapy (prednisolone > 7.5 mg/day for > 3 months)

Low body mass index (< 19 kg/m^2)

Age (women over 65; men over 70 years)

Parental history of hip fracture

Disease known to be associated with secondary osteoporosis (e.g. rheumatoid arthritis, coeliac disease,hyperparathyroidism, Cushing's syndrome, etc.)

Radiographic evidence of osteopenia and/or vertebral farctures

Previous low-trauma fracture, particularly hip, wrist and spine, in adults

Loss of height, thoracic kyphosis (after radiographic confirmation of vertebral fracture)

Monitoring response to therapy

Table 7.3. DXA artefacts causing errors in estimation of BMD

Artefacts causing overestimation of BMD:

Spinal degeneration and hyperostosis (osteophytes)

Vertebral fracture

Extraneous calcification (lymph nodes, aortic calcification)

Sclerotic metastases

Vertebral haemangioma

Ankylosing spondylitis

Overlying metal (navel rings, surgical rods/plates, Myodil)

Poor positioning of femoral neck (inadequate internal rotation)

Excessive body weight

Strontium ranelate therapy

Vertebroplasty/kyphoplasty

Artefacts causing underestimation of BMD:

Laminectomy

Lytic metastases

Low body weight

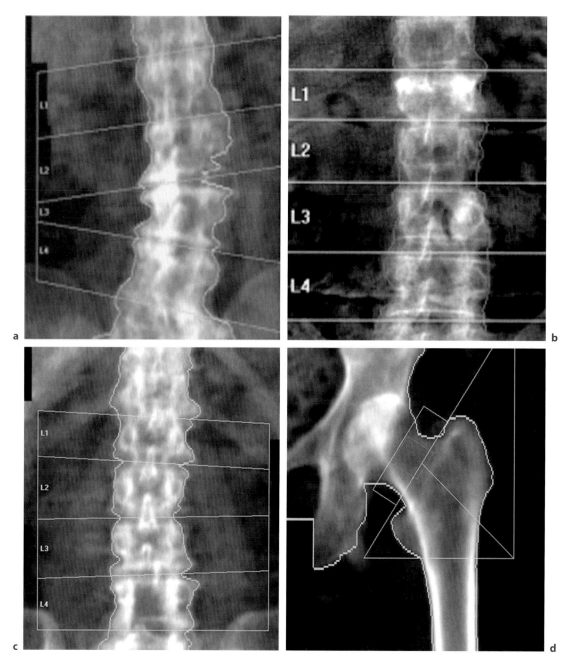

Fig. 7.5a–d. Artefacts on DXA: lumbar spine. **a** Degenerative disc disease and marginal osteophytes on the right at L2/3 and L3/4 falsely elevated BMD at these levels. **b** Vertebral fracture of L1. BMD at this level will be falsely elevated (same BMC as non-fractured vertebra, but in a smaller projected area, giving higher apparent BMD). **c** Laminectomy L4. The removal of the laminae and spinous process will falsely reduce the BMD of this vertebra. The DXA images must always be carefully scrutinised for such artefacts, and the affected vertebra excluded from analysis. If a vertebral fracture has occurred between sequential DXA measurements, then the results from that vertebra must be excluded from all scans to calculate change in BMD. For diagnosis there must be at least two vertebrae available for analysis, and must not be made on a single vertebra. **d** Proximal femur: the lesser trochanter is prominent, indicating inadequate internal rotation of the femur. This will cause foreshortening of the femoral neck and hence overestimation of BMD (same BMC as well-positioned femoral neck, in a smaller projected area)

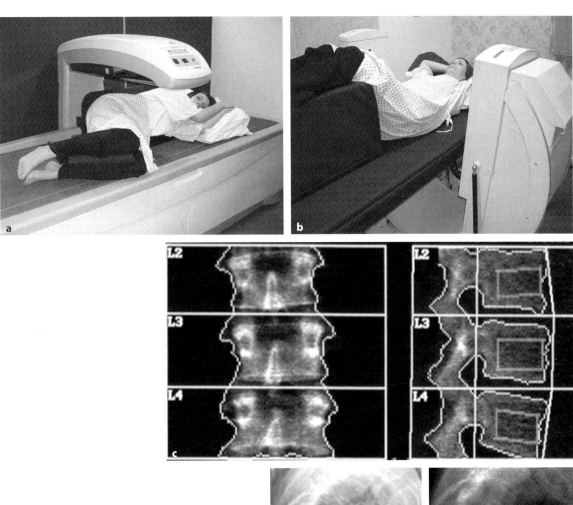

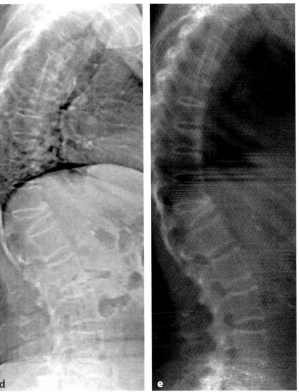

Fig. 7.6a–e. Lateral DXA of the spine. **a** With a fixed arm scanner the patient has to be repositioned into the lateral decubitus. **b** With a "C" arm scanner the patient can remain in the supine position as the arm of the scanner can be rotated (as illustrated) through 90° (**c**) from bone densitometry in two planes (PA and lateral projections) calculations can be made of volumetric BMD (g/cm^3) (bone mineral apparent density BMAD). The lateral DXA gives a measurement that is predominantly trabecular bone (*oblong box*) and therefore is not so affected by degenerative spinal changes as is the PA measurement. However, ribs may overlie L1 and L2, and the iliac crest may overlie L4, leaving only one vertebra (L3) for analysis. The precision of BMD measurement from lateral spinal DXA is poorer than for PA DXA, so that it is not generally used in clinical practice. **Vertebral fracture assessment:** can be made on DXA scanners on (**d**) single energy and (**e**) dual energy images (grade 3 severe crush fracture of T12) at much lower radiations doses (1/100th to 1/50th) than those in conventional spinal radiographs; some of the thoracic vertebrae are better seen on dual, that single, energy images. Six point morphometry (MXA) and visual assessment of the vertebrae can be made

otherwise the patient has to be repositioned in the lateral decubitus position, which limits its clinical practicality and precision (CV=2.8%–5.9% in lateral decubitus position, 1.6%–2% in the supine position) (Fig. 7.6). L3 may be the only vertebra in which lateral DXA can be measured, as L1 and L2 may have ribs superimposed, and L4 is overlain by the iliac crest. So although lateral DXA may be a more sensitive predictor of vertebral fracture than PA spinal DXA, its limited precision and impracticality means that it is not often performed in clinical practice (GUGLIEMI et al. 1994; DEL RIO et al. 1995; JERGAS et al. 1995).

Because of these artefacts on PA DXA scans of the lumbar spine, it has been suggested that in the more elderly population (over 65 years) only the proximal femur (femoral neck, total hip) should be scanned (KANIS and GLUER 2000). However, monitoring change is performed optimally in the lumbar spine, if there are no artefacts (GLUER 1999).

7.4.3
Sources of Error

Spinal scoliosis may make DXA scans of the spine difficult to analyse, and it may prove impossible to perform DXA if the patient is not able to lie flat on the scanner table (e.g. if the patient is in cardiac failure, has severe chronic obstructive airways disease or thoracic kyphosis), or if pain or deformity makes positioning problematic.

As DXA uses the soft tissues as a reference, errors in BMD can arise if the patient is excessively under- or overweight. Some manufacturers (GE/Lunar) used to apply a weight correction to the results provided (Z-score), although it is preferable that this is not applied.

7.5
Interpretation of Results

When a BMD measurement has been made in a patient, this has to be interpreted as normal or abnormal and a report formulated that will be of assistance to the referring clinician (MILLER et al. 1996). For this it is essential that age-, sex- and ethnically-matched reference data are available. The scanner manufacturer supplies such normal reference databases. These databases are predominantly, but not exclusively, drawn from a white, Caucasian, American-based population (based on 7,000–10,000 individuals). There is a paucity of appropriate reference ranges for children and certain ethnic minorities (e.g. Asians). A patient's results can be interpreted in terms of the standard deviations (SD) from the mean of either sex-matched peak bone mass (PBM) (T-score) or age-matched BMD (Z-score) (PARFITT 1990). Alternative methods of interpretation are as a percentage or percentile of expected PBM, either sex- and age-matched or just sex-matched.

The World Health Organisation (WHO) has defined osteoporosis in terms of bone densitometry. A T-score of less than –2.5 defines osteoporosis (WORLD HEALTH ORGANISATION 1994). This was arbitrarily defined as the level of BMD in post-menopausal women that identified approximately 30% of that population as having osteoporosis in their lifetime (this is thought to be the percentage of post-menopausal women who would suffer a vertebral fracture in their lifetime). The definition applied to DXA measurements made in the lumbar spine, the proximal femur and the distal third of the forearm. The definition does not apply to other techniques (e.g. quantitative computed tomography QCT, quantitative ultrasound QUS) or other anatomical sites (e.g. calcaneus) (GRAMPP et al. 1997; FAULKNER et al. 1999; MILLER 2000), nor is it yet confirmed to be applicable to younger women and men. Until PBM has been reached (i.e. in children and young adults up to approximately 25 years) interpretation can be made only by comparison to the age-matched mean (Z-score) (FAULKNER et al. 1993; NATIONAL OSTEOPOROSIS SOCIETY 2004; INTERNATIONAL SOCIETY FOR CLINICAL DENSITOMETRY 2005). Variations in the mean and standard deviation of reference ranges may alter the number of patients identified as osteoporotic (AHMED et al. 1997); in DXA of the hip, use of the NHANES reference database is preferred for white Caucasians (LOOKER et al. 1998).

In calculating change over time, the absolute BMD values (g/cm^2) have to be used. To be statistically significant the change in BMD has to be 2.77 multiplied by precision; in longitudinal studies in an individual patient one needs to leave an intervening period of at least 18–24 months between measures to ensure significant change, unless large changes in BMD are anticipated, such as may occur following organ transplantation together with large doses of glucocorticoids (GLUER 1999).

7.6
Applications

7.6.1
Clinical

7.6.1.1
Diagnosis of Osteoporosis

Osteoporosis is defined as "a condition characterised by reduced bone mass and deterioration of bone structure", and is the most common of the metabolic bone diseases. DXA is currently the most widely available bone densitometric technique for the diagnosis of osteoporosis, although its availability in different countries varies. Central DXA scanners cost approximately 80,000 EUR to 160,000 EUR, depending on the sophistication and versatility of scan functions; dedicated peripheral DXA scanners are less expensive (approximately 30,000 EUR), smaller and portable, with the potential for use in a community, rather than a hospital, setting. For clinical diagnosis the lumbar spine and proximal femur are scanned; forearm scanning can be performed on either central or dedicated peripheral scanners. Although the ionising radiation from these DXA scanners is low, ionising radiation regulations apply to their installation and operation. Dedicated and highly motivated technical staff with appropriate training will ensure high quality of positioning of the patient and good precision of the results.

Different manufacturers use different edge detection algorithms and analyse different ROIs for analysis in the hip (Fig. 7.2). For this reason, results from different scanners are not interchangeable. In longitudinal studies it is vital to use the same scanner and software programme. With technical developments it may become necessary to replace a scanner. In order to cross-calibrate between the old and the new scanner, scanning patients (approximately 100, with a spread of BMD from high to low) and phantoms (scanner manufacturer or European Spine Phantom) will generally allow the required calculations to be made (GENANT et al. 1994; KALENDER et al. 1995; HUI et al. 1997).

7.6.1.2
Prediction of Fracture

DXA BMD measurements made in any skeletal site (central and peripheral) are predictive of fracture,

Table 7.4. Relative risk (RR) of fracture per 1 SD decrease in BMD (measured by photon absorptiometry) below age-adjusted mean (MARSHALL et al. 1996)

BMD site	Forearm	Hip	Vertebral	All
Radius, distal	1.8	2.1	2.2	1.5
Radius, ultradistal	1.7	1.8	1.7	1.4
Hip	1.4	2.6	1.8	1.6
Lumbar spine	1.5	1.6	2.3	1.5
Calcaneus	1.6	2.0	2.4	1.5
All	1.6	2.0	2.1	1.5

with the risk of fracture increased in individuals with the lower BMD. The relative risk of fracture in various skeletal sites for every 1-SD reduction in age-adjusted mean BMD were published in a meta-analysis study and are given in Table 7.4 (MARSHALL et al. 1996). This reduction in BMD in predicting fracture is as good as a rise of 1-SD in blood pressure is in predicting stroke, and a 1-SD rise in cholesterol is in predicting myocardial infarction. Site-specific measurements are best in predicting fracture in that particular anatomical place.

7.6.1.3
Decisions for Treatment

Although there is consensus on the definition of osteoporosis in terms of bone densitometry (WHO T-Score less than –2.5), there is as yet no consensus on levels of BMD which justify therapeutic intervention which are cost-effective. This is perhaps not surprising, since it is the individual patient that is being treated, not the bone density result, and age is such a strong independent predictor of fracture (ROYAL COLLEGE OF PHYSICIANS 2000). Other factors (e.g. age, previous low trauma fracture over age 50, parental hip fracture, glucocorticoid therapy, rheumatoid arthritis, smoking, alcohol consumption) contribute to prediction of fracture risk; the WHO will shortly publish algorithms for calculating 10 year fracture risk for patients which will make the decision to instigate therapy more cost-effective (KANIS 2002; BORGSTROM et al. 2006; KANIS et al. 2006)

7.6.1.4
Monitoring Change with Time and Treatment

DXA is used to monitor the change in BMD to assess disease progression and the efficacy of therapy. As the rate of change in BMD, under most circumstances, is relatively slow, it is essential that an adequate interval of time exists between BMD assessments (GLUER 1999). A statistically significant change in BMD has to be greater than 2.77 times the precision of the technique. The rate of change will vary at different skeletal sites, and will be influenced by the ratio of cortical to trabecular bone, as trabecular bone is some eight-fold more metabolically active than cortical bone (EASTELL et al. 1998). As the distal forearm is predominantly cortical bone, this is not a sensitive site for monitoring change in BMD (BOUXSEIN et al. 1999); however, bone may be lost preferentially from this site in parathyroid overactivity (WISHART et al. 1990). DXA of the lumbar spine and total hip (precision 1%) are generally used for monitoring change, and an interval of approximately 2 years should be left between measurements, unless rapid loss of bone is suspected. Excessive changes in weight between measurements may artefactually account for apparent changes in BMD (PATEL et al. 1997)

7.6.2
Research and Advances in Clinical Applications

There are other scanning facilities on central scanners, which currently remain as research applications. These include whole-body scanning for total and regional BMC, lean muscle and fat mass (PIETROBELLI et al. 1996; TOTHILL and HANNAN 2000). Software programs are available for measuring BMD around prostheses following hip and knee arthroplasty (SOININVAARA et al. 2000; WILKINSON et al. 2001). There is an increasing demand for dedicated software programmes for DXA applicable to bone specimens and small animals in which scanning is now feasible (GRIFFIN et al. 1993; KASTL et al. 2002). Applications of DXA to other established and novel anatomical sites (hand, mandible) have been described (HORNER et al. 1996; HAUGEBERG and EMERY 2005; DRAGE et al. 2007). Although there may be no specific commercial software program available for scanning such sites, programs available for scanning conventional sites (e.g. forearm) can be used, with analysis being performed by hand-placed ROIs; these would not be as precise as automated ROIs.

Anatomical measurements can also be derived from DXA. The hip axis length (HAL) has been found to be predictive of hip fracture; the normal HAL in post-menopausal women is 10.5 ± 0.62 cm; an HAL of 11.0 cm increased hip fracture two-fold, and an HAL of 11.5 cm increased the risk four-fold. The HAL is the distance from the inner margin of the bony pelvis to the lateral border of the femur along a line drawn through the midline of the femoral neck, and parallel to its margins (FAULKNER et al. 1994). There will be some magnification of the hip geometry with fan-beam scanners, so that corrections have to be applied (YOUNG et al. 2000). Structural components of the proximal femur (size and shape), in combination with BMD, has been found to improve fracture risk prediction (GREGORY et al. 2004, 2005). The hip structure analysis (HSA) method has been introduced to extract geometric strength information from hip DXA (Fig. 7.2), by making mathematical calculations of the distribution of calcium in DXA cross-sections in the femoral neck, trochanteric region and proximal femoral shaft (BECK 2007) and has been applied retrospectively in several large research studies. Its application in clinical practice is still to be defined.

Lateral views of the thoracic and lumbar spine (T4–L4) can be obtained with fan-beam scanners, using dual- or single-energy scanning, and with the patient either in the supine ("C" arm scanners) or lateral decubitus position (Fig. 7.6). From these a visual assessment can be made as to whether or not vertebral fractures are present, and they have the potential for morphometric assessment of vertebral shape (REA et al. 1998, 2000, 2001; GENANT et al. 2000; LINK et al 2004; FERRAR et al 2005). The latter is currently time-consuming, with the requirement of considerable operator interaction, and so is not often used in clinical practice. Such morphometric analysis has the potential for automation by the application of computer analysis techniques (e.g. active shape models) that may make them more practical for use in a clinical setting (SMYTH et al. 1999; ROBERTS et al 2007). If it proves that DXA can be applied to the assessment of vertebral shape and fracture, this would have several advantages over conventional radiography, including exposing the patient to a lower dose of ionising radiation and avoiding the problems resulting from the divergent X-ray beam of radiography that can distort vertebral shape, causing apparent bi-concavity of the endplates (LEWIS and BLAKE 1995). DXA uses a lateral scan projection method, with simultaneous movement of the X-ray source and detectors along the spine, so the X-ray beam is always parallel to the vertebral endplates and avoids the 'bean can' artefact of vertebral endplates due to the parallax effect of radiographs.

Research studies may involve different scanners in multiple centres. To make the results comparable it is necessary to cross-calibrate between scanners with phantoms (e.g. scanner manufacturer's and European Spine Phantom). To combine results from different scanners, standardised bone mineral density (sBMD) is provided by most manufacturers or can be calculated (NORD 1992; GENANT et al. 1994; KALENDER et al. 1995; HUI et al. 1997). In bone densitometry generally, and in research studies in particular, quality assurance programmes must be rigorous (FAULKNER and MCCLUNG 1995).

7.7
Peripheral DXA (pDXA)

A number of small, portable DXA scanners have been available for application to peripheral sites, generally the forearm and the calcaneus (Fig. 7.3). BMD measurements in these sites can be as predictive of fractures in all sites as the more conventional measurements in central sites (Table 7.4). The forearm measurements are particularly predictive of wrist fractures; the calcaneus measurements are particularly predictive of spine fractures, even in the elderly, in whom spinal DXA is confounded by degenerative disease (MARSHALL et al. 1996; CHENG et al. 1997; NATIONAL OSTEOPOROSIS SOCIETY 2001).

Although the WHO criterion for the diagnosis of osteoporosis (T-Score less than –2.5) is applicable to the distal third of the forearm, it is not to the calcaneus. T-Scores between –1.0 and –1.5 for BMD in the calcaneus have been suggested as more appropriate in this site, but the definitive threshold for diagnosis has still to be determined and may be device specific (PACHECO et al. 2002).

It has been suggested that pDXA measurements could be used in a triage approach using device specific thresholds which define patients who have osteoporosis of the spine or hip with 90% sensitivity and 90% specificity (NATIONAL OSTEOPOROSIS SOCIETY 2001; PATEL et al. 2004), and such device specific thresholds have been published (BLAKE et al. 2005). However, such an approach may not be cost-effective (HARRISON and ADAMS 2006).

For monitoring change in BMD, the forearm site, being predominantly cortical bone, is not a sensi-

tive site; the calcaneus, being 95% trabecular bone, offers more potential for this purpose.

7.8
DXA in Children and Adjustments for Size Dependency

DXA, with its low radiation dose and good precision, offers a tool to study the growing skeleton (BLAKE et al. 2006b). However, there are some limitations of the technique, including a paucity of appropriate reference data and the size dependency of DXA (GILSANZ 1998, VAN RIJN et al. 2003).This is a particular problem in children, in whom the bones change markedly in size and shape during growth, especially during puberty, and in patients whose disease might result in them being small in stature or having slender, small bones (e.g. chronic illness, cystic fibrosis, growth hormone deficiency, Turner's syndrome) (HOLMES et al. 1994; GILSANZ 1998; FEWTRELL et al. 2003; NATIONAL OSTEOPOROSIS SOCIETY 2004; BACHRACH 2005; SANCHEZ and GILSANZ 2005; BRENNAN et al. 2005; SAWYER et al. 2006). To overcome this limitation, to some extent, bone mineral apparent density (BMAD) can be calculated in the spine (KATZMAN et al. 1991). One approach involves the calculation of bone mineral apparent density (BMAD) by dividing BMC by the three-dimensional bone volume derived from its two-dimensional projected bone area (BA). The BMAD of the lumbar spine (LS) is estimated by modelling it as a cube ($BMAD_{LS}= BMC_{LS}/BA_{LS}^{1.5}$) (CARTER et al. 1992) or as a cylinder ($BMAD_{LS}= BMC_{LS} \times [4/(\pi \times$ bone width of LS)]) (KROGER et al. 1992). Reference data for BMAD for children 6–17 years using Hologic 4500 Discovery scanners have been published (WARD et al. 2007). At the mid-femoral shaft and the femoral neck, it has been showed that the age and height dependence of BMD_a at the mid-femoral shaft and the femoral neck disappeared when the data were expressed as BMAD, assuming that these skeletal sites are cylinders (LU et al. 1996).

Another approach for correcting DXA for size involves the estimation of a 'size adjusted, BMC', which is calculated using a regression, or a multivariate, statistical model (PRENTICE et al. 1994) to adjust BMC for cofounders, such as projected bone area, overall body height and weight (surrogates for bone size) and Tanner stages of sexual development (WARNER et al. 1998). 'Size adjusted BMC' is often used in research studies, for example when comparing BMC in a group of children with a disease to healthy controls. However, body height and weight might not completely control for all relevant differences in size and shape of the skeletal region of interest. Differences in bone size and shape may have important implications for bone strength, independently of adjusted or unadjustedd BMC/BMD$_a$.

MØLGAARD et al. (1997) proposed a three-step approach for the evaluation of whole body BMC in children, which seeks to determine: (a) is the child's height appropriate for age? ('short bones'); (b) is the bone size (bone area) appropriate for height? ('narrow bones'); (c) is the BMC appropriate for bone area? ('light, undermineralised bones'). These analyses are used to calculate standard deviation scores by reference to local gender and ethnic specific reference data for these parameters. This approach allows the clinician to separately determine if the child's skeletal fragility is due to reduction in the size of the bones or the amount of BMC within the periosteal envelope, or both these factors. An alternative approach is to interpret bone mineral content (BMC) in relation to lean tissue mass (LTM) which is a major predictor of BMC. An algorithm for interpreting whole body DXA scans using a four step approach has been published (HOGLER et al. 2003): 1) BMD or BMC for age, 2) height for age, 3) LTM for height, 4) BMC/LTM ratio for height with normative data for this using a Lunar DPX-L scanner. A similar approach is proposed by CRABTREE et al. (2004).

Quantitative CT has some important advantages in children, as it provides separate measurements of cortical and trabecular bone, and true volumetric density (mg/cm^3), so is not size-dependent. Quantitative CT is therefore an important tool in assessing BMD in the developing skeleton, and is applied to the central (T12–L3) and peripheral (usually forearm, but also tibia) skeleton (NATIONAL OSTEOPOROSIS SOCIETY 2004; WARD et al. 2006).

There are some DXA reference data for the spine, but most of these are based on chronological age and do not take into account the pubertal staging of the child, which is crucial to changes in size and density of the developing skeleton (FAULKNER et al. 1993). For these reasons DXA in children should probably still be regarded as a research tool rather than an established clinical service. Those referring children for bone densitometry, and those performing the measurements and providing interpretation of the results, need to have experience in the field and

be aware of the limitations of the technique. Nonetheless, the method is being increasingly applied to the investigation of bone in children, including neonates (SALLE et al. 1992; Koo et al. 2004).

7.9 Conclusions

DXA offers a precise and reasonably accurate technique for measuring BMD in both central and peripheral skeletal sites, using very small doses of radiation (in the region of levels of natural background radiation). DXA is currently regarded as the "gold standard" for BMD measurements for the diagnosis of osteoporosis. However, there are some important limitations ["areal" density, size dependency, measurement of integral (cortical and trabecular) bone], of which users and operators need to be aware. Good precision is dependent on scanners being operated by skilled and appropriately trained staff, and quality assurance protocols being in place. DXA can be used to diagnose osteoporosis using the WHO threshold (T-Score –2.5 or below in lumbar spine L1–4; femoral neck and total hip), to predict fractures, to contribute to the decision on patient management and therapeutic intervention, and to monitor change in BMD (except in the forearm). There is potential for visual assessment and MXA to determine whether or not vertebral fractures are present, an important element in defining the most appropriate management of patients at risk of osteoporosis. There are increasing, and varied, applications of DXA in research studies in novel sites, and in both humans and animals.

References

Adams JE (1998) Single- and dual-energy X-ray absorptiometry. In: Genant HK, Guglielmi G, Jergas M (eds) Bone densitometry and osteoporosis. Springer, Berlin Heidelberg New York, p 305–334

Adams JE (2008) Metabolic and endocrine skeletal disease. In: Grainger & Allison's Diagnostic Radiology, 5th Edition. Vol 2, Sect 5 Musculoskeletal Chap 49. Churchill Livingstone Elsevier, Philadelphia, p 1083–1113

Ahmed AIH, Blake GM, Rymer JM, Fogelman I (1997) Screening for osteoporosis and osteopenia: do the accepted normal ranges lead to overdiagnosis? Osteoporos Int 7:432–438

Bachrach LK (2005) Assessing bone health in children: who to test and what does it mean? Pediatr Endocrinol Rev 2(S3):332–336

Beck TJ (2007) Extending DXA beyond bone mineral density: understanding hip structure analysis. Curr Osteoporos Rep 5:49–55

Blake GM, Fogelman I (1997) Technical principles of dual energy X-ray absorptiometry. Semin Nucl Med 27:210–228

Blake GM, Fogelman I (2007a) The role of DXA bone density scans in the diagnosis and treatment of osteoporosis. Postgrad Med J 83:509–517

Blake GM, Fogelman I (2007b) The correction of BMD measurements for bone strontium content. J Clin Densitom 10:259–265

Blake GM, Wahner HW, Fogelman I (1999) The evaluation of osteoporosis: dual energy X-ray absorptiometry and ultrasound in clinical practice. Martin Dunitz, London

Blake GM, Chinn DJ, Steel SA, Patel R, Panayiotou E, Thorpe J, Fordham JN, National Osteoporosis Society Bone Densitometry Forum (2005) A list of device-specific thresholds for the clinical interpretation of peripheral X-ray absorptiometry examinations. Osteoporos Int 16:2149–2156

Blake GM, Knapp KM, Spector TD, Fogelman I (2006a) Predicting the risk of fracture at any skeletal site: are all bone mineral density measurement sites equally effective? Calcif Tiss Int 78:9–17

Blake GM, Naeem M, Boutros M (2006b) Comparison of effective dose to children and adults from dual energy X-ray absorptiometry examinations. Bone 38:935–942

Borgstrom F, Johnell O, Kanis JA, Jonsonn B, Rehnberg C (2006) At what hip fracture risk is it cost-effective to treat? International intervention thresholds for the treatment of osteoporosis. Osteoporos Int 17:1459–1471

Bouxsein ML, Parker RA, Greenspan SL (1999) Forearm bone mineral densitometry cannot be used to monitor response to alendronate. Osteoporos Int 10:505–509

Brennan BM, Mughal Z, Roberts SA, Ward K, Shalet SM, Eden TO, Will AM, Stevens RF, Adams JE (2005) Bone mineral density in childhood survivors of acute lymphoblastic leukaemia treated without cranial irradiation. J Clin Endocrinol Metab 90:689–694

Cameron JR, Sorenson J (1963) Measurement of bone mineral density in vivo: an improved method. Science 142:230–232

Carter DR, Bouxsein ML, Marcus R (1992) New approaches for interpreting projected bone densitometry data. J Bone Miner Res 7:137–145

Cheng S, Suominen H, Sakari-Rantala R, Laukkanen P, Avikainen V, Heikkinen E (1997) Calcaneal bone mineral density predicts fracture occurrence: a five-year follow-up study in elderly people. J Bone Miner Res 12:1075–1082

Compston J (2005) Guidelines for the management of osteoporosis: the present and the future. Osteoporos Int 16:1173–1176

Compston JE, Cooper C, Kanis JA (1995) Bone densitometry in clinical practice. Br Med J 310:1507–1510

Cooper C (1996) Epidemiology and definition of osteoporosis. In: Compston JE (ed) Osteoporosis: new perspectives on causes, prevention and treatment. Royal College of Physicians of London p 1–10

Crabtree NJ, Kibirige MS, Fordham J, Banks LM, Muntoni F, Chinn D, Boivin CM, Shaw NJ (2004) The relationship between lean body mass and bone mineral content in paediatric health and disease. Bone 35:965–972

Cullum ID, Ell PJ, Ryder JP (1989) X-ray dual photon absorptiometry: a new method for the measurement of bone density. Brit J Radiol 62:587–592

de Laet CE, Van Hout BA, Burger H, Weel AE, Hofman A, Pols HA (1998) Hip fracture prediction in elderly men and women: validation in the Rotterdam study. J Bone Miner Res 13:1587–1593

Del Rio L, Pons F, Huguet M, Setoain FJ (1995) Anteroposterior versus lateral bone mineral density of spine assessed by dual X-ray absorptiometry. Eur J Radiol 22:407–412

Drage NA, Palmer RM, Blake GM, Wilson R, Crane F, Fogelman I (2007) A comparison of bone mineral density in the spine, hip and jaw of edentulous subjects. Clin Oral Implants Res 18:496–500

Dunn WL, Wahner HW, Riggs BL (1980) Measurement of bone mineral content in human vertebrae and hip by dual photon absorptiometry. Radiology 136:485–487

Eastell R, Wahner HW, O'Fallon WM, Amadio PC, Melton LJ 3rd, Riggs BL (1989). Unequal decrease in bone density of the lumbar spine and ultradistal radius in Colles' and vertebral fracture syndromes. J Clin Invest 83:168–174

Engelke K, Gluer CC (2006) Quality and performance measures in bone densitometry: part 1: errors and diagnosis. Osteoporos Int 17:1283–1292

Engelke K, Gluer CC (2006) Quality and performance measures in bone densitometry: part 2: fracture risk. Osteoporos Int 17:1449–1458

Eiken P, Kolthoff N, Barenholdt O, Hermansen F, Pors Nielsen S (1994) Switching from pencil-beam to fanbeam. II. Studies in vivo. Bone 15:671–676

European Communities/European Foundation for Osteoporosis (1998) Building strong bones and preventing fractures. Summary report on osteoporosis in the European Community – action for prevention. European Communities/European Foundation for Osteoporosis, Germany, p 3–12

Faulkner KG, McClung MR (1995) Quality control of DXA instruments in multicenter trials. Osteoporos Int 5:218–227

Faulkner KG, Gluer CC, Majumdar S, Lang P, Engelke K, Genant HK (1991) Non-invasive measurements of bone mass, structure and strength: current methods and experimental techniques. Am J Radiol 157:1229–1237

Faulkner RA, Bailey DA, Drinkwater DT, Wilkinson AA, Houston CS, McKay HA (1993) Regional and total body bone mineral content, bone mineral density, and total body tissue composition in children 8–16 years of age. Calcif Tissue Int 53:7–12

Faulkner KG, McClung M, Cummings SR (1994) Automated evaluation of hip axis length for predicting hip fracture. J Bone Miner Res 9:1065–1070

Faulkner KG, von Stetten E, Miller P (1999) Discordance in patient classification using T-score. J Clin Densitom 2:343–350

Ferrar L, Jiang G, Eastell R, Peel NF (2003) Visual identification of vertebral fractures in osteoporosis using morphometric X-ray absorptiometry. J Bone Miner Res 18:933–938

Ferrar L, Jiang G, Adams J, Eastell R (2005) Identification of vertebral fractures: an update. Osteoporos Int 16:717–728

Fewtrell MS; British Paediatric and Adolescent Bone Group (2003) Bone densitometry in children assessed by dual X-ray absorptiometry: uses and pitfalls. Arch Dis Child 88:795–798

Fogelman I, Blake GM (2005) Bone densitometry: an update. Lancet 366(9503):2068–2070

Franck H, Munz M, Scherrer M (1995) Evaluation of dual-energy X-ray absorptiometry bone mineral measurement – comparison of a single-beam and fan beam design: the effect of osteophytic calcification on spine bone mineral density. Calcif Tissue Int 56:192–195

Frohn J, Wilken T, Falk S, Strutte HJ, Kollath J, Hor G (1991) Effect of aortic sclerosis on bone mineral measurements by dual-photon absorptimetry. J Nucl Med 32:259–262

Genant HK, Grampp S, Glueer CC, Faulkner KG, Jergas M, Engelke K, Hagiwara S, van Kuijk C (1994) Universal standardisation for the dual X-ray absorptiometry: patient and phantom cross-calibration results. J Bone Miner Res 9:1503–1514

Genant HK, Engelke K, Fuerst T, Gluer CC, Grampp S, Harris ST, Jergas M, Lang T, Lu Y, Majumdar S, Mathur A, Takada M (1996) Noninvasive assessment of bone mineral and structure: state of the art. J Bone Miner Res 11:707–730

Genant HK, Li Y, Wu CY, Shepherd JA (2000) Vertebral fractures in osteoporosis: a new method for clinical assessment. J Clin Densitom 3:281–290

Gilsanz V (1998) Bone density in children: a review of the available techniques and indications. Eur J Radiol 26:177–182

Gluer CC (1999) Monitoring skeletal changes by radiological techniques. J Bone Miner Res 14:1952–1962

Gluer CC, Blake G, Blunt BA, Jergas M, Genant HK (1995) Accurate assessment of precision errors: how to measure the reproducibility of bone densitometry techniques. Osteoporos Int 5:262–270

Goh JC, Low SL, Bose K (1995) Effect of femoral rotation on bone mineral density measurements with dual energy X-ray absorptiometry. Calcif Tissue Int 57:340–343

Grampp S, Jergas M, Gluer CC, Lang P, Brastow P, Genant HK (1993) Radiologic diagnosis of osteoporosis: current methods and perspectives. Radiol Clin North Am 31(5):1131–1145

Grampp S, Genant HK, Mathur A, Lang P, Jergas M, Takada M, Gluer CC, Lu Y, Chavez M (1997) Comparisons of non-invasive bone mineral measurements in assessing age-related loss, fracture discrimination and diagnostic classification. J Bone Miner Res 12:697–711

Gregory JS, Testi D, Stewart A, Undrill PE, Reid DM, Aspden RM (2004) A method of assessment of the shape of the proximal femur and its relationship to osteoporotic hip fracture. Osteoporos Int 15:5–11

Gregory JS, Stewart A, Undrill PE, Reid DM, Aspden RM (2005) Bone shape, structure and density as determinants of osteoporotic hip fracture: a pilot study investigating the combination of risk fracture. Invest Radiol 40:591–597

Griffin MC, Kimble R, Hopfer W, Pacifici R (1993) Dual-energy X-ray absorptiometry of the rat: accuracy, precision and measurement of bone loss. J Bone Miner Res 8:795–800

Griffiths MR, Noakes KA, Pocock NA (1997) Correcting the magnification error of fan beam densitometers. J Bone Miner Res 12:119–123

Guglielmi G, Grimston SK, Fischer KC, Pacifici R (1994) Osteoporosis: diagnosis with lateral and posteroanterior dual X-ray absorptiometry compared with quantitative CT. Radiology 192:845–850

Harrison EJ, Adams JE (2006) Application of a triage approach to peripheral bone densitometry reduces requirement for central DXA, but is not cost effective. Calc Tiss Int 79:199–206

Haugeberg G, Emery P (2005) Value of dual-energy X-ray absorptiometry as a diagnostic tool in early rheumatoid arthritis. Rheum Dis Clin North Am 31:715–728

Holmes SJ, Economou G, Whitehouse RW, Adams JE, Shalet SM (1994) Reduced bone mineral density in patients with adult onset growth hormone deficiency. J Clin Endocrinol Metab 78:669–674

Hogler W, Briody J, Woodhead HJ, Chan A, Cowell CT (2003) Importance of lean mass in the interpretation of total body densitometry in children and adolescents. J Pediatr 143:81–88

Horner K, Devlin H, Alsop CW, Hodgkinson IM, Adams JE (1996) Mandibular bone mineral density as a predictor of skeletal osteoporosis. Br J Radiol 69:1019–1025

Huda W, Morin RL (1996) Patient doses in bone densitometry Br J Radiol 69:422–425

Hui SL, Gao S, Zhou XH, Johston CC Jr, Lu Y, Gluer CC, Grampp S, Genant HK (1997) Universal standardisation of bone density measurements: a method with optimal properties for calibration among several instruments. J Bone Miner Res 12:1463–1470

International Society for Clinical Densitometry (2005) 342 North Main Street, West Hartford CT06117-2507 USA; www.ISCD.org

Jaovisidha S, Sartoris DJ, Martin EM, De Maeseneer M, Szollar SM, Deftos LJ (1997) Influence of spondylopathy on bone densitometry using dual energy X-ray absorptiometry. Calcif Tissue Int 60:424–429

Jergas M, Breitenseher M, Gluer CC, Black D, Lang P Grampp s, Engelke K, Genant HK (1995) Which vertebrae should be assessed using lateral dual-energy X-ray absorptiometry of the lumbar spine. Osteoporos Int 5:196–204

Kalender WA (1992) Effective dose values in bone mineral measurements by photon absorptiometry and computed tomography. Osteoporos Int 2:82–87

Kalender WA, Felsenberg D, Genant HK, Dequeker J, Reeve J (1995) The European Spine Phantom: a tool for standardisation and quality control in spinal bone mineral measurement by DXA and QCT. Eur J Radiol 20:83–92

Kanis JA (2002) Diagnosis of osteoporosis and assessment of fracture risk. Lancet 359(9321):1929–1936

Kanis JA, Delmas P, Burckhardt P, Cooper C, Torgerson D (1997) Guidelines for diagnosis and management of osteoporosis: EFFO report. Osteoporos Int 7:390–406

Kanis JA, Gluer C, for the Committee of the Scientific Advisors, International Osteoporosis Foundation (2000) An update in the diagnosis and assessment of osteoporosis with densitometry. Osteoporos Int 11:192–202

Kanis JA, Johnell O, Oden A, Johansson H, Eisman JA, Fujiwara S, Kroger H, Honkanen R, Melton LJ Jr, O'Neill T, Reeve J, Silman A, Tenenhouse A (2006) The use of multiple sites for the diagnosis of osteoporosis. Osteoporos Int 17:527–534

Kastl S, Sommer T, Klein P, Hohenberger W, Engelke K (2002) Accuracy and precision oof bone mineral density and bone mineral content in the excised rat humeri using fan beam dual-energy X-ray absorptiometry. Bone 30:243–246

Katzman DK, Bachrach LK, Carter DR, Marcus R (1991) Clinical and anthropometric correlates of bone mineral acquisition in healthy adolescent girls. J Clin Endocrinol Metab 73:1332–1339

Kelly TL, Slovik DM, Schoenfeld DA, Neer RM (1988) Quantitative digital radiography versus dual photon absorptiometry of the lumbar spine. J Clin Endocrinol Metab 67:839–844

Keen R (2007) Osteoporosis: strategies for prevention and management. Best Pract Res Clin Rheumatol 21:109–122

Kim J, Shen W, Gallagher D, Jones A Jr, Wang Z, Wang J, Heshka S, Heymsfield SB (2006) Total-body skeletal muscle mass: estimation by dual-energy X-ray absorptiometry in children and adolescents Am J Nutr 84:1014–1020

Koo WW, Hockman EM, Hammami M (2004) Dual energy X-ray absorptiometry measurements in small subjects: conditions affecting clinical measurements. J Am Coll Nutr 23:212–219

Kroger H, Kotaniemi A, Vainio P, Alhava E (1992) Bone densitometry of the spine and femur in children by dual-energy X-ray absorptiometry. Bone Miner 17:75–85

Kroger H, Huopio J, Honkanen R, Tuppurainen M, Puntila E, Alhava E, Saarikoski S (1995) Prediction of fracture risk using axial bone mineral density in a perimenopausal population: a prospective study. J Bone Miner Res 10:302–306

Laskey MA, Crisp AJ, Compston JE, Khaw KT (1993) Heterogeneity of spine bone density. Br J Radiol 66:480–483

Lewis MK, Blake GM (1995) Patient dose in morphometric X-ray absorptiometry Osteoporos Int 5:281–282

Lewis MK, Blake GM, Fogelman I (1994) Patient doses in dual X-ray absorptiometry. Osteoporos Int 4:11–15

Link TM, Guglielmi G, van Kuijk C, Adams JE (2005) Radiologic assessment of osteoporotic fracture: diagnostic and prognostic implications. Eur Radiol 15:1521–1532

Lu PW, Cowell CT, Lloyd-Jones SA, Briody J, Howman-Giles R (1996) Volumetric bone mineral density in normal subjects, aged 5–27 years. J Clin Endocrinol Metab; 81:1586–1590

Looker AC, Wahner HW, Dunn WL, Calvo MS, Harris TB, Heyse SP, Johnston CC Jr, Lindsay R (1998) Updated data on proximal femur bone mineral levels of US adults. Osteoporos Int 8:468–489

Lu PW, Cowell CT, Lloyd-Jones SA, Briody JN, Howman-Giles R (1996) Volumetric bone mineral density in normal subjects, aged 5–27 years. J Clin Endocrinol Metab 81:1586–1590

Marshall D, Johnell O, Wedel H (1996) Meta-analysis of how well measures of bone density predict occurrence of osteoporotic fractures. Br Med J 312:1254–1259

Melton LJ, Eddy DM, Johnson CC (1990) Screening for osteoporosis. Ann Intern Med 112:516–528

Melton LJ 3rd, Atkinson EJ, O'Fallon WM, Wahner HW, Riggs BL (1993) Long-term fracture prediction by bone mineral assessed at different skeletal sites. J Bone Miner Res 8:1227–1233

Meunier PJ (2001) Anabolic agents for treatment of postmenopausal osteoporosis. J Bone Spine 68:576–581

Miller P (2000) Controversies in bone mineral density diagnostic classification. Calcif Tissue Int 66:317–319

Miller P, Bonnick SL Rosen CJ (1996) Consensus of an international panel on the clinical utility of bone mass measurements in the detection of low bone mass in the adult population. Calcif Tissue Int 58:207–214

Mølgaard C, Thomsen BL, Prentice A, Cole TJ, Michaelsen KF (1997) Whole body bone mineral content in healthy children and adolescents. Arch Dis Child 76:9–15

National Osteoporosis Society (2001) Position statement on the use of peripheral X-ray absorptiometry in the managament of osteoporosis. National Osteoporosis Society, Camerton, Bath, UK, p 1–15

National Osteoporosis Society (2004) A practical guide to bone densitometry in children. National Osteoporosis Society, Camerton, bath, BA2 0PJ, UK

Njeh CF, Apple K, Temperton DH, Boivin CM (1996) Radiological assessment of a new bone densitometer: the Lunar expert. Br J Radiol 69:335–340

Nord RH (1992) Work in progress: a cross-calibration study of four DXA instruments designed to culminate in intermanufacturer standardization. Osteoporos Int 2:210–211

Orwoll ES, Oviatt SK, Mann T (1990) The impact of osteophytic and vascular calcifications on vertebral mineral density measurements in men. J Clin Endocrinol Metab 70:1202–1207

Pacheco EM, Harrison EJ, Ward KA, Lunt M, Adams JE (2002) Detection of osteoporosis by dual energy X-ray absorptiometry (DXA) of the calcaneus: is the WHO criterion applicable? Calcif Tissue Int 70:475–482

Parfitt AM (1990) Interpretation of bone densitometry measurements: disadvantages of a percentage scale and a discussion of some alternatives. J Bone Miner Res 5:537–540

Patel R, Blake GM, Herd RJM, Fogelman I (1997) The effect of weight change on DXA scans in a 2 year prospective clinical trial of cyclical etidronate therapy. Calcif Tissue Int 61:393–399

Patel R, Blake GM, Fogelman I (2004) An evaluation of the United Kingdom Osteoporosis Society position statement on the use of peripheral dual-energy X-ray absorptiometry. Osteoporos Int 15:497–504

Peel N, Eastell R (1993) Measurement of bone mass and turnover. Baillieres Clin Rheumatol 7:479–498

Peel N, Johnson A, Barrington NA, Smith TW, Eastell R (1993) Impact of anomalous vertebral segmentation on the measurements of bone mineral density. J Bone Miner Res 8:719–723

Poole KE, Compston JE (2006) Osteoporosis and its management. BMJ 333(7581):1251–1256

Pietrobelli A, Formica C, Wang Z, Heymsfield SB (1996) Dual-energy X-ray absorptiometry body composition model: review of physical concepts. Am J Physiol 271(6 Pt 1) E941–951

Prentice A, Parsons TJ, Cole TJ (1994) Uncritical use of bone mineral density in absorptiometry may lead to size-related artifacts in the identification of bone mineral determinants. Am J Clin Nutr; 60:837–842

Prince RL (2007) Calcium and vitamin D – for whom and when. Menopause Int 13:35–37

Quek ST, Peh WC (2002) Radiology of osteoporosis. Semin Musculoskelet Radiol 6:197–206

Rea JA, Steiger P, Blake GM, Fogelman I (1998) Optimizing data acquisition and analysis of morphometric X-ray absorptiometry. Osteoporos Int 8:177–183

Rea JA, Li J, Blake GM, Steiger P, Genant HK, Fogelman I (2000) Visual assessment of vertebral deformity by X-ray absorptiometry: a highly predictive method to exclude vertebral deformity. Osteoporos Int 11:660–668

Rea JA, Chen MB, Li J, Marsh E, Fan B, Blake GM, Steiger P, Smith IG, Genant HK, Fogelman I (2001) Vertebral morphometry: a comparison of long-term precision of morphometric X-ray absorptiometry and morphometric radiography in normal and osteoporotic subjects. Osteoporos Int 12:158–166

Roberts MG, Cootes TF, Pacheco EM, Adams JE (2007) Quantitative fracture detection on Dual Energy X-ray Absorptiometry (DXA) images using shape and appearance models. Acad Radiol 14:1166–1178

Royal College of Physicians (1999) Osteoporosis: guidelines for prevention and treatment. Royal College of Physicians, London, UK, p 63–70

Royal College of Physicians (2000) Osteoporosis: clinical guidelines for prevention and treatment. Update on pharmacological interventions and an algorithm for management. Royal College of Physicians, London, UK, pp 1–16

Salle BL, Braillon P, Glorieux FH, Brunet J, Cavero E, Meunier PJ (1992) Lumbar bone mineral content measured by dual energy X-ray absorptiometry in newborns and infants. Acta Paediatr 81:953–958

Sambrook P, Cooper C (2006) Osteoporosis. Lancet 367 (9527):2010–2018

Sawyer AJ, Bachrach LK, Fung EB (Eds) (2006) Bone densitometry in growing patients; guidelines for clinical practice. Humana Press http://www.humanapress.com

Sanchez MM, Gilsanz V (2005) Pediatric DXA measurements Pediatr Endocrinol Rev 2 Suppl 3:337–341

Schott AM, Cormier C, Hans D, Favier F, Hausherr E, Dargent-Molina P, Delmas PD, Ribot C, Sebert JL, Breart G, Meunier PJ (1998) How hip and whole-body bone mineral density predict hip fracture in elderly women: the EPIDOS Prospective Study. Osteoporos Int 8:247–254

Sievanen H, Oja P, Vuori I (1992) Precision of dual energy x-ray absorptiometry in determining bone mineral density and content of various skeletal sites. J Nucl Med 33:1137–1142

Smyth PP, Taylor CJ, Adams JE (1999) Vertebral shape: automatic measurement with active shape models. Radiology 211:571–578

Soininvaara T, Kroger H, Jurvelin JS, Miettinen H, Suomalainen O, Alhava E (2000) Measurement of bone density around total knee arthroplasty using fan-beam dual energy X-ray absorptiometry. Calcif Tissue Int 67:267–272

Tothill P, Hannan WJ (2000) Comparison between Hologic QDR 1000 W, QDR 4500A, and Lunar Expert dual-energy X-ray absorptiometry scanners for measuring total bone and soft tissues. Ann N Y Acad Sci 904:63–71

van Rijn RR, van der Sluis IM, Link TM, Grampp S, Guglielmi G, Imhof H, Glüer C, Adams JE, van Kuijk C (2003) Bone densitometry in children: a critical appraisal. Eur Radiol 13:700–710

van Staa TP, Dennison EM, Leufkens HG, Cooper C (2001) Epidemiology of fractures in England and Wales. Bone 29:517–522

Vokes T, Bachman D, Baim S, Binkley N, Broy S, Ferrar L, Lewiecki EM, Richmand B, Schousboe J; International Society of Clinical Densitometry (2006) Vertebral fracture assessment: the 2005 ISCD Official Positions. J Clin Densitom 9:37–46

Ward KA, Mughal Z, Adams JE (2006) Tools for measuring bone in children and adolescents. In: Bone densitometry in growing patients; guidelines for clinical practice. Editors: Sawyer AJ, Bachrach LK, Fung EB Humana Press http://www.humanapress.com pp 15–40

Ward KA, Ashby RL, Roberts SA, Adams JE, Mughal MZ (2007) UK reference data for the Hologic QDR Discovery dual energy X-ray absorptiometry scanner in healthy children aged 6–17 years. Arch Dis Child 92:53–59

Warner JT, Cowan FJ, Dunstan FD, Evand WD, Webb DK, Gregory JW (1998) Measured and predicted bone mineral content in healthy boys and girls aged 6–18 years: adjustment for body size and puberty. Acta Paediatr 87:244–249

Wilkinson JM, Peel NF, Elson RA, Stockley I, Eastell R (2001) Measuring bone mineral density of the pelvis and proximal femur after total hip arthroplasty. J Bone Joint Surg Br 83:283–288

Wilson CR, Fogelman I, Blake GM, Rodin A (1991) The effect of positioning on dual-energy X-ray absorptiometry of the proximal femur. Bone Miner 13:69–76

Wishart J, Horowitz M, Need A, Nordin BE (1990) Relationship between forearm and vertebral mineral density in postmenopausal women with primary hyperparathyroidism. Arch Intern Med 150:1329–1331

World Health Organisation Study Group (1994) Assessment of fracture risk and its application to screening for postmenopausal osteoporosis. World Health Organisation, Geneva, Switzerland (WHO Technical Report Series 843)

Young JT, Carter K, Marion MS, Greendale GA (2000) A simple method of computing hip axis length using fan-beam densitometry and anthropomorphic measurements. J Clin Densitom 3:325–331

Vertebral Morphometry

Giuseppe Guglielmi and Daniele Diacinti

CONTENTS

G. Guglielmi, MD
Professor of Radiology, University of Foggia, Viale Luigi Pinto, 71100 Foggia, Italy
D. Diacinti, MD
Department of Clinical Sciences, University "La Sapienza", Roma, Italy

8.1 Introduction

Vertebral fractures are the most common of all osteoporotic fractures and are present in a significant percentage (25%) of the population over the age of 50, resulting in >400,000 in the US and >1 million in Europe per year (Cooper 1995; Cummings and Melton 2002; Davies et al. 1996; Finnern and Sykes 2003; Ismail et al. 1999; Jackson et al. 2000; Melton LJ III 1997; O'Neill et al. 1996; Roy et al. 2003). Vertebral fractures are associated with an increased mortality rate (Center et al. 1999; Kado et al. 1999) and loss of independence and impaired quality of life (Burger et al. 1997; Fink et al. 2003; Nevitt et al. 1998; Schlaich et al. 1998).

Even asymptomatic vertebral fractures could have clinical consequences for the patient because of the increased, approximately five-fold risk of future fractures that may be symptomatic (Lindsay et al. 2001). For these reasons the prevention of future fractures for patients with vertebral fractures has been considered the endpoint in clinical trials on osteoporosis therapy (Chesnut III et al. 2004; Ettinger et al. 1999; Liberman et al. 1995; Mc Closkey et al. 2001; Neer et al 2001; Reid et al. 2000). It is in the accurate diagnosis of asymptomatic vertebral fractures that radiologists make perhaps the most significant contribution to osteoporotic patient care. In everyday clinical practice, the qualitative reading of spinal radiographs is still the standard tool to identify vertebral fractures. The assessment by radiologists of conventional radiographs of the thoracic and lumbar spine in lateral and anterior-posterior (AP) projections generally is uncomplicated, allowing the identification of moderate and severe vertebral fractures, as wedge, end-plate (mono-or biconcave), and crush fractures (Fig. 8.1). Since the majority of vertebral fractures appear as mild vertebral deformities without visible discontinuity of bone architecture, often occurring in the absence of specific trauma and remaining asymptomatic, the visual

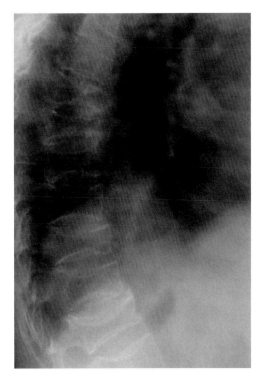

Fig. 8.1. Multiple vertebral fractures: crushing, wedging and biconcavity

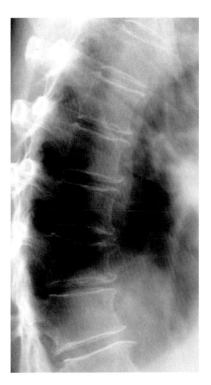

Fig. 8.2. Visual SQ assessment of vertebral fractures: moderate wedging (grade 2 with 25%–40% reduction in anterior height) of T9

radiological approach may lead to disagreement about whether a vertebra is fractured (HEDLUND and GALLAGHER 1988). In an effort to improve the accuracy of the diagnosis of vertebral fractures the semiquantitative assessment (SQ) and the quantitative measurement of vertebral heights (e.g., vertebral morphometry) were introduced more than a decade ago for the definition of vertebral fractures.

8.2
Visual Semiquantitative (SQ) Method

In this approach the conventional radiographs are evaluated by skeletal radiologists or experienced clinicians in order to identify and classify the vertebral fractures (GENANT et al. 1993). Vertebrae T4–L4 are graded by visual inspection and without direct vertebral measurement as normal (grade 0), mild but "definite" fracture (grade 1 with approximately 20%–25% reduction in anterior, middle, and/or posterior height and 10%–20% reduction in area), moderate fracture (grade 2 with approximately 25%–40%

reduction in any height and 20%–40% reduction in area), and severe fracture (grade 3 with approximately 40% or greater reduction in any height and area) (Fig. 8.2). Additionally, a grade 0.5 was used to designate a borderline deformed vertebra that was not considered to be a definite fracture (Table 8.1).

Incident fractures are defined as those vertebrae that show a higher deformity grade on the follow-up radiographs. The SQ method is a simple but standardized approach that provides reasonable reproducibility, sensitivity, and specificity, allowing excellent agreement for the diagnosis of prevalent and incident vertebral fractures to be achieved among trained observers using a semiquantitative method (GENANT et al. 1996).

However, this method has some limitations. In cases of subtle deformities (some mild wedges in the midthoracic region and bowed endplates in the lumbar region) the distinction between borderline deformity (grade 0.5) and definite mild (grade 1) fractures can be difficult and sometimes arbitrary (Fig. 8.3). Another limitation, relatively unimportant, of visual SQ assessment is the poor reproducibility or concordance in distinguishing the three grades of prevalent fractures.

Table 8.1. Semiquantitative (SQ) grading scheme

Fractures	Grading	Vertebral heights	Area
Absent	0	Normal	Normal
Uncertain	0.5	"Borderline"	"Borderline"
Mild	1	Reduction of 20%–25%	Reduction of 10%–20%
Moderate	2	Reduction of 25%–40%	Reduction of 20%–40%
Severe	3	Reduction >40%	Reduction >40%

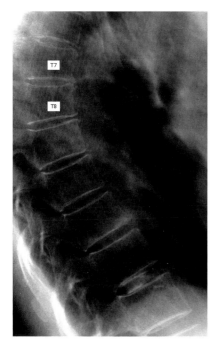

Fig. 8.3. Limits of visual SQ method: "borderline" deformities (grado 0.5) or definite mild fracture (grade 1 with 20%–25% reduction in anterior height) of T7 and T8?

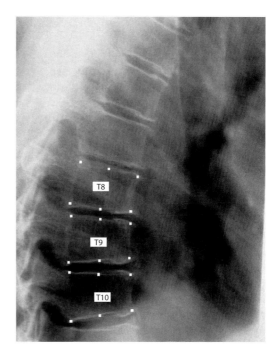

Fig. 8.4. MRX: measurement of vertebral heights showed mild wedging of T8 (ha/hp=0.80), T9 (ha/hp=0.78) and T10 (ha/hp=0.74)

8.3
Vertebral Morphometry

Quantitative vertebral morphometry involves making measurements of vertebral body heights. In fact, these measurements may be made on conventional spinal radiographs (MRX, morphometric X-ray radiography) or on absorptiometry images (MXA, morphometric X-ray absorptiometry).

8.3.1
Morphometric X-Ray Radiography (MRX)

This technique was introduced as early as 1960 by BARNETT and NORDIN, who used a transparent rule to measure vertebral heights on conventional lateral radiographs of the thoracolumbar spine. Before performing the measurement of vertebral heights, the reader has to identify the vertebral levels; to make this easier, T12 and L1 should be seen on both the lateral thoracic and lumbar radiographs. The vertebral bodies should be marked so that they can be more easily identified in other reading sessions or when compared with follow-up radiographs. On lateral radiographs, with six-point placement – the most widely used technique (JERGAS and SAN VALENTIN 1995) – the four corner points of each vertebral body from T4 to L5 (or L4, because of the highly variable shape of L5) and additional points in the middle of the upper and lower endplates are manually marked (Fig. 8.4).

8.3.2
Digital Morphometric X-Ray Radiography (MRX)

More than a decade ago some investigators (DIACINTI et al. 1995b; NICHOLSON et al. 1993) developed a computerized method to assess the vertebral dimensions from digital images of spine radiographs, captured by means of a scanner. Post-processing of the digital images can highlight the endplate and the four corners of vertebral bodies allowing points to be placed more precisely. After the radiographs have been digitized, the operator manually chooses the four corners of a vertebra. The software automatically determines the midpoints between anterior and posterior corner points of the upper and lower endplates. The operator then selects the true midpoints by moving the calipers along a vertical line joining the vertebral endplates. The x and y coordinates of each point are stored in the computer, which calculates the posterior, middle, and anterior heights (H_p, H_m, H_a) of each vertebra, from T4 to L5 and specific indices derived from height measurements for defining vertebral deformities. More recently a semi-automated software solution based on a statistical model-based vision approach, has been commercialized (MorphoXpress, P&G Pharmaceuticals, Rusham Park, Egham, UK). (Fig. 8.5)This system has several advantages, one of which consists in the fact that the statistical shape models approach by applying simple constraints on the parameters, generates shape used to describe the underlying image which will always remain within physically reasonable bounds (SMYTH et al. 1999; COOTES and TAYLOR 2001). Another advantage of this approach is given by the improvement of the workflow and in the overall positive results in terms of diagnostic accuracy (2.1% CV) and precision (1.68% CV) (unpublished data).

8.3.3
Limits of MRX

MRX enables quantitative assessment of thoracic and lumbar spine with a relatively good reproducibility; however, it is important that the radiographs are performed according to standardized procedures (BANKS et al. 1995) to achieve good quality as well as to allow comparisons of vertebral dimensions between individuals and between multiple radiographs of the same individual. Firstly, it is important that the films are exposed properly, because

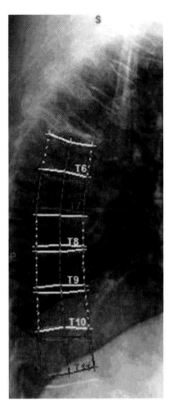

Fig. 8.5.
MORPHO-X-EXPRESS report

the image quality may have a substantial impact on the manual point placement process. Furthermore, because of the vertebral distortion due to the cone beam geometry the same centering of the X-ray beam (e.g., T7 and L3) should be used. Identification of vertebral levels on radiographs of lumbar and thoracic spine may be difficult at times (e.g., anatomic variants of the lumbosacral transition or the thoracolumbar junction). Manual point placement is carried out according to HURXTHAL (1968), who proposed excluding the uncinate process at the posterosuperior border of the thoracic vertebrae and the Schmorl's nodes and osteophytes from vertebral height measurement. When the outer contours of the endplate are not superimposed (incorrect patient positioning or severe scoliosis) the middle points are placed in the centre between the upper and the lower contour.

In the case of serial X-rays it is important to use the same focus to film distance to avoid the apparent decrement of vertebral heights. In fact, a 10.2 cm increase in tube-to-film distance results in a 6.4% decrease in measured posterior height, a 5.5% decrease in measured anterior height, and a 3.5% decrease in measured vertebral area (GALLAGHER et al. 1988).

Thus it is necessary, primarily, that the radiographs are good quality; furthermore, the vertebral morphometry should be performed by trained observers for spine image analyses, resulting in good inter-observer measurement precision (GARDNER et al. 2001).

8.3.4
Morphometric X-Ray Absorptiometry (MXA)

To overcome some limitations of MRX, a new technique called morphometric X-ray absorptiometry (MXA) has been developed by the two major manufacturers of dual-energy X-ray absorptiometry (DXA) equipment: Hologic, Inc. (Waltham, Mass.) and General Electric/Lunar (Madison, Wis.) (ADAMS 1997; STEIGER and WAHNER 1994). In Hologic systems, two views of the thoracic and lumbar spine are acquired: a posteroanterior (PA) scan and a lateral scan. The PA image is acquired in order to visualize spinal anatomy such as scoliosis, to determine the centerline of the spine. This information is used in subsequent lateral scans to maintain a constant distance between the centre of the spine and the X-ray tube for all subjects at all visits, regardless of patient position or degree of scoliosis, thus eliminating the geometric distortion (BLAKE et al. 1994). Each lateral scan covers a distance of 46 cm , imaging the vertebrae from L4 to T4. The GE/Lunar scanner determine the starting position of the lateral morphometry scan by positioning a laser spot 1 cm above the iliac crest. The scan range for the GE/Lunar systems is determined by measuring the length between the iliac crest and the armpit. The lateral scan can be acquired using a single-energy X-ray beam with a very short scan time (12 s). However, the analysis may be affected by soft tissue artifacts in the image caused by the prominent imaging of lung structures. These artifacts are absent from the dual-energy scan, which, however, takes between 6 min (array mode) and 12 min (fast and high definition modes). After the scan, the program automatically identifies vertebral levels and indicates the centres of the vertebrae. The six-point placement for the determination of the vertebral heights is semiautomated. The operator uses a mouse pointing device to specify the 13 locations of the anterior inferior corner of the vertebrae from L4 to T4. Then the MXA software computes the positions of the remaining five vertebral points for each. To guide the operator during image analysis of follow-up scans the vertebral endplate markers from the previous scan are superimposed on the current scan improving long-term precision. After the analysis is finished, a final report is displayed. It gives information on the measured vertebral body heights and their ratios, and includes an assessment of the patient's fracture status based on normative data and different models for fracture assessment using quantitative morphometry (Fig. 8.6).

8.3.5
Limits of MXA

The principal source of error for MXA is the relatively limited spatial resolution of the lateral spine scans obtained by DXA technique compared to conventional radiographs, which use a fast screen to provide a spatial resolution of approximately 5 lp/mm. However in the new DXA scanners, Discovery (Hologic, Inc.) and Prodigy (GE/Lunar, Inc.) the spatial resolution has been improved by a factor of two, achieved by doubling the number of detectors and by even finer collimation of the X-ray beam. Another major limitation of the MXA is the limited visualization in the single-energy images of the upper thoracic spine (T4 and T5) and thoracolumbar junction as a result of overlying soft-tissue and bony (ribs, shoulder blade) structures. Dual-energy images are able to visualize the entire spine, but may result in very noisy images that do not allow a clear distinction of anatomic structures. In adipose patients the MXA images may prove very noisy because the increased soft-tissue thickness reduces the photon flux significantly.

8.4
Comparison Between MRX and MXA

Both MRX and MXA have good precision, the intra-operator CV ranging from 1.2% for MXR to 3.4% for MXA, while the interoperator CV ranges from 1.9% to 5.3% according to various authors (ADAMS 1997; BLAKE et al. 1997; HARVEY et al. 1998). For MXA the precision obtained with two systems, Hologic and GE/Lunar, is similar (CRABTREE et al. 2000; FERRAR et al. 2001). MXA overcome some of the patient-positioning and exposure factor problems inherent in conventional radiography. In fact the scanner arm of some models of densitometers can be rotated 90°, so that lateral scans can be obtained with the patient in the supine position without repositioning. A fur-

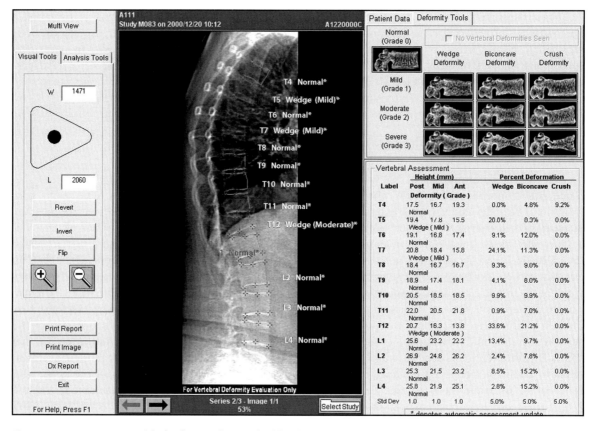

Fig. 8.6. MXA scan report with the data on the vertebral height measurements

ther advantage of MXA when using the scanning fan-beam geometry of DXA devices is the absence of distortions and magnification effects inherent in the standard X-ray technique (KALENDER and EIDLOTH 1991). The main attraction of MXA is that the effective dose-equivalent to the patient is considerably lower than for conventional radiography (LEWIS and BLAKE 1995; NJEH et al. 1999). While MXA is able to assess the entire spine in a single image, in conventional radiography radiographs of the lumbar and thoracic spine have to be taken separately, so the identification of the vertebral levels to perform MXR may be difficult at times. Furthermore, the improved image spatial resolution in the new DXA scanners allows better visualization of the upper thoracic vertebrae (REA et al. 1998). Table 8.2 summarizes advantages and limitations of MRX and MXA. There have been various comparative studies carried out (EDMONDSTON et al. 1999; FERRAR et al. 2000; REA et al. 1998, 2000a; STEIGER et al. 1994) that have found excellent agreement between qualitative and quantitative radiographic assessment using fan-beam dual-energy DXA images,

particularly for moderate and severe deformities in osteoporotic populations. A large proportion of vertebrae are not visualized sufficiently for analysis on MXA scans and this reduces the number of vertebral fractures identified, particularly in the upper thoracic spine. However, other authors (REA et al. 1998) have shown that high-speed fan-beam DXA imaging was feasible in a clinical population, allowing visualization of a substantial proportion of the vertebrae, using a rapid (10-s) single-energy imaging mode during suspended respiration.

8.5
Morphometric Vertebral Fractures

Because there is no "gold standard" of deformity, it may sometimes be difficult to discriminate the osteoporotic vertebral fracture from a normal variant of vertebral shape or from a vertebral deformation that may have occurred long ago (KLEEREKOPER

Table 8.2. Comparative characteristics of radiographs vs. fan-beam DXA in spine imaging

Parameter	Radiographs	Fan-beam DXA
Image resolution	5 lp/mm	0.5–1 lp/mm
Radiation dose	800 µSv	< 10 µSv
Lateral images required	2	1
Imaging geometry	Cone-beam	Fan-beam
Cone beam distortion	Yes	No
Patient positioning	Lateral	Supine
Patient anatomy (scoliosis, obesity)	Possible Compensation	Not possible Compensation
Vertebrae visualized	All from T4 to L5	Poorly visualized T4–T6

and Nelson 1992). Furthermore, there is variation in vertebral size and shape at different levels of the spine; the anterior and posterior vertebral height increases from T3 to L2, but for L3–L5 the posterior height is lower than the anterior height (Djoumessi et al. 2004). Vertebral size also varies between individuals: large people tend to have larger vertebrae (Johnell et al. 1997). Therefore, to identify a fracture, ratios of vertebral heights for individual vertebrae are compared with the normal values for that vertebra.

8.5.1
Morphometric Reference Data

Several approaches have been developed to determine the reference values of vertebral bodies heights. Some authors have used a sample of premenopausal women, assuming that the prevalence of vertebral fractures is very low in this population (Smith-Bindman et al. 1991).This approach may not be feasible for many studies because it involve radiation exposure for fertile women. Moreover, it has been demonstrated that vertebral heights change significantly with age, showing rates of loss of 1.2–1.3 mm/year (Cline et al. 1989; Diacinti et al. 1995a; Nicholson et al. 1993). Age-related decrease of vertebral heights influences the definition of the normal range of vertebral shape, since a deformity which may be in excess of 2SD from the mean in younger subjects may be well within this limit 20 years later. Other authors (Evans et al. 1993; Melton et al. 1989) have selected a subsample of postmenopausal women in which all vertebrae have been judged to be normal (unfractured) on the radiographs by an expert reader. A third approach for defining normal vertebral dimensions uses the values of a population that includes postmenopausal

women with and without vertebral fractures (Black et al. 1991).

Also, in a large study (Rea et al. 1998) the authors have shown that reference ranges of vertebral heights derived from MRX studies may not be applicable to MXA, in view of the observed differences between their MXA mean values when compared with MRX values reported in the earlier studies (Gallagher and Hedlund 1989; Hermann et al. 1993). The differences observed led to a tendency for lower MXA critical values for detection of vertebral deformities, suggesting the use of technique-specific reference ranges. However, reference ranges are not generally applicable to different populations, genders, or ages, because the differences in vertebral size are too large (O'Neill et al. 1994) and some true fractures may be found within the normal range for the population. The preliminary report of an Italian multicentre study (Diacinti et al. 2005) showed that vertebral heights of 569 "normal" Italian women measured from T4–L4 using VFA on Lunar Prodigy (GE Healthcare) densitometers in all vertebrae were significantly smaller than the existing values collected from "normal" American women.

For this reason reference ranges should be established in the population under study, using the same technique, and derived from "normal" subjects or by "data trimming" of a population-based-sample.

8.5.2
Morphometric Algorithms of Vertebral Fracture

There is still disagreement about establishing a threshold of height reduction which would allow unequivocal discrimination between vertebral fractures, deformities, and normal shape (Ziegler et al. 1996). Various morphometric algorithms to define vertebral fractures have therefore been developed.

MELTON et al. (1989) introduced an "adjusted algorithm" based on analysis of vertebral height ratios corrected by an adjustment factor. A vertebral body was fractured if any of three height ratios – anterior to posterior height (H_a/H_p for wedge), middle to posterior height (H_m/H_p for biconcavity) and posterior to posterior height of adjacent vertebra (rH_p for crush) – was reduced by more than 15% compared to the normal ratio for that level. The method developed by EASTELL et al. (1991) classified vertebral fractures by type of deformity (wedge, biconcavity, or crush) and further by degree of deformity as grade 1 or grade 2 based on vertebral height ratios below 3SD or 4SD of a respective normal range for that vertebral level. This approach fails when three or more consecutive posterior deformities are present, and for this reason McCLOSKEY et al. (1993) suggested using a predicted posterior height (H_{pp}) that represents the mean of up to four individual predicted posterior heights for each vertebra. Thus, it is not possible to measure accurately the true and false positive rates of various morphometric definitions of vertebral fractures because there is no "gold standard" for defining a vertebral fracture. In fact, results show wide discordances between the studies on the prevalence of vertebral fractures, ranging from 33% to 85% (SMITH-BINDMAN et al. 1991; GRADOS et al. 2001) and clinical trials have also shown that the estimated incidence of new vertebral fractures in postmenopausal osteoporosis varies markedly, from 6 to 83 fractures per 100 patient years (NEVITT et al. 1999; LUNT et al. 2002; HOCHBERG et al. 1999). In particular, less stringent criteria (e.g., -2SD) result in too many false positive results, because they identify as fractures some deformities that may represent developmental abnormalities. By contrast, a more stringent cutoff level, such as 4SD, results in a lower false positive rate (MELTON et al. 1998).

8.5.3
Can Vertebral Morphometry Predict a Vertebral Fracture?

The number of vertebral fractures may not be representative of the severity of spinal osteoporosis, especially in the case of biconcavity fractures, which represent deformations of only the endplate. For this reason, some methods have been developed to estimating the deformity of overall thoracic and lumbar spine. MINNE et al. (1988) and SAUER et al. (1991) developed the Spine Deformity Index (SDI)

to quantify spinal deformity and assess progression of vertebral deformation during follow-up. Other authors (MAZZUOLI et al. 1998) introduced new morphometric indices to quantify the spinal deformity, namely, sums of anterior, middle and posterior heights (AHS, MHS, PHS) of the respective 14 vertebral body heights from T4 to L5. There is a strong correlation between these indices and the lumbar bone mineral density (L-BMD), suggesting their use as fracture risk indices.

Irregularity in the curvature of the spine can be quantified as the integrated average of the ratios of the anterior to posterior vertebral heights of adjacent vertebrae. This Spinal Curvature Irregularity Index (SCII) is a measure of the 'smoothness' of the spinal curvature. A large SCII is correlated with the presence of vertebral deformities (ZEBAZE et al. 2004).

8.6
Comparison of Semiquantitative (SQ) Visual and Quantitative Morphometric Assessment of Vertebral Fractures

A vertebral deformity is not always a vertebral fracture, but a vertebral fracture is always a vertebral deformity. There are many causes of vertebral deformities, and the correct differential diagnoses for them can be achieved only by visual inspection and expert interpretation of a radiograph. The quantitative morphometry is unable to distinguish osteoporotic vertebral fractures by vertebral deformities due to other factors, such as degenerative spine and disc disease. This limitation is a characteristic of any method of quantitative morphometry, but the limited spatial resolution of the DXA images in MXA may increase this problem (GENANT and JERGAS 2003). On the other hand, MRX, with its superior image quality, has the potential for qualitative reading of the radiographs to aid the differential diagnosis. In fact, although it is recognized that the visual interpretation of radiographs is subjective, it is also true that an expert eye can better distinguish between true fractures and vertebral anomalies than can quantitative morphometry. For example, the distinction between a fractured endplate and the deformity associated with Schmorl's nodes can only be made visually by an experienced observer; as is the case for the diagnosis of the wedge-shaped appearance caused by remodeling of the vertebral bodies in degenerative disc disease (LENCHIK et al. 2004).

Some comparative studies (GENANT et al. 1996; BLACK et al. 1995; WU et al. 2000) found a high concordance between different quantitative morphometric approaches and visual semiquantitative evaluation for prevalent vertebral fractures defined as moderate or severe. In these cases there was a strong association with clinical parameters (bone mineral density, height loss, back pain, incidence of subsequent deformities).

8.7
Instant Vertebral Assessment (IVA) by DXA

Recently the visual semiquantitative (SQ) method for identification of vertebral fractures has applied to images of the spine acquired by fan-beam DXA devices. This method is called "instant vertebral assessment "(IVA) by Hologic and "vertebral fracture assessment" (VFA) by GE/Lunar (Fig. 8.7). IVA has been compared with SQ evaluation of spinal radiographs demonstrating good agreement (96.3%, $k = 0.79$) in classifying vertebrae as normal or deformed in the 1978 of 2093 vertebrae deemed analyzable on both the DXA scans and conventional radiographs (REA et al. 2000b). IVA showed good sensitivity (91.9%) in the identification of moderate/severe SQ deformities and an excellent negative predictive value (98%) to distinguish subjects with very low risk of vertebral fractures from those with possible fractures. The disagreement between the IVA and the SQ method resulted from the poor image quality, particularly in the upper thoracic vertebrae that were not visualized sufficiently for analysis. Although some vertebral fractures were missed by IVA, all patients with prevalent vertebral fractures were identified; therefore, for the identification of patients with fracture, visual assessment of DXA scans had 100% sensitivity and specificity (FERRAR et al. 2003). This means that if IVA had

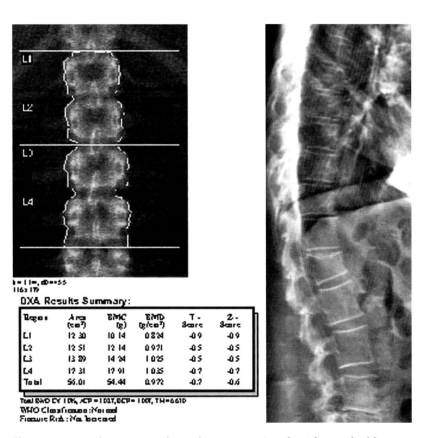

Fig. 8.7. Integrated assessment of BMD for osteoporosis and IVA for vertebral fracture. A 57-year-old female with normal BMD (lumbar spine T-score –0.7 and proximal femur T-score –0.8), and moderate fracture of L2

been used as a diagnostic pre-screening tool at the first assessment, all the patients with prevalent vertebral fracture would have been correctly referred for radiography to confirm the diagnosis. Also, the "normal" subjects can then be excluded prior to performing conventional radiographs and further time-consuming and costly methods of vertebral deformity assessment such as SQ by an experienced radiologist and/or quantitative morphometry. So, with its low radiation and good precision, IVA could be utilized to identify vertebral fractures in populations affected by conditions different from osteoporosis, but with high vertebral fracture risk, i.e. liver or kidney transplant patients (GIANNINI et al. 2001; MAZZAFERRO et al. 2005).

8.8
Conclusion

A combination of semiquantitative visual and quantitative morphometric methods may be the best approach to fracture definition, as suggested by the NATIONAL OSTEOPOROSIS FOUNDATION (1998) and by KANIS et al. (2002). Currently, there is no consensus on which morphometric technique should be used, or how to evaluate patients at risk of osteoporosis. MRX, based upon assessment of conventional radiographs, has, unlike MXA, the potential for qualitative reading of the radiographs by a trained radiologist or highly experienced clinician who can distinguish between vertebral anomalies and true fractures and detect technical artifacts on the films which might increase the errors on quantitative morphometry.

However, in view of the relatively low radiation dose to the patient and the excellent agreement with the visual SQ method for the identification of vertebral deformities, the visual or morphometric assessment of lateral DXA spine images may have the potential for use as a prescreening tool. If all vertebrae are visualized adequately by lateral DXA images and classified as normal by IVA or MXA, the patient could be classified as normal. If all vertebrae are not visualized by DXA and if one or more deformities are detected by IVA or MXA, it will be necessary to acquire conventional radiography to check for further prevalent deformities and to identify the nature of the deformity. The availability of a rapid, low-dose method for assessment of vertebral frac-

tures, using advanced fan-beam DXA devices, provides a practical means for integrated assessment of BMD and vertebral fracture status. This approach allows the identification of most osteoporotic vertebral fractures, even asymptomatic ones, in patients with low BMD, thus improving selection of candidates for therapeutic intervention.

References

Adams JE (1997) Single and dual energy X-ray absorptiometry. In: Guglielmi G, Passariello R, Genant HK (eds) Bone densitometry: an update. Eur Radiol 7[Suppl 2]:S20–S31

Banks LM, van Kuijk C, Genant HK (1995) Radiographic technique for assessing osteoporotic vertebral fracture. In: Genant HK, Jergas M, van Kuijk C (eds) Vertebral fracture in osteoporosis. University of California Osteoporosis Research Group, San Francisco, pp 131–147

Barnett E, Nordin BEC (1960) Radiographic diagnosis of osteoporosis: new approach. Clin Radiol 11:166–174

Black DM, Cummings SR, Stone K et al (1991) A new approach to defining normal vertebral dimensions. J Bone Miner Res 6:883–892

Black DM, Palermo L, Nevitt MC et al (1995) Comparison of methods for defining prevalent vertebral deformities: the study of osteoporotic fractures. J Bone Miner Res 10:890–902

Blake GM, Rea JA, Fogelman I (1997) Vertebral morphometry studies using dual-energy X-ray absorptiometry. Semin Nucl Med 27:276–290

Blake GM, Jagathesan T, Herd RJM, Fogelman I (1994) Dual X-ray absorptiometry of the lumbar spine: the precision of paired anteroposterior/lateral studies. Br J Radiol 67:624–630

Burger H, Van Daele PLA, Gashuis K et al (1997) Vertebral deformities and functional impairment in men and women. J Bone Miner Res 12:152–157

Center JR, Nguyen TV, Schneider D et al (1999) Mortality after all major types of osteoporotic fractures in men and women: an observational study. Lancet 353:878–882

Chesnut CH III, Skag A, Christiansen C et al (2004) Effects of oral ibandronate administered daily or intermittently on fracture risk in postmenopausal osteoporosis. J Bone Miner Res 19:1241–1249

Cline MG, Meredith KE, Boyer JT et al (1989) Decline in height with age in adults in a general population sample: estimating maximum height and distinguishing birth cohort effect from actual loss of stature with aging. Hum Biol 61:415–425

Cooper C (1995) Epidemiology of vertebral fractures in western populations. Spine: 8 State of art reviews 8:1–11

Cootes TF, Taylor CJ (2001) Statistical models of appearance for medical image analysis and computer vision. Proc SPIE Medical Imaging 3:138–147

Crabtree N, Wright J, Walgrove A et al (2000) Vertebral morphometry: repeat scan precision using the Lunar Expert-XL and the Hologic 4500A. A study for the 'WISDOM' RCT of hormone replacement therapy. Osteoporos Int 11:537–543

Cummings SR, Melton LJ (2002) Epidemiology and outcomes of osteoporotic fractures. Lancet 359:1761–1767

Davies KM, Stegman MR, Heaney RP et al (1996) Prevalence and severity of vertebral fracture: The Saunders County Bone Quality Study. Osteoporos Int 6:160–165

Diacinti D, Acca M, D'Erasmo E et al (1995) Aging changes in vertebral morphometry. Calcif Tissue Int 57:426–429

Diacinti D, Acca M, Tomei E (1995) Metodica di radiologia digitale per la valutazione dell'osteoporosi vertebrale. Radiol Med 91:1–5

Diacinti D, Francucci C, Fiore C et al (2005) Italian preliminary reference data of normal vertebral dimensions for Morphometric X-ray Absorptiometry (MXA): Normal Morphometric Dexa (NORMODEXA) Study. Bone 36[Suppl 2]:S351

Djoumessi RMZ, Maalouf G, Wehbe J et al (2004) The varying distribution of intra- and intervertebral height ratios determines the prevalence of vertebral fractures. Bone 35:348–356

Eastell R, Cedel SL, Wahner H et al (1991) Classification of vertebral fractures. J Bone Miner Res 6:207–215

Edmondston SJ, Price RI, Valente B et al (1999) Measurement of vertebral body height: ex vivo comparison between morphometric X-ray absorptiometry, morphometric radiography and direct measurements. Osteoporosis Int 10:7–13

Ettinger B, Black DM, Mitlak BH et al (1999) Reduction of vertebral fracture risk in postmenopausal women with osteoporosis treated with raloxifene: results from a 3-year randomised clinical trial – Multiple Outcomes of Raloxifene Evaluation (MORE) Investigators. JAMA 282:637–645

Evans SF, Nicholson PHF, Haddaway MJ et al (1993) Vertebral morphometry in women aged 50–81 years. Bone Miner 21:29–40

Ferrar L, Jiang G, Barrington NA et al (2000) Identification of vertebral deformities in women: comparison of radiological assessment and quantitative morphometry using morphometric radiography and morphometric X-ray absorptiometry. J Bone Miner Res 15:575–585

Ferrar L, Jiang G, Eastell R (2001) Short-term precision for morphometric X-ray absorptiometry. Osteoporos Int 12:710–715

Ferrar L, Jiang G, Eastell R et al (2003) Visual identification of vertebral fractures in osteoporosis using morphometric X-ray absorptiometry. J Bone Miner Res 18:933–938

Fink HA, Ensrud KE, Nelson DB et al (2003) Disability after clinical fracture in postmenopausal women with low bone density: The Fracture Intervention Trial (FIT). Osteoporos Int 14:69–76

Finnern HW, Sykes DP (2003) The hospital cost of vertebral fractures in the EU: estimates using national datasets. Osteoporos Int 14:429–436

Gallagher JC, Hedlund LR, Stoner S et al (1988) Vertebral morphometry: normative data. Bone Miner 4:189–196

Gardner JC, von Ingersleben G, Heyano SL et al (2001) An interactive tutorial-based training technique for vertebral morphometry. Osteoporosis Int 12:63–70

Genant HK, Jergas M (2003) Assessment of prevalent and incident vertebral fractures in osteoporosis research. Osteoporos Int 14 [Suppl 3]:S43–S55

Genant HK, Wu CY, van Kuijk C et al (1993) Vertebral fracture assessment using a semiquantitative technique. J Bone Miner Res 8:1137–1148

Genant HK, Jergas M, Palermo L et al (1996) Comparison of semiquantitative visual and quantitative morphometric assessment of prevalent and incident vertebral fractures in osteoporosis. J Bone Miner Res 11:984–996

Giannini S, Nobile M, Dalle Carbonare L et al (2001) Vertebral morphometry by X-ray absorptiometry before and after liver transplant: a cross-sectional study. Eur J Gastroenterol Hepatol 13:1201–1207

Grados F, Roux C, de Vernejoul MC et al (2001) Comparison of four morphometric definitions and a semiquantitative consensus reading for assessing prevalent vertebral fractures. Osteoporos Int 12:716–722

Harvey SB, Hutchinson KM, Rennie EC et al (1998) Comparison of the precision of two vertebral morphometry programs for the Lunar Expert-XL imaging densitometer. Br J Radiol 71:388–398

Hedlund LR, Gallagher JC (1988) Vertebral morphometry in diagnosis of spinal fractures. Bone Miner 5:59–67

Hermann AP, Brixen K, Andresen J et al (1993) Reference values for vertebral heights in Scandinavian females and males. Acta Radiologica 34:48–52

Hochberg MC, Ross PD, Black D et al (1999) Larger increases in bone mineral density during alendronate therapy are associated with a lower risk of new vertebral fractures in women with postmenopausal osteoporosis. Fracture Interventional Trial Research Group. Arthritis Rheum 42:1246–1254

Hurxthal LM (1968) Measurement of vertebral heights. AJR Am J Roentgenol 103:635–644

Ismail AA, Cooper C, Felsenberg D et al (1999) Number and type of vertebral deformities: epidemiological characteristics and relation to back pain and height loss. European Vertebral Osteoporosis Study Group. Osteoporos Int 9:206–213

Jackson SA, Tenenhouse A, Robertson L and the CaMos Study Group (2000) Vertebral fracture definition from population-based data: preliminary results from the Canadian Multicenter Osteoporosis Study (CaMos). Osteoporos Int 11:680–687

Jergas M, San Valentin R (1995) Techniques for the assessment of vertebral dimensions in quantitative morphometry. In: Genant HK, Jergas M, van Juijk C (eds) Vertebral fracture in osteoporosis. University of California Osteoporosis Research Group, San Francisco, pp 163–188

Johnell O, O'Neill T, Felsenberg D et al (1997) Anthropometric measurements and vertebral deformities. European Vertebral Osteoporosis Study (EVOS) Group. Am J Epidemiol 146:287–293

Kado DM, Browner WS, Palermo L et al (1999) Vertebral fractures and mortality in older women: study of osteoporotic fractures research group. Arch Intern Med 159:1215–1220

Kalender WA, Eidloth H (1991) Determination of geometric parameters and osteoporosis indices for lumbar vertebrae from lateral QCT localizer radiographs. Osteoporos Int 1:197–200

Kanis JA, Black D, Cooper C et al (2002) A new approach to the development of assessment guidelines for osteoporosis. Osteoporos Int 13:527–536

Kleerokoper M, Nelson DA. (1992) Vertebral fracture or vertebral deformity? Calcif Tissue Int 50:5–6

Lenchik LL, Rogers LF, Delmas PD et al (2004) Diagnosis of osteoporotic vertebral fractures: importance of recognition and description by radiologists. AJR Am J Roentgenol 183:949–958

Lewis MK, Blake GM. (1995) Patient dose in morphometric X-ray absorptiometry (letter). Osteoporos Int 5:281–282

Liberman UA, Weiss SR, Broll J et al (1995) Effect of oral alendronate on bone mineral density and the incidence of fractures in postmenopausal osteoporosis. N Engl J Med 333:1437–1443

Lindsay R, Silverman S, Cooper C et al (2001) Risk of new vertebral fracture in the year following a fracture. JAMA 285:320–323

Lunt M, Ismail AA, Felsenberg D et al (2002) Defining incident vertebral deformities in population studies: a comparison of morphometric criteria. Osteoporos Int 13:809–815

Mazzaferro S, Diacinti D, Proietti E et al (2006) Morphometric X ray absorptiometry in the assessment of vertebral fractures in renal transplant patients. Nephrol Dial Transplant 21:466–471

Mazzuoli GF, Diacinti D, Acca M et al (1998) Relationship between spine bone mineral density and vertebral body heights. Calcif Tissue Int 62:486–490

Mc Closkey EV, Spector TD, Eyres KS et al (1993) The assessment of vertebral deformity: a method for use in population studies and clinical trials. Osteoporos Int 3:138–147

Mc Closkey E, Selby P, de Takats D et al (2001) Effects of clodronate on vertebral fracture risk in osteoporosis: a 1 year interim analysis. Bone 28:310–315

Melton LJ III (1997) Epidemiology of spinal osteoporosis. Spine 22[Suppl 1]:2S–11S

Melton LJ III, Kan SH, Frye MA et al (1989) Epidemiology of vertebral fractures in women. Am J Epidemiol 129:1000–1010

Melton LJ III, Egan KS, O'Fallon WM et al (1998) Influence of fracture criteria on the outcome of a randomized trial of therapy. Osteoporos Int 8:184–191

Minne HW, Leidig C, Wuster CHR et al (1988) A newly developed spine deformity index (SDI) to quantitative vertebral crush fractures in patients with osteoporosis. Bone Miner 3:335–349

National Osteoporosis Foundation (1998) Osteoporosis: review of the evidence for prevention, diagnosis and treatment and cost-effectiveness analysis. Osteoporos Int 8 [Suppl 4]:S1–S85

Neer RM, Arnaud CD, Zanchetta JR et al (2001) Effect of parathyroid hormone (1-34) on fractures and bone mineral density in postmenopausal women with osteoporosis. N Engl J Med 344:1434–1441

Nevitt MC, Ettinger B, Black DM et al (1998) The association of radiographically detected vertebral fractures with back pain and function: a prospective study. Ann Intern Med 128:793–800

Nevitt MC, Ross PD, Palermo L et al (1999) Association of prevalent vertebral fractures, bone density, and alendronate treatment with incident vertebral fractures: effect of number and spinal location of fractures. Bone 25:613–619

Nicholson PHF, Haddaway MJ, Davie MWJ et al (1993) A computerized technique for vertebral morphometry. Physiol Meas 14:195–204

Nicholson PHF, Haddaway MJ, Davie MWJ et al (1993) Vertebral deformity, bone mineral density, back pain and height loss in unscreened women over 50 years. Osteoporos Int 3:300–307

Njeh CF, Fuerst T, Hans D et al (1999) Radiation exposure in bone mineral density assessment. Appl Radiat Isot 50:215–236

O'Neill T.W., D.Felsenberg D, Varlow J et al (1996) The prevalence of vertebral deformity in European men and women: The European Vertebral Osteoporosis Study. J Bone Miner Res 11:1010–1018

O'Neill TW, Varlow J, Felsenberg D et al (1994) Variation in vertebral heights ratios in population studies. J Bone Miner Res 9:1895–1907

Rea JA, Steiger P, Blake G et al (1998) Optimizing data acquisition and analysis of morphometric X-ray absorptiometry. Osteoporos Int 8:177–183

Rea JA, Chen MB, Li J et al (2000a) Morphometry X-ray absorptiometry and morphometric radiography of the spine: a comparison of prevalent vertebral deformity identification. J Bone Miner Res 15:564–574

Rea JA, Li J, Blake GM et al (2000b) Visual assessment of vertebral deformity by X-ray absorptiometry: a highly predictive method to exclude vertebral deformity. Osteoporos Int 11:660–668

Reid DM, Hughes RA, Laan RFJM et al (2000) Efficacy and safety of daily risedronate in the treatment of corticosteroid-induced osteoporosis in men and women: a randomized trial European Corticosteroid-Induced Osteoporosis Treatment Study. J Bone Miner Res 15:1006–1013

Roy DK, O'Neill TW, Finn JD, Lunt M, Silman AJ et al (2003) Determinants of incident vertebral fracture in men and women: results from the European prospective Osteoporosis Study (EPOS). Osteoporos Int 14:19–26

Sauer P, Leidig G, Minne HW et al (1991) Spine Deformity Index (SDI) versus other objective procedures of vertebral fracture identification in patients with osteoporosis: a comparative study. J Bone Miner Res 6:227–238

Schlaich C, Minne HW, Bruckner T et al (1998) Reduced pulmonary function in patient with spinal osteoporotic fractures. Osteoporos Int 8:261–267

Smith-Bindman R, Cummings SR, Steiger P et al (1991) A comparison of morphometric definitions of vertebral fracture. J Bone Miner Res 6:25–34

Smyth PP, Taylor CJ, Adams JE (1999) Vertebral shape: automatic measurement with active shape models. Radiology 211:571–578

Steiger P, Cummings SR, Genant HK, Weiss H and the Study of Osteoporotic Fractures Research Group (1994) Morphometric X-ray absorptiometry of the spine: correlation in vivo with morphometric radiography. Osteoporos Int 4:238–244

Steiger P, Wahner H (1994) Instruments using fan-beam geometry. In: Wahner H, Fogelman I (eds) The evaluation of osteoporosis. Dual energy X-ray absorptiometry in clinical practice. Martin Dunitz, Ltd., London; pp 281–288

Wu C, van Kuijk C, Jiang Y et al (2000) Comparison of digitized images with original radiography for semiquantitative assessment of osteoporotic fractures. Osteoporos Int 11:25–30

Zebaze R, Maalouf G, Maalouf N, Seeman E (2004) Loss of regularity in the curvature of the thoracolumbar spine: a measure of structural failure. J Bone Miner Res 19:1099–1104

Ziegler R, Scheidt-Nave C, Leidig-Bruckner G (1996) What is a vertebral fracture? Bone 18:169–177

Spinal Quantitative Computed Tomography

Rick R. van Rijn and Cornelis van Kuijk

CONTENTS

9.1
Introduction

Since its development by Sir Godfrey N. Hounsfield (1919–2004) and Allan M. Cormack (1924–1998), computed tomography (CT) rapidly became a widely used imaging technique in diagnostic radiology (Cormack 1973; Hounsfield 1973). Currently it is ubiquitously available and used for a multitude of indications. CT imaging shows cross-sectional human anatomy and additionally provides a three-dimensional dataset which can be used for image reconstruction and analysis in several planes or three-dimensional settings. With modern multi-row detector CT (MDCT) systems and associated imaging software, it enables an inside look into the patient.

In skeletal radiology, CT is used to study bone pathology ranging from traumatic lesions to bone neoplasms. In addition to morphologic information, CT also provides information about the attenuation of the tissues studied. Attenuation can be enhanced by using contrast media and in this way additional information can be acquired. The attenuation values can be extracted from the raw CT data from which the image is reconstructed. These values can also be used to estimate the density of tissues. In spinal quantitative computed tomography (QCT), it is these values that play a role in the assessment of bone mineral density (BMD) (Cann and Genant 1980; Kalender et al. 1987). QCT is a relatively inexpensive technique; the estimated cost is $20,000 for a calibration phantom and image analysis software which can be used on standard CT systems which are available worldwide.

9.2
Technique

9.2.1
Basic Principles

In CT a two-dimensional map of attenuation values is reconstructed from a dataset, acquired when the X-ray tube rotates around the patient. These attenuation values are measured in several directions and are presented in Hounsfield units (HU) according to the equation:

$$HU = 1000 \cdot (\mu_T - \mu_w)/\mu_w$$

R. R. van Rijn, MD, PhD
Department of Radiology, Academic Medical Center, University of Amsterdam, Meibergdreef 9, 1105 AZ Amsterdam, The Netherlands
C. van Kuijk, MD, PhD
Department of Radiology, University Medical Center 'St. Radboud' Nijmegen, Geert Grooteplein-Zuid 10, 6525 GA Nijmegen, The Netherlands

where HU is the CT number in Hounsfield units, μ_T is the linear attenuation coefficient of the tissue and μ_w is the linear attenuation coefficient of water.

By definition the CT number of water is 0 HU and tissues with an attenuation coefficient lower than that of water, e.g. fat and air, have a negative CT number (the HU of air is set at –1000). The CT number of bone, with a higher coefficient, will be positive.

In spinal QCT a calibration standard is used to recalculate the CT numbers to bone mineral equivalent values. Usually a calibration phantom made of different concentrations of calcium hydroxyapatite in water-equivalent plastic is used. The mean CT numbers of the different compounds are measured and plotted against the concentrations using linear regression. The mean CT numbers measured in objects of interest can then be recalculated to bone mineral equivalent values, usually in milligrams of calcium hydroxyapatite per millilitre.

9.2.2
Spinal QCT Scanning Protocol

9.2.2.1
Dedicated QCT Technique

The patient is placed supine on the CT table and a cushion is placed under the knees to reduce the lumbar lordosis. The calibration standard is placed

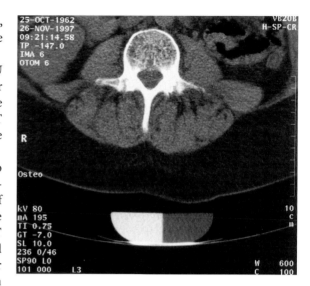

Fig. 9.2. Axial view with calibration device under the patient

under the lumbar spine. A lateral scanogram (topogram) is made from approximately T12 to S1 (Fig. 9.1). This is used to position the axial slices through the mid-vertebral levels of three to four consecutive lumbar vertebral bodies, where vertebral bodies showing a fracture are omitted from the analysis. The axial scans are made perpendicular to the axis of the spine (Fig. 9.2). Usually a low-dose technique is used (80 kVp, 140 mAs), with a slice thickness of 10 mm.

9.2.2.2
Analysis

The axial images can be automatically analyzed with commercially available software either on-line or off-line. Within the vertebral bodies regions of interest are defined and the attenuation values are determined and recalculated to bone equivalent values. The region of interest is usually confined to the inner vertebral body that contains solely trabecular bone (Fig. 9.3). Trabecular bone has a high metabolic turnover, and changes in mineralization or in the amount of bone will be measurable more easily with techniques that can selectively measure trabecular bone. This makes QCT unique as a modality for estimating true BMD.

A spinal QCT study, including imaging and analysis, takes less than 10 min, while patient scanning can be performed much faster. The effective dose equivalent is approximately 60–100 mSv, comparable to that of a standard X-ray of the chest.

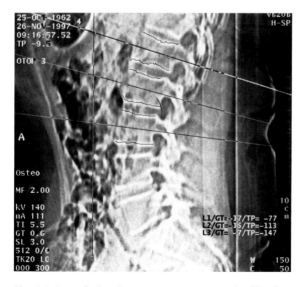

Fig. 9.1. Lateral view (scanogram or topogram) of lumbar spine with slice positioning at L1–L3

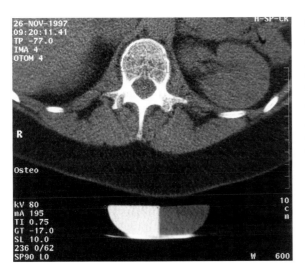

Fig. 9.3. Axial view with regions of interest placed automatically in vertebral body and within the cortical rim

9.2.2.3
Use of Clinical CT

An increasing number of patients undergo CT for clinical indications outside the field of bone densitometry. Therefore, interest has risen to use these non-dedicated CT scans for bone densitometry purposes (BODEN et al. 1989; GUDMUNDSDOTTIR et al. 1993; HOPPER et al. 2000; LINK et al. 2004). With modern day multiple detector CT (MDCT) scanners a complete volume of the abdomen is routinely scanned. This volume dataset can then be used to provide both three-dimensional reconstructions of complete vertebral bodies as well as targeted two-dimensional reconstructions of parts of vertebral bodies. Major differences compared to dedicated QCT measurements include, firstly, the angulation of the tube – the gantry will not be tilted to obtain an axial slice perpendicular to the spinal axis. Secondly, the CT tube settings will be significantly higher as most clinical studies in adults will use 120 kv and mAs values ranging from 180 to 260. A caveat for the use of clinical CT studies is in order: as post-contrast CT will significantly increase the BMD since hematopoietic bone marrow will enhance and increase the measured HU.

Whichever scan technique is used, it is important that the scanning protocol is never changed, especially when patients are followed over time.

9.2.2.4
Analysis

In 1989 BODEN et al. proposed using internal references, e.g. muscle and fat, to assess BMD on clinical CT scans of the abdomen (BODEN et al. 1989). As muscle and subcutaneous fat have known linear attenuation coefficients it is possible to calibrate the HU. Several years later GUDMUNDSDOTTIR et al. (1993) reported on the use of these internal references in 187 healthy women. Although it has shown to correlate significantly with QCT using an external reference phantom (r=0.96) this technique has not been widely adopted.

LINK et al. (2004) reported on a study of 20 cadaver vertebrae; in their study a significant difference between QCT and helical CT BMD was found. However, a significantly strong correlation between these two measurements was found and the authors present a conversion factor to derive BMD-QCT values from helical CT. In their in-vivo study they made use of a calibration standard which is routinely used in QCT. As this calibration standard is relatively thin it can be fitted within a standard CT mattress and does not interfere with patient comfort. The analysis of the helical CT data is identical to QCT and can be performed on-line or off-line using automated software.

9.2.2.5
Volumetric QCT

In 1999 LANG et al. proposed the use of three-dimensional vertebral data in order to eliminate the influence of slice positioning and bone rotation errors, such as those seen in patients with scoliosis, inherent to single-slice QCT on BMD assessment. Using dedicated software a 3D image of the lumbar vertebrae is generated (Fig. 9.4). Using the 3D dataset the influence of orientation along the Z-axis can be reduced and a volumetric BMD, encompassing approximately 70% of the total vertebral body volume, can be computed.

9.3
Interpretation of Data

The results of QCT studies are expressed as bone equivalent values, usually expressed in milligrams of

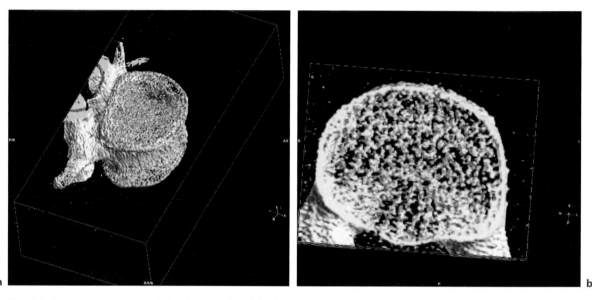

a   b

Fig. 9.4a,b 3D reconstruction of a lumbar vertebra (**a**). The cutaway slice (**b**) shows the cortex and trabecular structure of the vertebral body

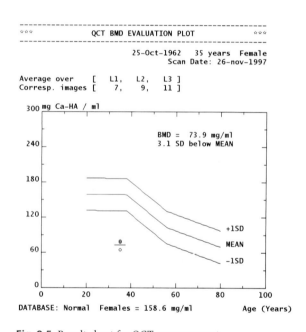

```
***            QCT BMD EVALUATION PLOT           ***
------------------------------------------------------
                        25-Oct-1962    35 years  Female
                            Scan Date: 26-nov-1997

Average over   [  L1,   L2,   L3 ]
Corresp. images [   7,    9,   11 ]
```

Fig. 9.5. Result sheet for QCT measurement

```
***          QCT BMD EVALUATION RESULTS          ***
------------------------------------------------------
                        25-Oct-1962    35 years  Female
                            Scan Date: 26-nov-1997

                    Bone mineral density
                    [mg Ca-HA / ml]:

corresp. image       trabecular          cortical
------------------------------------------------------
[T12]
[ L1]           7         79.3             235.4
[ L2]           9         77.6             272.5
[ L3]          11         64.6             288.2
[ L4]
[ L5]
------------------------------------------------------

average                  73.9 +- 8.1      265.4 +- 27.1
```

Fig. 9.6. QCT result placed in normogram

calcium hydroxyapatite per millilitre (Fig. 9.5). They are given per vertebral body as well as a mean value for all vertebral bodies measured. These values are compared to normative data (Fig. 9.6). The results of the measurements are usually presented both in the form of absolute values and as Z-scores and T-scores, i.e. compared to normative data. Based on the T-score the osteoporotic status of the patient can be assessed using the WHO guidelines (T-score

< –2.5 equals osteoporosis, T-score between –2.5 and –1.0 equals osteopenia and a T-score > –1.0 is considered to be normal).

Normative data are gender- and race-specific, as both factors influence BMD accrual (Yu et al. 1999). Women have a different BMD curve over age compared to men. In women accelerated bone loss is observed in the years immediately after the onset of menopause, superimposing the normal physiologic bone loss that occurs in both men and women in aging. Absolute normal BMD values are race-dependent, as black men and women have higher BMD values and Asian men and women have lower BMD values compared to white men and women.

It has been shown that low bone density increases fracture risk. Both biomechanical in vitro studies and clinical in vivo studies comparing patients with and without osteoporotic fractures show that there is a convincing risk gradient: the lower the BMD the higher the risk of bone fracture (HAIDEKKER et al. 1999).

The reported reproducibility of QCT measurements is in the range of 2%. With this level of precision a 5.6% or higher difference in bone density over time in a single patient is significant. Measured accelerated bone loss in immediately postmenopausal women is 5%–10% in the first years as measured with spinal QCT. Some treatments have been shown to increase bone density by 5%–10% (WIMALAWANSA 2000). These losses and gains are much larger than those seen with other techniques, such as dual- and single-energy X-ray absorptiometry (DXA, SXA). This is due to the selective trabecular measurement with QCT, which makes this technique very sensitive in measuring changes in a relatively short follow-up period.

Reproducibility is influenced by CT scanner variability (which is why scan techniques should be standardized), by operator variability (which is why the analysis is automated with minimal operator interaction), and by patient variability (the patient should not move during scanning). The accuracy of the measurement is influenced by the choice of calibration material as well as by unsuspected changes in vertebral marrow content (the same is true for DXA) (KUIPER et al. 1996). One should be aware of the fact that both myelofibrosis and marrow changes in hematopoietic disorders can affect the measurements.

9.4
Comparison with Other Techniques

Spinal QCT has been shown to be superior in discriminating between patients with and those without osteoporosis compared to other bone densitometry techniques (BERGOT et al. 2001; GENANT et al. 1985; GRAMPP et al. 1997; ITO et al. 1997). It has also been argued that due to its selective trabecular measurement spinal QCT is very sensitive to changes in bone density. This implies that using QCT will enable the clinician to assess the efficacy of osteoporosis treatment in an earlier stage, enabling him to either prolong or change the treatment regimen and to motivate the patient (since osteoporosis as a disease does not have direct consequences on the patient's health, therapy compliance has been reported to be low) (McCOMBS et al. 2004).

Furthermore, QCT is insensitive to factors that confound DXA data, such as degenerative disease of the spine and extraspinal calcifications, such as atherosclerosis of the aorta, in the scanning path of DXA (GUGLIELMI et al. 2005). Like DXA, but unlike SXA and to a lesser extend quantitative ultrasound, QCT can measure those skeletal parts that are predisposed to fractures in the osteoporotic syndrome, such as the vertebral bodies, distal radius and hip.

Although spinal QCT is used all over the world, it has not achieved the impact that DXA measurements have had on the study of the osteoporotic syndrome and its multiple proposed therapies. One aspect that plays a role in this under-utilisation is the fact that CT machines are used in a wide variety of clinical settings and problems; given the time constraints and the clinical implications most departments of radiology will choose to use their CT systems for other clinical applications than bone densitometry. DXA on the other hand is a relatively cheap technique dedicated (though not proven to be better) to bone densitometry.

9.5
Dual-Energy QCT

The CT technique most widely used is a single-energy technique as discussed above. However, it has been shown that single-energy QCT is liable to accuracy errors due to the marrow fat content within the vertebral bodies, as it lowers the average attenuation values and thus causes underestimation of bone mineral density. For this reason, dual-energy techniques have been developed that use either pre-postprocessing or post-processing methods to improve the accuracy of the measurement at the cost of decreased reproducibility. These techniques are not widely used (VAN KUIJK et al. 1990).

References

Bergot C, Laval-Jeantet AM, Hutchinson K, Dautraix L, Caulin F, Genant HK (2001) A comparison of spinal quantitative computed tomography with dual energy X-ray absorptiometry in European women with vertebral and nonvertebral fractures. Cacif Tissue Int 68:74–82

Boden SD, Goodenough D, Stockham CD, Dina T, Allman RM (1989) Precise measurement of vertebral bone density using computed tomography without the use of an external reference phantom. J Digit Imaging 2:31–38

Cann CE, Genant HK (1980) Precise measurement of vertebral mineral content using computed tomography. J Comput Assist Tomogr 4:493–500

Cormack AM (1973) Reconstruction of densities from their projections, with applications in radiological physics. Phys Med Biol 18:195–207

Genant HK, Ettinger B, Cann CE, Reiser U, Gordan GS, Kolb FO (1985) Osteoporosis: assessment by quantitative computed tomography. Othop Clin N Amer 16:557–568

Grampp S, Genant HK, Mathur A, Lang P, Jergas M, Takada M, Gluer CC, Chavez M (1997) Comparison of noninvasive bone mineral measurements in assessing age related loss, fracture discrimination, and diagnostic classification. J Bone Miner Res 12:697–711

Gudmundsdottir H, Jonsdottir B, Kristinsson S, Johannesson A, Goodenough D, Sigurdsson G (1993) Vertebral bone density in Icelandic women using quantitative computed tomography without on external reference phantom. Osteoporosis Int 3:84–89

Guglielmi G, Floriani I, Torri V, van Kuijk C, Genant HK, Lang TF (2005) Effect of spinal degenerative changes on volumetric bone mineral density of the central skeleton as measured by quantitative computed tomography. Acta Radiol 46:269–275

Haidekker MA, Andresen R, Werner HJ (1999) Relationship between structural parameters, bone mineral density and fracture load in lumbar vertebrae, based on high-resolution computed tomography, quantitative computed tomography and compression tests. Osteopororis Int 9:443–440

Hopper KD, Wang MP, Kunselman AR (2000) The use of clinical CT for baseline bone density assessment. J Comp Assisst Tomogr 24:869–899

Hounsfield GN (1973) Computerized transverse axial scanning (tomography). Br J Radiol 46:1016

Ito M, Hayashi K, Ishida Y, Uetani M, Yamada M, Ohki M, Nakamu T (1997) Discrimination of spinal fractures with various bone mineral measurements. Calcif Tiss Int 60:11–15

Kalender WA, Klotz E, Suess C (1987) Vertebral bone mineral analysis: an integrated approach with CT. Radiology 164:419–423

Kuiper JW, van Kuijk C, Grashuis JL, Ederveen AGH, Schütte HE (1996) Accuracy and the influence of marrow fat on quantitative CT and dual-energy X-ray absorptiometry measurements of the femoral neck in vitro. Osteoporosis Int 6:23–30

Lang TF, Li J, Harris ST, Genant HK (1999) Assessment of vertebral bone mineral density using volumetric quantative CT. J Comp Assisst Tomogr 23:130–137

Link TM, Koppers BB, Bauer J, Lu Y, Rummeny EJ (2004) In vitro and in vivo spiral CT to determine bone mineral density: initial experience in patients at risk for osteoporosis. Radiology 231:805–811

McCombs JS, Thiebaud P, McLaughlin-Miley C, Shi J (2004) Compliance with drug therapies for the treatment and prevention of osteoporosis. Maturitas 48:271–287

van Kuijk C, Grashuis JL, Steenbeek JM, Schütte HE, Trouerbach WT (1990) Evaluation of postprocessing dual-energy methods in quantitative computed tomography. Part II: Practical aspects. Invest Radiol 25:882–889

Wimalawansa SJ (2000) Prevention and treatment of osteoporosis: efficacy of combination of hormone replacement therapy with other antiresorptive agents. J Clin Densitom 3:187–201

Yu W, Qin M, van Kuijk C, Meng X, Cao J, Genant HK (1999) Normal changes in spinal bone mineral density in a Chinese population: assessment by quantitative computed tomography and dual-energy X-ray absorptiometry. Osteopororis Int 9:179–187

pQCT: Peripheral Quantitative Computed Tomography

Sven Prevrhal, Klaus Engelke, and Harry K. Genant

CONTENTS

S. Prevrhal, PhD
Musculoskeletal Quantitative Imaging Research Group, University of California, San Francisco, 185 Berry Street, Suite 350, San Francisco, CA 94107, USA
K. Engelke, PhD
Institute of Medical Physics, University of Erlangen, Henkestr. 91, 91052 Erlangen, Germany
and Synarc, Hamburg, Germany
H. K. Genant, MD
Osteoporosis and Arthritis Research Group, University of California, San Francisco, 505 Parnassus Avenue, San Francisco, CA 94143-0628, USA
and Synarc, San Francisco, USA

10.1
Introduction

Peripheral quantitative computed tomography (pQCT) for the forearm was introduced shortly after CT for medical imaging and several years before the development of spinal QCT (Genant and Boyd 1977; Rüegsegger 1974), as a volumetric extension to Cameron's projectional technique for bone mineral measurements (Cameron and Sorenson 1963). Compared to single photon absorptiometry (SPA), the advantages of pQCT are obvious: separate assessment of trabecular and cortical bone and determination of true volumetric density instead of areal bone mineral density (BMD).

However, despite the advantage of an early start and constant improvements in technology, for example replacing isotope sources with x-ray tubes, the clinical impact of pQCT in the field of osteoporosis has been rather small compared to projectional techniques such as SPA or DXA or volumetric assessment by spinal QCT. This may be explained in part by the late commercialization of pQCT. In particular, in the United States pQCT devices are rarely used for the assessment of osteoporosis in patients. Therefore, only a limited amount of data is available for pQCT.

Moreover, pQCT has never been integrated into large prospective studies largely because of this limited accessibility. While forearm BMD as measured by DXA is a confirmed predictor of forearm and hip fractures, the association of pQCT with fracture risk can currently only be inferred from cross-sectional data. Several studies using either DXA (Tucci et al. 1996) or pQCT (Schneider et al. 1999) indicate that, compared to the spine and femur, the forearm is less sensitive to treatment effects. It is known that appendicular cancellous bone is metabolically less active than the spongiosa at the axial skeleton, which might be explained by the lower appendicular hematopoietic tissue.

On the other hand, volumetric pQCT is not affected by bone shape and size, as are areal density measurements. This is important when determining BMD in the growing skeleton, when assessing biomechanical parameters such as cross-sectional moments of inertia, or when measuring cortical bone thickness. The contribution of these parameters to fracture risk prediction has not been fully evaluated yet, but the importance of compact bone may have been underestimated in the past and has recently gained more attention with the introduction of anabolic therapeutic agents such as parathyroid hormone (PTH). pQCT has a clear advantage over peripheral SXA and DXA in the differential assessment of their effects on the cortical and trabecular bone.

Two recent developments in technology have further increased the interest in forearm measurements. Firstly, a new in-vivo ultra-high spatial resolution device has been introduced for the assessment of structural parameters of the trabecular network to complement densitometric information. Secondly, the introduction of multidetector row technology in whole-body clinical CT scanners along with the increase in spatial resolution of these detectors has turned these devices into a potential alternative to pQCT, a term still reserved for the much smaller dedicated forearm and distal leg scanners. Whole-body scanners are widely available and offer very short scan times for true volumetric data acquisition, but typically data processing is only available as third-party software on offline workstations.

In this chapter, we will first briefly review the pQCT technology and introduce the devices most commonly used today. Then we will concentrate on the diagnostic performance of pQCT, with emphasis on the classical application of bone densitometry. Finally, new and emerging applications of pQCT will be discussed. The advantages of separating cortical from trabecular bone will be illuminated. Comparisons of pQCT with other established methods such as DXA will be included in most sections. The new developments discussed in the last paragraph will be introduced, but naturally the literature is still sparse.

Another application of pQCT is osteoporosis research in small laboratory animals, which is widely used in preclinical trials for the development of treatment strategies and pharmacological research (CAPOZZA et al. 1995; LALLA et al. 1998; SATO et al. 1995; SRIVASTAVA et al. 2000). Dedicated devices have been designed for small animals; however, this is an application beyond the scope of this chapter, which is limited to investigations in humans.

10.2
Bone Densitometry with pQCT

10.2.1
Overview and Scan Procedure

Peripheral QCT (pQCT) denotes quantitative computed tomography performed of the peripheral appendicular skeleton, usually at the distal forearm to assess trabecular and cortical BMD of the radius and ulna. Applications to the tibia and the proximal femur have also been reported. In contrast to spinal QCT, which utilizes clinical whole-body CT scanners and special analysis software, pQCT is performed with dedicated, more compact scanners with smaller gantries. As with spinal QCT, the average volumetric BMD inside a certain region of interest (ROI) is determined. BMD results, which are reported in milligrams per cubic centimeter, are calculated from the CT values using a calibration standard that, in the case of pQCT, is measured separately from the patient.

Patient examination starts with a projectional localizer scan (scout view). Tube and detector are fixed in the anterior–posterior position while the limb is inserted into the gantry. The scout view is used to locate the correct position of a single CT slice (single-slice mode) or of a scan range consisting of multiple slices (multislice mode). The tomogram(s) are usually analyzed automatically by segmenting cortical and trabecular regions and computing BMD results separately and jointly for both compartments. Although imaging multiple slices increases measurement time and radiation exposure, this mode offers higher precision because BMD results are averaged over a larger volume. Figure 10.1 shows two representative cross-sectional pQCT images.

To optimally evaluate trabecular bone in single-slice mode, the scan should be positioned ultra-distally at 4% of the ulnar length proximal to the radial endplate, as measured between the proximal end of the olecranon and distal edge of the ulnar styloid. On most machines, the operator only has to specify the radial endplate and the software will calculate the correct position. Multislice scans usually cover the radius from 4% to 10% of the ulnar length. On some scanners, an ultra-distal and a second, more proximally located region can be selected.

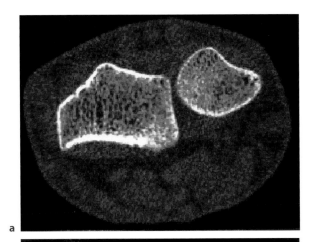
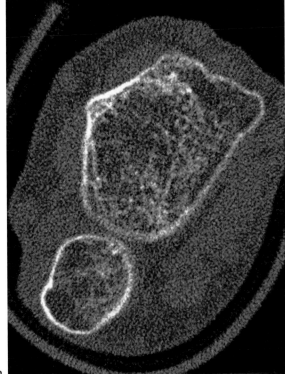

Fig. 10.1a,b. Two representative cross-sectional pQCT images of the distal forearm. **a** XCT-2000, **b** DensiScan 1000

10.2.2
Devices and Modes of Operation

Initially, pQCT devices used ^{125}I photon sources for radiation generation (HANGARTNER et al. 1987; RÜEGSEGGER 1974). While some of those scanners are still in use, all modern scanners employ X-ray tubes. Unlike DXA, pQCT is a single-energy technique. An X-ray energy for which the attenuation discrimination between fat/water and bone mineral

is optimized must be selected. The oil-cooled X-ray tubes are typically operated at 45–60 kV, resulting in effective energies of 30–45 keV after prefiltering to reduce beam hardening effects. In this energy range, the ratio of soft tissue to bone absorption is relatively low. Tube currents are on the order of 0.2–0.4 mA.

Table 10.1 lists the devices most commonly used in clinical routine and research applications along with some of their most important features. All scanners in the table have been or are commercially available. There are also a few dedicated laboratory scanners optimized for special applications, for example for very high precision (HANGARTNER 1993) or for thin-slice high-resolution investigations. The majority of clinical and research pQCT data has been collected with the devices listed in the table, in particular with the XCT-960. There are approximately 1,000 of these machines and the differently calibrated but otherwise identical XCT-900 in use today, most of them in Europe. The scientific literature mainly reports on these two types and more recently on the XCT-2000. We will explicitly note if a citation is based on another device.

All scanners listed in Table 10.1 are second-generation small-angle fan beam CT scanners with a limited number of detector elements that employ a slice-by-slice translation-rotation scan sequence. Although their scan speeds are slow compared to modern-day whole-body CTs, scan times are acceptable for the peripheral skeleton, where motion artifacts can easily reduced by proper fixation of arms or legs.

Some pQCT scanners such as the DensiScan 1000 have also been used to image the lower limb, in particular the tibia. However, because of the rather slow age- and treatment-related BMD changes at this skeletal location, this measurement mode has not found much use, and the literature is sparse (GROLL et al. 1999; RITTWEGER et al. 2000; SIEVÄNEN et al. 1998). The XCT-3000 also allows for assessment of the humerus (BRAUN et al. 1998) and may potentially be used to image the femoral shaft in slim people. Positioning the more proximal femur in elderly and obese patients can be difficult.

The applied effective dose in peripheral QCT is very low and comparable to axial DXA scans. Operator exposure is negligible, and additional radiation shielding is not required under current occupational dose limits in most countries.

Although currently the term "pQCT" is used in conjunction with the dedicated devices discussed above, clinical whole-body scanners can also used

Table 10.1. Technical details (manufacturer data) of the most widely distributed pQCT scanners

Model	DensiScan 1000	XCT 900/960[a]	XCT 2000/2000L[d]	XCT 3000	XtremeCT
Tube energy (kV)	50	45–49	45–69	45–60	60
Tube current (μA)	300	140	180	200–400	1000
Pixel size (μm)	80–300	300[a]	200–800	200–2000[b]	40–250[c]
Entrance dose/slice (μSv)	125	30	60	90	0.05[e]
Scan time/slice (min)	1–3	3	1.5	1.5	0.03
Slice thickness (mm)	1–1.5	2.4	2.1	2.2	0.08
Currently manufactured?	No	No	Yes	Yes	Yes
Company	Scanco	Stratec	Stratec	Stratec	Scanco

[a] Some scanners of the XCT900/960 line were equipped with serial scanning capabilities and smaller pixel sizes
[b] Data from (BRAUN et al. 1998)
[c] 100 μm at 10% MTF
[d] Compared to the XCT 2000 the currently manufactured XCT2000 L offers better positioning capabilities
[e] Due to very low slice thickness

for peripheral appendicular measurements. Compared to pQCT scanners, they offer a number of advantages. In particular, the tube intensity is much higher and with newer multirow detector technology several slices are scanned simultaneously, so true 3D data acquisition can be performed in seconds. For example a 10-cm scan of the complete distal forearm using 1-mm slice thickness takes typically less than 30 s. On most scanners, slice thickness can even be decreased to 0.5–0.7 mm. The principal advantage of such a scan is that changes in shape and bone mineral can be analyzed continuously from the ultra-distal to the one-third site. Effective dose values will increase from less than 1 μSv in the case of single-slice pQCT scanners to approximately 20–50 μSv, but these values are still negligible compared to the average annual background radiation of about 2,500 μSv in Europe and the US.

As whole-body scanners are not dedicated to quantitative BMD analysis, similar to spine or proximal femur scans, a calibration phantom must be scanned simultaneously with the patient in order to calibrate the Hounsfield units (HU) delivered by the scanner to BMD values. So far, whole-body scanners are not widely used for peripheral BMD measurements because the scanner manufacturers do not provide integrated analysis software, and because of the generally greater interest in central skeletal assessment. Third-party programs requiring image transfer to external analysis workstations must be used and so far no program exploiting the full potential of these scans is available. This is a clear disadvantage compared to the fully integrated pQCT scanners.

The XtremeCT is a novelty in pQCT because of its very high spatial resolution: 100 μm at 10% modulation transfer function (MTF) (see below). It can be used to assess not only bone mineral density and geometrical parameters, but also nearly histomorphometry-equivalent parameters of trabecular structure of the forearm and the tibia. Like many micro-CT devices, it is a cone-beam scanner equipped with a micro focus tube that delivers 1-mA output at 60 kVp and can scan the region of interest within 3 min and with under 5 μSv effective dose.

10.2.3
Spatial Resolution and Its Impact on the Assessment of Cortical Bone

Investigations of differential effects of age-related changes or pharmaceutical interventions on cortical and trabecular bone compartments, studies of bone development in children, and research in bone biomechanics make the cortex an interesting target for pQCT analysis. However, accurate segmentation and analysis of cortical bone requires that the imaging pQCT system have sufficient spatial resolution

It is important to understand that the pixel size in the reconstructed images and spatial resolution are two different issues. Unfortunately, scientific publications as well as manufacturers often report pixel sizes for spatial resolution. There are three main reasons: (1) pixel sizes may be easier to comprehend than parameters specifying the spatial resolution; (2) pixel sizes are easier to determine; and (3) pixel sizes are almost always smaller than the spatial resolution. However, their improper use can easily lead to misstating resolution of a given system.

Spatial resolution can be given as the full width half maximum value of the point spread function of the imaging system (FWHM$_{PSF}$) or as the 2%, 5%, or 10% value of its Fourier transform, the modulation transfer function (MTF) (WEBB 1998). In contrast, pixel sizes can be chosen arbitrarily during image reconstruction and do not characterize spatial resolution. The three-dimensional spatial resolution of course depends on the slice thickness as well. Few CT and almost no pQCT scanners have isotropic resolution. Therefore, the resolution in the reconstructed plane is often reported separately from the resolution perpendicular to this plane. This is very important in the ultra-distal radius because of its tapered geometry (SCHLENKER and VONSEGGEN 1976). An insufficiently low slice thickness can easily cause partial volume artifacts in the cortex at this location.

If the spatial resolution is too low, neither cortical thickness nor cortical density can be measured accurately. Moreover, it becomes irresolvable whether an observed change in cortical BMD is caused by a true change in BMD or a change in cortical thickness. PREVRHAL et al. showed that cortical density can be determined accurately as long as the thickness is larger than approximately four times the spatial resolution. Cortical thickness measurements are accurate until the thickness is smaller than the spatial resolution (PREVRHAL et al. 1999).

In pQCT systems used for densitometric measurements, in-plane pixel sizes vary from 80–100 μm (DensiScan 1000, XCT 2000) to approximately 300 μm (XCT 900/960). The manufacturers do not often report the more meaningful MTF values; therefore Table 10.1 lists pixel sizes only. Slice thickness varies from less than 1 mm up to 2.5 mm. Laboratory devices with even better spatial resolution are currently reserved for research (MÜLLER et al. 1996).

Accuracy studies using phantoms showed a decrease in measured cortical BMD at true cortical thickness values below 4 mm on an XCT-960 (AUGAT et al. 1998b) and below 2 mm on an XCT-2000 (BINKLEY and SPECKER 2000). For the XCT-960, the BMD underestimation amounted to 40% at a thickness of 1 mm. However, in the same phantom the decrease in cortical bone mineral content (BMC) amounted to only 6%, indicating segmentation effects. Indeed a (changeable) global threshold is used on the XCT scanners to separate cortical from trabecular bone and from soft tissue. Changing this threshold obviously changes results for cortical thickness and BMD (HASEGAWA et al. 2000), but there is no objective strategy for selecting one or several specific thresholds. Newer XCT software versions offer different user-selectable contour-finding modes for both cortical and trabecular bone, and predictably, the accuracy then becomes dependent on that choice in addition to the threshold. In the same study, however, it was found that the lower thresholds offered on these systems are too low (ASHE et al. 2006). Also, global partial volume correction schemes (RITTWEGER et al. 2004) typically rely on certain assumptions on shape and density of the objects that may not always be true, in particular if the object dimensions approach the spatial resolution of the scanner. Better approaches for segmenting the cortical bone using local relative thresholds or gradient techniques have been published (PREVRHAL et al. 1999).

Limitations in spatial resolution probably explain some of the controversial findings on differential age-related bone loss in cortical and trabecular bone. In cross-sectional studies on healthy women, some authors reported higher trabecular than cortical losses (BOONEN et al. 1997; NIJS et al. 1998; QIN et al. 2000), others comparable losses (GATTI et al. 1996; GRAMPP et al. 1995; HASEGAWA et al. 1997), but one longitudinal study observed higher trabecular than cortical loss (HERNANDEZ et al. 1997).

10.2.4
Standardization and Quality Control

Scanner comparability is important when upgrading devices, when comparing results from an individual patient scanned on different machines, or when comparing results in multicenter clinical trials using a variety of equipment. Cross-calibration of forearm densitometry including pQCT, DXA, and SPA scanners has been reported (PEARSON et al. 1994) using the European Forearm Phantom (EFP) (Fig. 10.2) (RÜEGSEGGER and KALENDER 1993) and a common normative database for forearm densitometry has been published (REEVE et al. 1996). However, forearm cross-calibration is much more difficult than cross-calibration at the spine. Even if only DXA devices are considered, analysis results vary substantially as there is no definition or agreement on a common ROI to be used on all scanners. Thus, it is not advisable to directly compare forearm results of an individual patient scanned on devices from different manufacturers (SHEPHERD et al. 2000a, b).

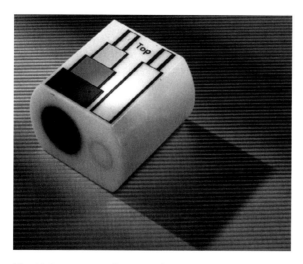

Fig. 10.2. European forearm phantom (EFP) used for the calibration of forearm densitometry

pQCT machines are typically stable enough to ensure that a baseline calibration at the factory using a standard phantom such as the EFP is sufficient. Although users are required to perform daily quality assurance by scanning a special phantom, these values are simply monitored and can trigger re-calibration as part of service maintenance, but are not used for daily re-calibration.

10.2.5
Precision and Accuracy

Tables 10.2 and 10.3 list published data for accuracy and precision of pQCT. Accuracy errors are systematic errors and describe the difference between the actual measurement and the true physical value. In densitometry, they are sometimes used interchangeably with the term "bias." Accuracy errors can be expressed in absolute or relative values. Precision, synonymous with reproducibility, is determined by random errors and describes a system's ability to consistently deliver the same results under unchanged measurement conditions. Precision is commonly reported either as root mean square standard deviation (SD) or as coefficient of variation (CV = SD / mean in %) of the repeated measurements.

When evaluating or comparing precision data, it is important to understand the nature of precision in densitometry. One must distinguish between phantom, in vitro, and in vivo precision, all of which can be measured with or without repositioning the phantom or subject between repeat scans, as well as

between short- and long-term precision. Consecutive phantom scans without repositioning typically yield minimum (short-term) precision errors, but more realistic errors can be obtained from short-term in vivo investigations with repositioning. In vivo short-term precision is given by the root mean square (RMS) SD or CV of repeat measurements from a number of subjects. To achieve sufficient statistical power, one should at least scan 27 subjects twice (or equivalently, 14 subjects three times each) (GLÜER et al. 1995).

The measurement of long-term precision in vivo is more complicated because the quantity one is interested in, for example BMD, may change within the subjects during the course of the measurements. One strategy to separate this effect from machine imprecision is to fit a regression line to the data of each individual separately and then pool the residual errors (GLÜER et al. 1995). In vivo precision is also affected by the choice of the individuals that are scanned. For example, it may be misleading to base the instrument's precision solely on young normals, since repositioning errors are larger in elderly and diseased patients. Reporting CVs instead of SDs facilitates the comparison of different devices but automatically increases apparent in vivo BMD precision errors in elderly people with lower BMD than younger people. If the SD is constant and absolute BMD decreases, CV increases. Therefore, one must be careful when comparing CVs of different devices or techniques. For instance, significantly different precision errors were found for cohorts of healthy premenopausal, healthy postmenopausal, and osteoporotic women (GRAMPP et al. 1995). We therefore included the mean age of the population samples in Table 10.3.

In clinical practice, high accuracy and precision are both important, the first for diagnosis, the latter for disease progression monitoring. Precision determines two important characteristics: The least significant change (LSC) and the monitoring time interval (MTI). LSC should be calculated using the long-term coefficient of variation of a technique (CV_{long}):

$$LSC = 1.96 \cdot (\sqrt{2} \cdot CV_{long})$$

Least significant change denotes the minimum true bone density change in a patient that can be measured by a densitometer with 95% confidence. In other words, if the change in the patient is smaller than the LSC then the chance of not detecting it will

Table 10.2. Accuracy of data published for pQCT derived from investigations of forearm specimens

Author	Device	No. of specimens	Parameter	Type of comparison	Results
TAKADA et al. 1996	XCT-960	7	BMC	Ash weight	$r=0.87$–0.95, CV$=9.7$–15.5% depending on number of slices
LOUIS et al. 1995b, 1996	XCT-960	27	Cortical thickness	Contact radiographs	$r=0.88$
			Cortical and total BMC	Neutron activation analysis, flame atomic absorption spectrometry	$r=0.86$–0.96, SEE$=7\%$–18%
AUGAT et al. 1998[a]	XCT-960	14	BMD	Whole-body QCT	$r^2>0.96$, RMSE$=6.2\%$
ASHE et al. 2006	XCT-2000	20[a]	BMC	Ash weight	Depending on resolution and edge detection

[a] Paired samples from ten donors

Table 10.3. Precision data in vivo published for pQCT at the forearm

Author	Device	Cohort	Short-term precision (with repositioning)[a]		Long-term precision[a]	
			In vitro	In vivo	In vitro	In vivo
BUTZ et al. 1994	XCT 900	$n=179$ age$=20$–79			- / - / 0.27	1.7 / 0.9 / 0.8
GUGLIELMI et al. 1997	XCT 900/960		- / - / 0.2-0.7		- / - / 0.2-0.7	
GUGLIELMI et al. 2000	XCT 960	$n=386$ age$=51$				1.6 / 0.9 / 0.8
GRAMPP et al. 1995	XCT 960	$n=20$ age$=31$		0.9 / 1.5 / 1.1		
GRAMPP et al. 1995	XCT 960	$n=20$ age$=62$		1.8 / 1.7 / 2.2		
GROLL et al. 1999	XCT 2000	$n=86$, cadaveric forearms, age$=80$	Distal radius 1.8 / - / 2.5 proximal radius - / 0.4–0.8 / 1.0–1.4 mid tibia - / 0.5 / 1.2 proximal/distal tibia 3.6 / - / 4.0			
TAKADA et al. 1996	XCT 960	$n=9$, cadaveric forearms	1.9 / - / 2.8			
SIEVÄNEN et al. 1998	XCT 3000	$n=19$ age$=32$	2.2 / 6.5 / -			
MÜLLER et al. 1989	DensiScan 1000			- / - / 0.3		
BOUTROY et al. 2005	XtremeCT[b]	$n=15$ age$=21$–47		0.9/1.7/1.0 3.0/3.2/2.8/1.2		

Exceptions are the studies of TAKADA (forearm specimen) and SIEVÄNEN (in vivo measurements at the femur and tibia)
[a] Values are given as %CV for trabecular / cortical / total BMD
[b] For the XtremeCT, %CV also given for TbN, TbTh, TbSp, and cTh

exceed 5%. If CV_{long} is unknown for the technique under consideration it may be replaced by short-term in vivo precision. MTI answers the question of the time between two measurements so that the change in a patient's bone density is at least equal to the LSC. MTI is calculated by:

$$MTI = LSC\ /\ (\%\ yearly\ rate\ of\ bone\ loss)$$

To be consistent, percent loss and precision values must be derived from the same cohort. The healthy postmenopausal population is most relevant for the calculation of LSC and MTI, but the fact that published precision data are often based on young healthy volunteers is a potential pitfall. MTI should be interpreted cautiously as the rate of bone loss may vary in a population. Since it is important to identify patients who lose bone rapidly it may be appropriate to use measurement intervals shorter than the MTI. LSC and MTI values for pQCT and other densito-metric techniques are given in Table 10.4.

10.2.6
Age-Related Changes

Age-related BMD changes in the healthy population are an important reference against which measurements of individual patients can be compared. The offset of an individual from the reference population is reported either as a Z-score (the difference from the age-matched population in units of standard deviations of this population) or as a T-score (the difference from the young healthy population at age 30, again in units of SD).

Figure 10.3 shows published normative data of pQCT in women compared to DXA at the forearm, spine, and hip. Besides the data shown in Fig. 10.3, a number of other authors have published age-related changes in a variety of cohorts. These data are sum-marized in Table 10.5.

The importance of the separate measurement of trabecular and cortical bone is supported by a small longitudinal study carried out by Ito et al. (1999b) using the DensiScan device. Age-related changes seen with forearm DXA were comparable to changes in pQCT total BMD, but were exceeded by pQCT tra-becular BMD. The latter were almost comparable to trabecular BMD changes in the spine, as observed by spinal QCT. As Table 10.5 suggests, devices may differ in their sensitivity to detect age-related changes.

With respect to the cortex, Russo et al. investi-gated cortical structural changes with aging at the tibia and found increasing porosity in both sexes. In men, both total and medullary cross-sectional area increased similarly with age, thereby leaving cortical area and moment of inertia constant. In women, the medullary cross-sectional area increased to a much larger extent, thereby diminishing cortical area and moment of inertia (Russo et al. 2006). Age at men-arche may influence the size of the medullary cavity of the distal radius as well (Rauch et al. 1999).

10.2.7
Fracture Discrimination and Response to Treatment

Data on fracture discrimination and response to treat-ment are relatively sparse. With respect to spinal frac-

Table 10.4. Least significant change (LSC) and monitoring time interval (MTI) for pQCT in comparison with other densi-tometric techniques

Technique and referenced literature	Precision (%)		LSC (%)		Loss (%/year)	MTI (years)	
	Min	Max	Min	Max		Min	Max
pQCT (trab.BMD) Grampp et al. 1995; Guglielmi et al. 2000; Reeve et al. 1997)	1.6	1.8	4.4	5.0	1.0	4.4	5.0
Axial QCT (Guglielmi et al. 1994; Kalender et al. 1989)	1.4	4	5.5	11.1	2.6	1.5	4.3
Spinal DXA (L1–4, PA) (Guglielmi et al. 1994) (loss from Hologic reference values)	0.5	1.5	1.4	4.2	0.78	1.8	5.3
Femoral neck DXA (Looker et al. 1998; Patel et al. 2000)	2.2	2.5	6.1	6.9	0.72	8.5	9.6

All values are drawn from healthy postmenopausal subjects, precision is long-term where available, short-term otherwise. Bone loss given in %/year is based on differences between age 50 and 70 and is given relative to the average value of the population at age 50. Values given here might thus deviate from the ones given in the cited publications

Table 10.5. Age-related BMD loss in women

Cohort	Sample size	Mean cohort age	Trabecular BMD BMD (mg/cm³)	% change /year	Cortical BMD BMD (mg/cm³)	% change /year	Total BMD BMD (mg/cm³)	% change /year	Device	Study type	Ethnicity	Reference
Premenopausal												
	29	36	195	-0.74	696	-0.65	442	-0.84	XCT 960	CS	Caucasian ?	Gatti et al. 1996
	40	31	192	-0.22	695	-0.22	360	-0.30	XCT 960	CS	?	Grampp et al. 1995
	91	-	191	0.38	-	-	374	0.35	XCT 960	CS	Caucasian	Guglielmi et al. 1997
	59	46	316	-1.46	1544	-0.51	701	-0.85	DensiScan 2000	CS	Chinese	Qin et al. 2000
	19	39	-	1.22[a]	-	-	-	2.83[a]	DensiScan 1000	Lg. (4 years)	Japanese	Ito et al. 1999b
	27	35	398	-	1180	-	398	-	XCT 3000	CS	Japanese	Horikoshi et al. 1999
Perimenopausal												
	169	-	186	0.63	-	-	363	0.04	XCT 960	CS	Caucasian	Guglielmi et al. 2000
	17	52	-	-4.92	-	-	-	-2.87	DensiScan 1000	Lg. (4 years)	Japanese	Ito et al. 1999b
Postmenopausal												
	53	63	173	-1.52	612	-1.46	417	-1.48	XCT 900	Lg. (1.8 years)	Caucasian ?	Hernandez et al. 1997
	129	75	171	-1.63	715	-1.72	-	-	XCT 900	CS	Caucasian ?	Boonen et al. 1997
	241	62	138	-0.77	517	-0.68	295	-0.89	XCT 960	CS	Caucasian ?	Gatti et al. 1996
	40	62	178	-0.21	665	-0.21	335	-0.29	XCT 960	CS	?	Grampp et al. 1995
	126	-	187	-0.46	-	-	356	-0.44	XCT 960	CS	Caucasian	Guglielmi et al. 2000
	275	68	188	-0.87	731	-0.38	-	-	XCT 960	CS	Caucasian ?	Nijs et al. 1998
	59	54	214	-2.21	1358	-0.85	548	1.77	DensiScan 2000	CS	Caucasian ?	
	12	56	-	-3.53	-	-	-	-2.63	DensiScan 1000	Lg. (4 years)	Japanese	Ito et al. 1999b
	38	62	-	-2.45	-	-	-	-1.58	DensiScan 1000	Lg. (4 years)	Japanese	Ito et al. 1999b
	33	64	126	-1.39[b]	1070	-0.29[b]	306	-0.85[b]	XCT 3000	CS	Japanese	Horikoshi et al. 1999

For better comparison, values were recalculated from the cited references and refer to age 30 for premenopausal and age 50 for peri- and postmenopausal women

[a] Not significant

[b] Based on both pre- and postmenopausal cohorts

CS cross-sectional, Lg longitudinal

Reference data (absolute values)

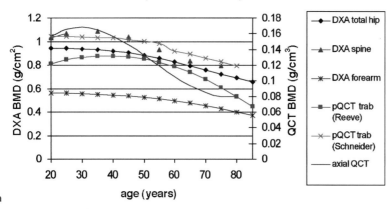

a

Reference data (T-scores)

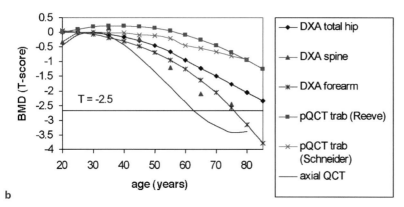

b

Fig. 10.3a,b. Comparison of age dependences of normative data for total BMD. **a** Absolute values, pQCT and axial QCT are scaled to the right plot axis, and DXA curves are scaled to the left plot axis; **b** T-scores. For pQCT data from Reeve et al. (1996) and Schneider et al. (1995) are shown. For lumbar (L1–L4) and forearm DXA (ulna + radius) hologic reference data are shown. For the total hip BMD NHANES data were used. Axial QCT reference data were used from Block et al. (1989)

ture discrimination, pQCT has been compared with several other densitometric techniques. In a small cross-sectional study that included young normal, postmenopausal, and osteoporotic (defined by spinal fracture) women, trabecular and cortical BMD of the osteoporotic subjects were significantly different from young normals, but not from postmenopausal normal subjects (Grampp et al. 1995). Different results were found in the multicenter European Quantitation of Osteoporosis Study (Kröger et al. 1999) that employed both Stratec and DensiScan devices that were cross-calibrated with the EFP. ROC analysis showed that pQCT BMD performed as well as spinal QCT in discriminating spinal fractures in women (32 fractured cases and 84 controls). The authors point out that the application of a diagnostic threshold of T-score = –2.5 as set forth by the WHO would have rendered pQCT insensitive to fracture in that population, while spinal QCT would have exhibited high sensitivity at the expense of specificity. This problem is also reflected in Figure 10.3b. It must be kept in mind that the WHO thresholds apply to neither QCT nor pQCT. Nijs et al. also found that ultra-distal trabecular BMD

discriminated better than the other pQCT parameters between women with and without spinal fractures, but did not include other densitometric devices in their study (Nijs et al. 1998).

There are very few pQCT studies dedicated to fracture discrimination at the forearm (Pludowski 1998; Wapniarz, 1997; Schneider et al. 2001). In a cross-sectional study, Schneider et al. investigated 214 women, 107 of them with Colles fractures, with an XCT 900 device. They reported similar odds ratios (5.3 and 5.1) of trabecular BMC and BMD for discriminating fracture, respectively. ORs for cortical parameters were below 3 per SD decrease (Schneider et al. 2001). Other forearm techniques such as SPA have proven to be highly predictive of Colles fractures (Eastell et al. 1989; Jensen et al. 1982; Nordin et al. 1987). SPA measurements have also shown long-term predictive power for hip fractures. The relative risk (RR) was 1.66 per 1 SD decrease in BMD (Duppe et al. 1997) compared to a RR of 2.4 reported for an 8-year follow-up using DXA at the femoral neck (Melton et al. 1993). It should be noted that absolute ORs cannot be compared across techniques because standardized odds ratios would be required (GLUER et al. 2006); however, these have not been reported for the studies above.

For monitoring osteoporosis treatment effects, the hip and the spine are the most important sites. The use of the forearm for this purpose is controversial (BARAN et al. 1997; BOUXSEIN et al. 1999; EASTELL 1998; HOSKING et al. 1998). However, pQCT has been used in several early studies to monitor treatment effects (DAMBACHER et al. 1986; HANGARTNER et al. 2001; MEDICI and RÜEGSEGGER 1990). More recently, Schneider et al. demonstrated in a subset of patients ($n = 89$) from the FOSIT trial that total but not trabecular BMD determined by pQCT significantly increased with treatment, while there was no change in the control group. Data were pooled from six centers, all using the XCT-900 scanner (SCHNEIDER 1996).

Inconsistent results have been reported for serial forearm DXA measurements. In a substudy of another large multicenter alendronate intervention trial, forearm DXA could not be used to monitor therapy (BOUXSEIN et al. 1999). Positive treatment effects were reported for ibandronate (RAVN et al. 1996), tibolone (BJARASON et al. 1996), calcitonin (NIELSEN 1994). and teriparatide (ZANCHETTA et al. 2003). The fracture intervention trial showed a 50% wrist fracture reduction in the alendronate treatment group accompanied by a 1.5% increase in distal forearm BMD vs controls as measured by DXA. However, in the same trial, the 50% hip fracture reduction was accompanied by a 4.7% increase in total femur BMD, also determined by DXA (BLACK et al. 1996). ITO et al. used pQCT (DensiScan) to monitor patients convalescing from hip surgery and found significant influence of corticosteroid treatment at the tibia (ITO et al. 1999a).

10.3
New Applications

10.3.1
Determination of Bone Strength and Geometry

The strength of a bone is determined by the properties of its tissue components and the spatial distribution of bone material. The trabecular structure cannot be assessed with densitometric equipment because of limitations in spatial resolution. Projectional techniques such as DXA are restricted to determination of an average bone mass or average aerial density

of the entire bone or at least a larger portion of it. The measurement of true volumetric bone density by QCT techniques and the separation of cortical and trabecular bone can be used to calculate geometrical parameters. To explain their principal usefulness, let us approximate a long bone diaphysis such as the mid radius by a hollow cylinder of uniform wall density, as shown in Figure 10.4. Under torsion, the failure torque T_f is proportional to the polar cross-sectional moment of inertia (CSMI) divided by the outer radius r_0. For the cylinder in Figure 10.4 with a cortical thickness Δ, the moment can be calculated as:

$$CSMI = \pi / 2 \cdot [r_0{}^4 - (r_0 - \Delta)^4]$$

With cortical thinning (decrease in Δ), the strength of the bone can be kept constant by periosteal expansion (increase in r_0). Volumetric cortical BMD as measured by pQCT would not be affected, although aerial BMD as measured by DXA would decrease, falsely indicating reduced bone strength. To take into account nonuniform bone density and a more realistic bone shape, parameters have been defined that combine cortical density and CSMI, such as the bone-strength index ($BSI = BMD_{cort} \cdot CSMI$) and the similarly calculated stress–strain index (SSI) (NIJS et al. 1998). The BSI showed an excellent correlation of $r = 0.94$ with fracture load in rats. In the same animals, the correlation between DXA and fracture load was $r = 0.7$ only (FERRETTI 1995). For the SSI a correlation of $r = 0.94$ with the product of muscle force and ulna length has been reported (ADAMI et al. 1999). Similar high correlations have been shown between

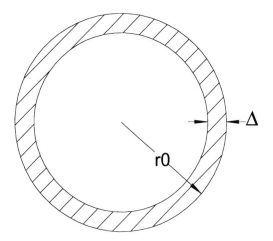

Fig. 10.4. Cylinder of uniform density as an approximation of long bones to demonstrate the cross-sectional moment of inertia (see text)

cortical area and fracture load at the 30% location of cadaveric forearms (Augat et al. 1996).

While these are impressive data, it must be remembered that they all were derived at a cortical site almost devoid of trabecular bone. However, osteoporotic fractures typically occur in trabecular-rich locations such as the distal radius. In the paper cited above, Augat et al. showed that for cortical area, the correlation with fracture load was lower at the distal 10% location than at the more proximal 30% location ($r = 0.71$ vs $r = 0.89$), but increased for trabecular BMD (10% location: $r = 0.72$; 30% location: $r = 0.55$). A similar trend was reported by Hudelmaier et al. (2004). In another forearm in vitro study, Spadaro et al. correlated SPA and QCT with fracture load. At the distal and the one-third sites, correlations were higher than 0.9 for SPA BMD. For the QCT cortical area, correlations of $r = 0.83$ (distal) and $r = 0.9$ (1/3) resulted. Cortical BMD determined by QCT did not correlate with fracture load at either site but trabecular BMD did ($r = 0.82$) (Spadaro et al. 1994). In contrast, Wu et al. found a correlation of $r = 0.61–0.67$ between fracture load and cortical BMD as determined by pQCT (Wu et al. 2000) and Louis et al. after removal of endosteal bone reported correlations of $r = 0.78$ for cortical density, of $r = 0.74$ for cortical thickness, and of $r = 0.87$ for cortical BMC with maximal stress in compression (Louis et al. 1995a). These studies differed in their biomechanical testing procedures, complicating a direct comparison. Spadaro's study might have been further hampered by the lack of spatial resolution of their CT device, which has a more severe effect on BMD than on thickness of the cortex. In vitro comparisons between pQCT and other densitometric techniques in predicting failure load of the radius using cadaveric specimens of the radius showed significant advantages compared to off-site measurements with DXA, QCT, or QUS but not compared to forearm DXA (Ashe et al. 2006; Lochmüller et al. 2002). A closer inspection of the contribution of geometrical parameters such as thickness or SSI in another sample of cadaveric forearms (Hudelmaier et al. 2004) showed that for pQCT the correlation of geometry with fracture load was not higher than with BMC. Again, correlation coefficients between pQCT and fracture load were as good as for DXA. However, there were much higher correlations (for pQCT as well as for forearm DXA) with bending moments ($r = 0.85–0.96$) than with failure loads ($r = 0.6–0.85$), indicating an influence of bone size that again emphasizes that a com-

parison of in vitro studies including bone strength measurements is difficult and that results should be interpreted carefully. Appropriate adjustments or corrections for bone size need to be employed for these in vitro studies, in part because in life, patients with larger bones also are heavier and bring larger forces to bear on the skeleton.

Lochmüller et al. have also published several in vitro studies correlating pQCT variables with other than forearm fractures and comparing correlation coefficients for fracture load across modalities, but a detailed discussion is beyond the scope of this contribution (Lochmüller et al. 2002, 2003). In in vivo studies, the indices BSI and SSI, which are derived from cortical bone geometry and mineral distribution (Adami et al. 1999), show a similar dependency on the measurement site as in in vitro studies discussed above: Nijs et al. found in a cross-sectional study that SSI at the proximal radius was almost as diagnostically sensitive for discriminating prevalent vertebral fracture as trabecular and total BMD at the ultra-distal radius (ROC = 0.72 vs 0.75). However, the SSI showed a much weaker diagnostic power at the ultra-distal site (Nijs et al. 1998). Augat et al. measured the 4% ultra-distal site in hip fracture cases and controls and found that SSI ranked behind all other pQCT parameters, although none of them had a significant odds ratio (Augat et al. 1998a). Also at the same site in the study by Schneider et al. already mentioned in Section 10.2.7 (Schneider et al. 2001), geometrical parameters such as cross-sectional moment of inertia and cortical area discriminated less well than trabecular BMC and BMD between patients with and without Colles fractures. In patients undergoing alendronate treatment, BSI showed a borderline significant ($p = 0.04$) increase of 4.7% vs baseline compared to a highly significant increase of 6.8% in total BMD after 24 months (Schneider et al. 1999).

More data are needed to better judge the value of the geometric parameters for fracture prediction. As mentioned earlier, accurate segmentation of the cortex is critical for the calculation of cortical BMD and thickness. This also applies to the determination of the CSMI, BSI, SSI, and other geometrical parameters. So far, these parameters were not shown to be more effective than BMD. The effect of potentially insufficient spatial resolution should be investigated thoroughly.

Differential effects on BMD and geometry have been reported in the growing skeleton, which will be discussed in Section 10.3.3 and in exercise studies. For example, athletic tennis players showed an increase in bone size of the dominant compared to the non-dominant arm and a corresponding increase in BMC but no change in volumetric BMD (HAAPASALO et al. 2000). Compared to controls, an increase in cortical area of the forearm and thus in bone strength was also shown in competitive weightlifters, whereas at the femur trabecular BMD but was increased without a change in bone size (HEINONEN et al. 2001).

Another emerging research area is the study of bone–muscle interactions. According to Wolff's law and the concept of the mechanostat introduced by Frost (FROST 1987, 1996), bone modeling and remodeling are a response to the external forces acting upon bone. Forces are applied through gravity or through muscles. This concept has evolved into the muscle–bone unit (SCHOENAU 2005a). Muscle forces cannot be measured directly by QCT, but muscle area in individual CT slices or muscle volume in 3D scans can be determined, exploiting the differences in absorption between muscle and fat and between muscle and bone. With pQCT, typically muscle area is measured (HASEGAWA et al. 2001; NEU et al. 2002), but obviously muscle area is only a surrogate parameter for muscle strength. Typical correlations of the two measures are moderate ($r = 0.5-0.8$) (HAKKINEN and HAKKINEN 1991; HAKKINEN et al. 1996). Also, if just global thresholds are used to differentiate muscle from surrounding fat and bone, segmentation errors affecting the accurate size determination may occur. Additional indices relating bone area (RITTWEGER et al. 2004) or BMC to muscle area (SCHOENAU et al. 2002a) have been developed; however, they have not been widely used so far. Most of the work related to muscle area has been done in children and therefore will be discussed in Section 10.3.3.

10.3.2
Trabecular Structure Assessment

The assessment of trabecular structure in vivo is extremely difficult due to the tiny size of the individual trabeculae. In the distal forearm, trabecular thickness ranges from 60 to 150 μm and trabecular separation from 300 to 1000 μm (SCHNITZLER et al. 1996). To quantify the trabecular network, two basic approaches can be identified: (1) improve the spatial resolution of the imaging device to assess individual trabeculae of the network or (2) use current high-end whole-body scanners and apply texture methods using statistical or fractal methods that do not depend on resolving individual trabeculae.

The first approach has been pursued successfully by RÜEGSEGGER and colleagues, who built a thin-slice high-resolution laboratory pQCT scanner for in vivo applications with an isotropic voxel size of 170 μm^3 (MÜLLER et al. 1994). MÜLLER et al. reported a high in-vivo reproducibility of about 1% (MÜLLER et al. 1996) achieved by careful matching of the acquired three-dimensional data sets (MÜNCH and RÜEGSEGGER 1993). When in vitro pQCT structure measurements were compared to μCT, the correlation of various three-dimensional structural parameters between the two systems was $r^2 > 0.9$, despite the lower resolution of the pQCT system. Therefore a dedicated segmentation threshold can be obtained for the pQCT by calibrating the pQCT bone volume fraction to the μCT bone volume fraction (LAIB and RÜEGSEGGER 1999). The group also introduced a number of new parameters to quantify the trabecular network, such as ridge number density (LAIB et al. 1997). Structural parameters determined from images measured with XCT-960 scanners were also used to predict mechanical strength of trabecular specimens taken from the spine (JIANG et al. 1998) and the femur (WACHTER et al. 2001). In both studies, correlations were weaker than for BMD, which is not surprising as the spatial resolution of the XCT-960 is too low to extract structural parameters.

The new XtremeCT is the first scanner to deliver the spatial resolution in all three dimensions that is needed to resolve individual trabeculae (albeit not their thickness, which must be inferred). While few studies using this device have been reported yet, KHOSLA et al. found that at a young age men have thicker trabeculae than women at the ultra-distal radius with greater trabecular bone volume to tissue volume, but similar trabecular number. Similar rates of decline of bone volume were seen in both sexes, but in men this was due to a reduction of trabecular width but not number, whereas in women trabecular number decreased but not thickness. This is interesting because it raises questions regarding the mechanisms involved in this comparable loss of bone mass (KHOSLA et al. 2006a). The thinning of trabeculae in men appears to be driven by insulin-like growth factor 1, whereas sex hormones govern the overall trabecular structure in both sexes (KHOSLA et al. 2006b).

Two-dimensional texture analysis, a method to estimate trabecular structure when spatial resolution is insufficient to resolve individual trabeculae but high enough to capture their overall orienta-

tion and density, has been described in some publications using forearm images of commercially
available pQCT and QCT scanners. GORDON et al.
skeletonized the trabecular texture derived from
2.5-mm-thick slices from an XCT-960 scanner and
calculated trabecular hole area and a connectivity index (GORDON et al. 1996). CORTET et al. used
1-mm-thick images of a clinical CT to obtain nine
parameters describing structure, among them the
Euler number, the trabecular bone pattern factor
(TBPF), and the fractal dimension (CORTET et al.
1999). Unlike GORDON, CORTET et al. derived their
parameters directly from the gray-scale images
rather than using global thresholds to binarize the
images.

The few clinical results reported from these new
approaches are encouraging, but to establish their
clinical relevance more in vivo data are needed, particularly from longitudinal studies. Textural techniques have been successfully used in two smaller
cross-sectional studies that were less sensitive to
positioning errors (CORTET et al. 1998; GORDON et
al. 1996) However, 2D analysis using single slices, in
particular, may be very susceptible to these errors
when serial measurements are performed. Furthermore, the use of thresholds for the calculation of
binary images prior to the structural analysis can be
difficult; their specific selection may heavily affect
the results.

A longitudinal study with 18 healthy postmenopausal women has been reported using the thin
slice laboratory scanner described above (LAIB et al.
1998). In this apparently homogeneous group, considerable differences in bone loss (no loss, reduction
of cortical thickness, trabecular thickness, or trabecular number, or combinations) were found. The
device has also been used for an in vivo load transfer
analysis in the distal radius using a high-resolution
finite element model (ULRICH et al. 1999).

pQCT is not the only promising method for structural analysis at the distal forearm. Both QCT as
discussed in Section 10.2.2 and MR using clinical
scanners challenge the future of pQCT in this arena.
Although research employing high-resolution axial
CT has only begun to show convincingly that it
lends itself to assessing bone architecture (PATEL et
al. 2005), a small cross-sectional study showed CT-
based spinal architecture to be as strongly associated
with fracture as spinal BMD (GORDON et al. 1998).
Furthermore, latest-generation multislice scanners
offer far better spatial resolution than the preceding
models. Figure 10.6 shows examples of four slices
extracted from a full 3D in vivo scan acquired on
a Somatom VZ (Siemens Erlangen). MR is joining
the field as well. Despite the difficulties with artifacts caused by the magnetic field inhomogeneities
at this scale, architectural parameters assessed by
high-resolution MR at the appendicular skeleton

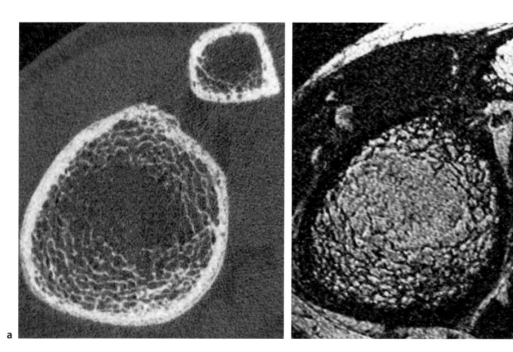

Fig. 10.5. a Trabecular bone specimen scanned by three-dimensional pQCT (XtremeCT). **b** Same location with micro-MR

were recently reported to add discriminatory power to bone density in a controlled cross-sectional study (see Fig. 10.5b) (MAJUMDAR et al. 1999). With the widening availability of 3.0 Tesla equipment, MRI may start to play a larger research role in trabecular structure assessment because of better resolution at the peripheral skeleton (PHAN et al. 2006) and the potential to reach the proximal femur (KRUG et al. 2005).

10.3.3
Study of Bone Development in Children

Because low peak bone density is a risk factor for osteoporotic fractures, it is important to understand and optimize bone growth. Currently DXA is used for most densitometric studies in children. To account for their relatively small size and weight, some DXA scan and analysis protocols have been adapted to infants and younger children (LEONARD et al. 1998; RUPICH et al. 1996), although longitudinal determination of BMD using DXA is complicated by bone size and shape, which are not constant (SCHONAU 1998b). Here peripheral QCT offers significant advantages over DXA. A number of cross-sectional as well as a few longitudinal studies have investigated the use of pQCT in children. Several of these have in particular addressed

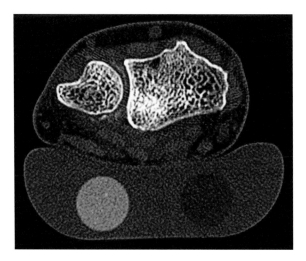

Fig. 10.6. In vivo scan of distal radius on a four-row axial CT scanner (Siemens Somatom VolumeZoom, Siemens, Erlangen, Germany; 120 kV, ultra-high resolution mode, 10-cm field of view). The forearm is scanned on a dedicated forearm QCT soft tissue equivalent calibration phantom containing two cylinders of water and bone (200 mg/cm³ HA) equivalent materials (QRM, Möhrendorf, Germany).

the bone–muscle interactions mentioned already in Section 10.3.1 (SCHONEAU 2005a, b; SCHONAU et al. 1996). Differential effects in growth pattern found between boys and girls during puberty and adolescence (NEU et al. 2001b; SCHONAU et al. 2002; SUMIK et al. 2006) and between distal radius and tibial shaft (WANG et al. 2005) demonstrate the power of a true volumetric assessment such a pQCT.

In two cross-sectional studies in children using pQCT at the forearm, trabecular and cortical bone density were found to be independent of age (FUJITA et al. 1999; SCHONAU 1998a). FUJITA et al. also included adults, but trabecular BMD did not change until the age of 25 (FUJITA et al. 1999). These two studies further showed significant increases in total and cortical bone area throughout childhood and adolescence. The results support the argument that increases in BMD measured with the projectional DXA technique are at least partly caused by a change in bone size and not only by a change in volumetric bone density. At a more diaphyseal site of the forearm, NEU et al. also included adults in their study (NEU et al. 2001b) and showed a 23% BMD increase in boys and a 48% increase in girls between 6 and 7 years of age and adulthood. Changes for BMC were different: 111% for girls and 140% for boys, again emphasizing the effect of change in shape and the importance of not just analyzing BMD. Muscle cross-sectional area and related bone muscle indices in children has been reported in (MacDONALD et al. 2005; SCHOENAU et al. 2000, 2001).

Most of the data presented in this section were generated at a predominantly cortical site of the forearm, but it still needs to be proven whether based on these results the concepts of bone growth can be generalized for the rest of the skeleton, or whether other mechanisms not assessable by pQCT contribute as well. As highlighted previously, the study of cortical bone is afflicted by spatial resolution. This is particularly true in children. At a location of 15% from the distal radial end, the young cortex has a thickness of around 1.7 mm (FUJITA et al. 1999). For accurate measurement of cortical thickness, these values are dangerously close to the spatial resolution limits for most of today's machines and probably prohibitive for an assessment of cortical density (PREVRHAL et al. 1999). As a consequence, published data on cortical density (FUJITA et al. 1999) should be reviewed with caution.

Limitations of cortical density measurements were confirmed in very young children (BINKLEY and SPECKER 2000) and in prepubertal children using a XCT 2000 scanner (SCHOENAU et al. 2002b). The average cortical thickness was 1.2 mm. This study found significant correlations of total radius cross-sectional area, cortical area, and cortical thickness with weight and height, but no gender differences. pQCT measurements in children have also been used for the assessment of osteogenesis imperfecta (MILLER and HANGARTNER 1999).

Although pQCT offers the advantage of 3D data acquisition, longitudinal bone growth needs to be accounted for, and it may be difficult to define a reference point that can be consistently applied across the study population, or, in the case of longitudinal studies, be re-applied. Consequently, NEU et al. had to define a different scan reference line to accommodate children whose radial growth plates were still open (NEU et al. 2001a).

10.4
Conclusions

Peripheral QCT offers good accuracy and precision for studying bone mineral density in the forearm, and recently, in the lower leg. However, bone density at these anatomical sites shows only weak effects of aging, resulting in very long monitoring time intervals. Furthermore, the appendicular skeleton may not correspond well enough with the lumbar spine and the proximal femur, the two most important fracture sites in clinical assessment of osteoporosis, to justify comprehensive diagnosis of skeletal status solely based on pQCT measurements. pQCT offers the ability to separately assess trabecular and cortical bone, which has been successfully explored in several cross-sectional and longitudinal studies. The use of this technique in addition to DXA should be of interest for pharmacological studies or research where differential effects on the two compartments are of concern. In the future, the use of pQCT to assess BMD at peripheral sites may be supplemented by axial CT whose latest-generation machines offer comparable spatial resolution to some of today's pQCT devices. The newest developments with augmented spatial resolution will reach marketability and improve pQCT's capacity to accurately assess cortical bone density and geometry.

References

Adami S, Gatti D, Braga V, Bianchini D, Rossini M (1999) Site-specific effects of strength training on bone structure and geometry of ultradistal radius in postmenopausal women [see comments]. J Bone Miner Res 14:120–124

Ashe MC, Khan KM, Kontulainen SA, Guy P, Liu D, Beck TJ, McKay HA (2006) Accuracy of pQCT for evaluating the aged human radius: an ashing, histomorphometry and failure load investigation. Osteoporos Int 17:1241–1251

Augat P, Reeb H, Claes LE (1996) Prediction of fracture load at different skeletal sites by geometric properties of the cortical shell. J Bone Miner Res 11:1356–1363

Augat P, Fan B, Lane NE, Lang TF, LeHir P, Lu Y, Uffmann M, Genant HK (1998a) Assessment of bone mineral at appendicular sites in females with fractures of the proximal femur. Bone 22:395–402

Augat P, Gordon CL, Lang TF, Iida H, Genant HK (1998b) Accuracy of cortical and trabecular bone measurements with peripheral quantitative computed tomography (pQCT). Phys Med Biol 43:2873–2883

Baran DT, Faulkner KG, Genant HK, Miller PD, Pacifici R (1997) Diagnosis and management of osteoporosis: guidelines for the utilization of bone densitometry. Calcif Tissue Int 61:433–440

Binkley TL, Specker BL (2000) pQCT measurement of bone parameters in young children: validation of technique. J Clin Densitom 3:9–14

Bjarnason NH, Bjarnason K, Haarbo J, Rosenquist C, Christiansen C (1996) Tibolone: prevention of bone loss in late postmenopausal women [see comments]. J Clin Endocrinol Metab 81:2419–2422

Black DM, Cummings SR, Karpf DB, Cauley JA, Thompson DE, Nevitt MC, Bauer DC, Genant HK, Haskell WL, Marcus R, Ott SM, Torner JC, Quandt SA, Reiss TF, Ensrud KE (1996) Randomised trial of effect of alendronate on risk of fracture in women with existing vertebral fractures. Fracture Intervention Trial Research Group. Lancet 348:1535–1541

Block JE, Smith R, Glüer CC, Steiger P, Ettinger B, Genant HK (1989) Models of spinal trabecular bone loss as determined by quantitative computed tomography. J Bone Miner Res 4:249–257

Boonen S, Cheng XG, Nijs J, Nicholson PH, Verbeke G, Lesaffre E, Aerssens J, Dequeker J (1997) Factors associated with cortical and trabecular bone loss as quantified by peripheral computed tomography (pQCT) at the ultradistal radius in aging women. Calcif Tissue Int 60:164–170

Boutroy S, Bouxsein ML, Munoz F, Delmas PD (2005) In vivo assessment of trabecular bone microarchitecture by high-resolution peripheral quantitative computed tomography. J Clin Endocrinol Metab 90:6508–6515

Bouxsein ML, Parker RA, Greenspan SL (1999) Forearm bone mineral density cannot be used to monitor response to alendronate therapy in postmenopausal women. Osteoporos Int 10:505–509

Braun MJ, Meta MD, Schneider P, Reiners C (1998) Clinical evaluation of a high-resolution new peripheral quantitative computerized tomography (pQCT) scanner for the bone densitometry at the lower limbs. Phys Med Biol 43:2279–2294

Butz S, Weuster C, Scheidt-Nave C, Geotz M, Ziegler R (1994) Forearm BMD as measured by peripheral quantitative computed tomography pQCT in a German reference population. Osteoporos Int 4:179–184

Cameron JR, Sorenson JA (1963) Measurement of bone mineral in vivo: an improved method. Science 142:230–232

Capozza R, Ma YF, Ferretti JL, Meta M, Alippi R, Zanchetta J, Jee WS (1995) Tomographic (pQCT) and biomechanical effects of hPTH(1–38) on chronically immobilized or overloaded rat femurs. Bone 17:233S–239S

Cortet B, Bourel P, Dubois P, Boutry N, Cotten A, Marchandise X (1998) CT scan texture analysis of the distal radius: influence of age and menopausal status. Rev Rhum Engl Ed 65:109–118

Cortet B, Dubois P, Boutry N, Bourel P, Cotten A, Marchandise X (1999) Image analysis of the distal radius trabecular network using computed tomography. Osteoporos Int 9:410–419

Dambacher MA, Ittner J, Ruegsegger P (1986) Long-term fluoride therapy of postmenopausal osteoporosis. Bone 7:199–205

Duppe H, Gardsell P, Nilsson B, Johnell O (1997) A single bone density measurement can predict fractures over 25 years. Calcif Tissue Int 60:171–174

Eastell R (1998) Treatment of postmenopausal osteoporosis. N Engl J Med 338:736–746

Eastell R, Riggs BL, Wahner HW, O'Fallon WM, Amadio PC, Melton LJD (1989) Colles' fracture and bone density of the ultradistal radius. J Bone Miner Res 4:607–613

Ferretti JL (1995) Perspectives of pQCT technology associated to biomechanical studies in skeletal research employing rat models. Bone 17:353S–364S

Frost HM (1987) Bone mass and the mechanostat: a proposal. Anat Rec 219:1–9

Frost HM (1996) Perspectives: a proposed general model of the mechanostat (suggestions from a new skeletal-biologic paradigm). Anat Rec 244:139–147

Fujita T, Fujii Y, Goto B (1999) Measurement of forearm bone in children by peripheral computed tomography. Calcif Tissue Int 64:34–39

Gatti D, Rossini M, Zamberlan N, Braga V, Fracassi E, Adami S (1996) Effect of aging on trabecular and compact bone components of proximal and ultradistal radius. Osteoporos Int 6:355–360

Genant HK, Boyd D (1977) Quantitative bone mineral analysis using dual energy computed tomography. Invest Radiol 12:545–551

Glüer CC, Blake G, Lu Y, Blunt BA, Jergas M, Genant HK (1995) Accurate assessment of precision errors: how to measure the reproducibility of bone densitometry techniques. Osteoporos Int 5:262–270

Gluer CC, Lu Y, Engelke K (2006) Quality and performance measures in bone densitometry: part 2. Fracture risk. Osteoporos Int 17:1449–1748

Gordon C, Lang T, Augat P, Genant H (1998) Image-based assessment of spinal trabecular bone structure from high-resolution CT images. Osteoporos Int 8:317–325

Gordon CL, Webber CE, Adachi JD, Christoforou N (1996) In vivo assessment of trabecular bone structure at the distal radius from high-resolution computed tomography images. Phys Med Biol 41:495–508

Grampp S, Lang P, Jergas M, Gluer CC, Mathur A, Engelke K, Genant HK (1995) Assessment of the skeletal status by peripheral quantitative computed tomography of the forearm: short-term precision in vivo and comparison to dual X-ray absorptiometry. J Bone Miner Res 10:1566–1576

Groll O, Lochmuller EM, Bachmeier M, Willnecker J, Eckstein F (1999) Precision and intersite correlation of bone densitometry at the radius, tibia and femur with peripheral quantitative CT. Skeletal Radiol 28:696–702

Guglielmi G, Grimston SK, Fischer KC, Pacifici R (1994) Osteoporosis: diagnosis with lateral and posteroanterior dual X-ray absorptiometry compared with quantitative CT. Radiology 192:845–850

Guglielmi G, Cammisa M, De Serio A, Giannatempo GM, Bagni B, Orlandi G, Russo CR (1997) Long-term in vitro precision of single slice peripheral Quantitative Computed Tomography (pQCT): multicenter comparison. Technol Health Care 5:375–381

Guglielmi G, De Serio A, Fusilli S, Scillitani A, Chiodini I, Torlontano M, Cammisa M (2000) Age-related changes assessed by peripheral QCT in healthy Italian women. Eur Radiol 10:609–614

Haapasalo H, Kontulainen S, Sievanen H, Kannus P, Jarvinen M, Vuori I (2000) Exercise-induced bone gain is due to enlargement in bone size without a change in volumetric bone density: a peripheral quantitative computed tomography study of the upper arms of male tennis players. Bone 27:351–357

Hakkinen K, Hakkinen A (1991) Muscle cross-sectional area, force production and relaxation characteristics in women at different ages. Eur J Appl Physiol Occup Physiol 62:410–414

Hakkinen K, Kraemer WJ, Kallinen M, Linnamo V, Pastinen UM, Newton RU (1996) Bilateral and unilateral neuromuscular function and muscle cross-sectional area in middle-aged and elderly men and women. J Gerontol A Biol Sci Med Sci 51:B21–B29

Hangartner TN (1993) The OsteoQuant: an isotope-based CT scanner for precise measurement of bone density. J Comput Assist Tomogr 17:798–805

Hangartner TN, Overton TR, Harley CH, van den Berg L, Crockford PM (1985) Skeletal challenge: an experimental study of pharmacologically induced changes in bone density in the distal radius, using gamma-ray computed tomography. Calcif Tissue Int 37:19–24

Hangartner TN, Battista JJ, Overton TR (1987) Performance evaluation of density measurements of axial and peripheral bone with x-ray and gamma-ray computed tomography. Phys Med Biol 32:1393–1406

Hasegawa Y, Kushida K, Yamazaki K, Inoue T (1997) Volumetric bone mineral density using peripheral quantitative computed tomography in Japanese women. Osteoporos Int 7:195–199

Hasegawa Y, Schneider P, Reiners C, Kushida K, Yamazaki K, Hasegawa K, Nagano A (2000) Estimation of the architectural properties of cortical bone using peripheral quantitative computed tomography [In Process Citation]. Osteoporos Int 11:36–42

Hasegawa Y, Schneider P, Reiners C (2001) Age, sex, and grip strength determine architectural bone parameters assessed by peripheral quantitative computed tomography (pQCT) at the human radius. J Biomech 34:497–503

Heinonen A, Sievanen H, Kannus P, Oja P, Vuori I (2002) Site-specific skeletal response to long-term weight training seems to be attributable to principal loading modality: a pQCT study of female weightlifters. Calcif Tissue Int 70:469–474

Hernandez ER, Revilla M, Seco-Durban C, Villa LF, Cortes J, Rico H (1997) Heterogeneity of trabecular and cortical postmenopausal bone loss: a longitudinal study with pQCT. Bone 20:283–287

Horikoshi T, Endo N, Uchiyama T, Tanizawa T, Takahashi HE (1999) Peripheral quantitative computed tomography of the femoral neck in 60 Japanese women. Calcif Tissue Int 65:447–453

Hosking D, Chilvers CED, Christiansen C, Ravn P, Wasnich R, Ross P, McClung M, Balske A, Thompson D, Daley M, Yates AJ (1998) Prevention of Bone Loss with Alendronate in Postmenopausal Women under 60 Years of Age. N Engl J Med 338:485–492

Hudelmaier M, Kuhn V, Lochmuller EM, Well H, Priemel M, Link TM, Eckstein F (2004) Can geometry-based parameters from pQCT and material parameters from quantitative ultrasound (QUS) improve the prediction of radial bone strength over that by bone mass (DXA)? Osteoporos Int 15:375–381

Ito M, Matsumoto T, Enomoto H, Tsurusaki K, Hayashi K (1999a) Effect of nonweight bearing on tibial bone density measured by QCT in patients with hip surgery. J Bone Miner Metab 17:45–50

Ito M, Nakamura T, Tsurusaki K, Uetani M, Hayashi K (1999b) Effects of Menopause on Age-Dependent Bone Loss in the Axial and Appendicular Skeletons in Healthy Japanese Women. Osteoporos Int 10:377–383

Jensen GF, Christiansen C, Boesen J, Hegedus V, Transbol I (1982) Epidemiology of postmenopausal spinal and long bone fractures. A unifying approach to postmenopausal osteoporosis. Clin Orthop 166:75–81

Jiang Y, Zhao J, Augat P, Ouyang X, Lu Y, Majumdar S, Genant HK (1998) Trabecular bone mineral and calculated structure of human bone specimens scanned by peripheral quantitative computed tomography: relation to biomechanical properties. J Bone Miner Res 13:1783–1790

Kalender WA, Felsenberg D, Louis O, Lopez P, Klotz E, Osteaux M, Fraga J (1989) Reference values for trabecular and cortical vertebral bone density in single and dual-energy quantitative computed tomography. Eur J Radiol 9:70–80

Khosla S, Melton LJ 3rd, Achenbach SJ, Oberg AL, Riggs BL (2006a) Hormonal and biochemical determinants of trabecular microstructure at the ultradistal radius in women and men. J Clin Endocrinol Metab 91:885–891

Khosla S, Riggs BL, Atkinson EJ, Oberg AL, McDaniel LJ, Holets M, Peterson JM, Melton LJ 3rd (2006b) Effects of sex and age on bone microstructure at the ultradistal radius: a population-based noninvasive in vivo assessment. J Bone Miner Res 21:124–131

Kröger H, Lunt M, Reeve J, Dequeker J, Adams JE, Birkenhager JC, Diaz Curiel M, Felsenberg D, Hyldstrup L, Kotzki P, Laval-Jeantet A, Lips P, Louis O, Perez Cano R, Reiners C, Ribot C, Ruegsegger P, Schneider P, Braillon P, Pearson J (1999) Bone density reduction in various measurement sites in men and women with osteoporotic fractures of spine and hip: the European quantitation of osteoporosis study. Calcif Tissue Int 64:191–199

Krug R, Banerjee S, Han ET, Newitt DC, Link TM, Majumdar S (2005) Feasibility of in vivo structural analysis of high-resolution magnetic resonance images of the proximal femur. Osteoporos Int 16:1307–1314

Laib A, Rüegsegger P (1999) Calibration of Trabecular Bone Structure Measurements of In Vivo Three-Dimensional Peripheral Quantitative Computed Tomography With 28-mm-resolution Microcomputed Tomography. Bone 24:35–39

Laib A, Hildebrand T, Heauselmann HJ, Reuegsegger P (1997) Ridge number density: a new parameter for in vivo bone structure analysis. Bone 21:541–546

Laib A, Hauselmann HJ, Ruegsegger P (1998) In vivo high resolution 3D-QCT of the human forearm. Technol Health Care 6:329–337

Lalla S, Hothorn LA, Haag N, Bader R, Bauss F (1998) Lifelong administration of high doses of ibandronate increases bone mass and maintains bone quality of lumbar vertebrae in rats. Osteoporos Int 8:97–103

Leonard MB, Feldman HI, Zemel BS, Berlin JA, Barden EM, Stallings VA (1998) Evaluation of low density spine software for the assessment of bone mineral density in children. J Bone Miner Res 13:1687–1690

Lochmuller EM, Burklein D, Kuhn V, Glaser C, Muller R, Gluer CC, Eckstein F (2002a) Mechanical strength of the thoracolumbar spine in the elderly: prediction from in situ dual-energy X-ray absorptiometry, quantitative computed tomography (QCT), upper and lower limb peripheral QCT, and quantitative ultrasound. Bone 31:77–84

Lochmuller EM, Lill CA, Kuhn V, Schneider E, Eckstein F (2002b) Radius bone strength in bending, compression, and falling and its correlation with clinical densitometry at multiple sites. J Bone Miner Res 17:1629–1638

Lochmuller EM, Muller R, Kuhn V, Lill CA, Eckstein F (2003) Can novel clinical densitometric techniques replace or improve DXA in predicting bone strength in osteoporosis at the hip and other skeletal sites? J Bone Miner Res 18:906–912

Looker AC, Wahner HW, Dunn WL, Calvo MS, Harris TB, Heyse SP, Johnston CC Jr, Lindsay R (1998) Updated data on proximal femur bone mineral levels of US adults. Osteoporos Int 8:468–489

Louis O, Boulpaep F, Willnecker J, Van den Winkel P, Osteaux M (1995a) Cortical mineral content of the radius assessed by peripheral QCT predicts compressive strength on biomechanical testing. Bone 16:375–379

Louis O, Willnecker J, Soykens S, Van den Winkel P, Osteaux M (1995b) Cortical thickness assessed by peripheral quantitative computed tomography: accuracy evaluated on radius specimens. Osteoporos Int 5:446–449

Louis O, Soykens S, Willnecker J, Van den Winkel P, Osteaux M (1996) Cortical and total bone mineral content of the radius: accuracy of peripheral computed tomography. Bone 18:467–472

MacDonald HM, Kontulainen SA, Mackelvie-O'Brien KJ, Petit MA, Janssen P, Khan KM, McKay HA (2005) Maturity- and sex-related changes in tibial bone geometry, strength and bone-muscle strength indices during growth: a 20-month pQCT study. Bone 36:1003–1011

Majumdar S, Link TM, Augat P, Lin JC, Newitt D, Lane NE, Genant HK (1999) Trabecular bone architecture in the distal radius using magnetic resonance imaging in subjects with fractures of the proximal femur. Magnetic Resonance Science Center and Osteoporosis and Arthritis Research Group. Osteoporos Int 10:231–239

Maughan RJ, Watson JS, Weir J (1984) Muscle strength and cross-sectional area in man: a comparison of strength-trained and untrained subjects. Br J Sports Med 18:149–157

Medici TC, Rüegsegger P (1990) Does alternate-day cloprednol therapy prevent bone loss? A longitudinal double-blind, controlled clinical study. Clin Pharmacol Ther 48:455–466

Melton LJd, Atkinson EJ, O'Fallon WM, Wahner HW, Riggs BL (1993) Long-term fracture prediction by bone mineral assessed at different skeletal sites. J Bone Miner Res 8:1227–1233

Miller ME, Hangartner TN (1999) Bone density measurements by computed tomography in osteogenesis imperfecta type I. Osteoporos Int 9:427–432

Müller A, Rüegsegger E, Rüegsegger P (1989) Peripheral QCT: a low-risk procedure to identify women predisposed to osteoporosis. Phys Med Biol 34:741–749

Müller R, Hildebrand T, Rüegsegger P (1994) Non-invasive bone biopsy: a new method to analyse and display the three-dimensional structure of trabecular bone. Phys Med Biol 39:145–164

Müller R, Hildebrand T, Hauselmann HJ, Rüegsegger P (1996) In vivo reproducibility of three-dimensional structural properties of noninvasive bone biopsies using 3D-pQCT. J Bone Miner Res 11:1745–1750

Münch B, Rüegsegger P (1993) 3-D repositioning and differential images of volumetric CT measurements. IEEE Trans Med Imag 12:509–514

Neu CM, Manz F, Rauch F, Merkel A, Schoenau E (2001a) Bone densities and bone size at the distal radius in healthy children and adolescents: a study using peripheral quantitative computed tomography. Bone 28:227–223

Neu CM, Rauch F, Manz F, Schoenau E (2001b) Modeling of cross-sectional bone size, mass and geometry at the proximal radius: a study of normal bone development using peripheral quantitative computed tomography. Osteoporos Int 12:538–547

Neu CM, Rauch F, Rittweger J, Manz F, Schoenau E (2002) Influence of puberty on muscle development at the forearm. Am J Physiol Endocrinol Metab 283:E103–E107

Nijs J, Westhovens R, Joly J, Cheng XG, Borghs H, Dequeker J (1998) Diagnostic sensitivity of peripheral quantitative computed tomography measurements at ultradistal and proximal radius in postmenopausal women. Bone 22:659–664

Nordin BE, Chatterton BE, Walker CJ, Wishart J (1987) The relation of forearm mineral density to peripheral fractures in postmenopausal women. Med J Aust 146:300–304

Patel PV, Prevrhal S, Bauer JS, Phan C, Eckstein F, Lochmuller EM, Majumdar S, Link TM (2005) Trabecular bone structure obtained from multislice spiral computed tomography of the calcaneus predicts osteoporotic vertebral deformities. J Comput Assist Tomogr 29:246–253

Patel R, Blake GM, Rymer J, Fogelman I (2000) Long-term precision of DXA scanning assessed over seven years in forty postmenopausal women. Osteoporos Int 11:68–75

Pearson J, Rüegsegger P, Dequeker J, Henley M, Bright J, Reeve J, Kalender W, Felsenberg D, Laval-Jeantet AM, Adams JE et al (1994) European semi-anthropomorphic phantom for the cross-calibration of peripheral bone densitometers: assessment of precision accuracy and stability. Bone Miner 27:109–120

Phan CM, Matsuura M, Bauer JS, Dunn TC, Newitt D, Lochmueller EM, Eckstein F, Majumdar S, Link TM (2006) Tra-

becular bone structure of the calcaneus: comparison of MR imaging at 3.0 and 1.5 T with micro-CT as the standard of reference. Radiology 239:488–496

Prevrhal S, Engelke K, Kalender W (1999) Accuracy limits for the determination of cortical width and density: the influence on object size and ct imaging parameters. Phys Med Biol 44:751–764

Qin L, Au SK, Chan KM, Lau MC, Woo J, Dambacher MA, Leung PC (2000) Peripheral volumetric bone mineral density in pre- and postmenopausal Chinese women in Hong Kong [In Process Citation]. Calcif Tissue Int 67:29–36

Rauch F, Klein K, Allolio B, Schonau E (1999) Age at menarche and cortical bone geometry in premenopausal women. Bone 25:69–73

Ravn P, Clemmesen B, Riis BJ, Christiansen C (1996) The effect on bone mass and bone markers of different doses of ibandronate: a new bisphosphonate for prevention and treatment of postmenopausal osteoporosis: a 1-year, randomized, double-blind, placebo-controlled dose-finding study. Bone 19:527–533

Reeve J, Kroger H, Nijs J, Pearson J, Felsenberg D, Reiners C, Schneider P, Mitchell A, Ruegsegger P, Zander C, Fischer M, Bright J, Henley M, Lunt M, Dequeker J (1996) Radial cortical and trabecular bone densities of men and women standardized with the European Forearm Phantom. Calcif Tissue Int 58:135–143

Rittweger J, Beller G, Ehrig J, Jung C, Koch U, Ramolla J, Schmidt F, Newitt D, Majumdar S, Schiessl H, Felsenberg D (2000) Bone-muscle strength indices for the human lower leg. Bone 27:319–326

Rittweger J, Michaelis I, Giehl M, Wusecke P, Felsenberg D (2004) Adjusting for the partial volume effect in cortical bone analyses of pQCT images. J Musculoskelet Neuronal Interact 4:436–441

Rüegsegger P (1974) An extension of classical bone mineral measurements. Ann Biomed Eng 2

Ruegsegger P, Kalender WA (1993) A phantom for standardization and quality control in peripheral bone measurements by pQCT and DXA. Phys Med Biol 38:1963–1970

Rupich RC, Specker BL, Lieuw AFM, Ho M (1996) Gender and race differences in bone mass during infancy. Calcif Tissue Int 58:395–397

Russo CR, Lauretani F, Seeman E, Bartali B, Bandinelli S, Di Iorio A, Guralnik J, Ferrucci L (2006) Structural adaptations to bone loss in aging men and women. Bone 38:112–118

Sato M, Kim J, Short LL, Slemenda CW, Bryant HU (1995) Longitudinal and cross-sectional analysis of raloxifene effects on tibiae from ovariectomized aged rats. J Pharmacol Exp Ther 272:1252–1259

Schlenker RA, VonSeggen WW (1976) The distribution of cortical and trabecular bone mass along the lengths of the radius and ulna and the implications for in vivo bone mass measurements. Calcif Tissue Res 20:41–52

Schneider P, Butz S, Allolio B, Börner W, Klein K, Lehmann R, Petermann K, Tysarczyk-Niemeyer G, Wüster C, Zander C et al (1995) Multicenter German reference data base for peripheral quantitative computer tomography. Technol Health Care 3:69–73

Schneider P, Reiners C, Cointry GR, Capozza RF, Ferretti JL (2001) Bone quality parameters of the distal radius as assessed by pQCT in normal and fractured women. Osteoporos Int 12:639–646

Schneider PF, Fischer M, Allolio B, Felsenberg D, Schroder U, Semler J, Ittner JR (1999) Alendronate increases bone density and bone strength at the distal radius in postmenopausal women. J Bone Miner Res 14:1387–1393

Schnitzler CM, Biddulph SL, Mesquita JM, Gear KA (1996) Bone structure and turnover in the distal radius and iliac crest: a histomorphometric study. J Bone Miner Res 11:1761–1768

Schoenau E (2005a) From mechanostat theory to development of the Functional Muscle-Bone-Unit. J Musculoskelet Neuronal Interact 5:232–238

Schoenau E (2005b) The functional muscle-bone unit: a two-step diagnostic algorithm in pediatric bone disease. Pediatr Nephrol 20:356–359

Schoenau E, Neu CM, Mokov E, Wassmer G, Manz F (2000) Influence of puberty on muscle area and cortical bone area of the forearm in boys and girls. J Clin Endocrinol Metab 85:1095–1098

Schoenau E, Neu CM, Rauch F, Manz F (2001) The development of bone strength at the proximal radius during childhood and adolescence. J Clin Endocrinol Metab 86:613–618

Schoenau E, Neu CM, Beck B, Manz F, Rauch F (2002a) Bone mineral content per muscle cross-sectional area as an index of the functional muscle-bone unit. J Bone Miner Res 17:1095–1101

Schoenau E, Neu CM, Rauch F, Manz F (2002b) Gender-specific pubertal changes in volumetric cortical bone mineral density at the proximal radius. Bone 31:110–113

Schonau E (1998a) The development of the skeletal system in children and the influence of muscular strength. Horm Res 49:27–31

Schonau E (1998b) Problems of bone analysis in childhood and adolescence. Pediatr Nephrol 12:420–429

Schonau E, Werhahn E, Schiedermaier U, Mokow E, Schiessl H, Scheidhauer K, Michalk D (1996) Influence of muscle strength on bone strength during childhood and adolescence. Horm Res 45 [Suppl 1]:63–66

Shepherd JA, Lu Y, Cheng X, Engelke K, Njeh C, Toschke J, Fuerst T, Genant HK (2000) Universal standardization of forearm bone densitometry: densitometry relationships. J Bone and Miner 17:734–745

Sievänen H, Koskue V, Rauhio A, Kannus P, Heinonen A, Vuori I (1998) Peripheral quantitative computed tomography in human long bones: evaluation of in vitro and in vivo precision [see comments]. J Bone Miner Res 13:871–882

Spadaro JA, Werner FW, Brenner RA, Fortino MD, Fay LA, Edwards WT (1994) Cortical and trabecular bone contribute strength to the osteopenic distal radius. J Orthop Res 12:211–218

Srivastava AK, Bhattacharyya S, Castillo G, Wergedal J, Mohan S, Baylink DJ (2000) Development and application of a serum C-telopeptide and osteocalcin assay to measure bone turnover in an ovariectomized rat model. Calcif Tissue Int 66:435–442

Sumnik Z, Land C, Coburger S, Neu C, Manz F, Hrach K, Schoenau E (2006) The muscle-bone unit in adulthood: influence of sex, height, age and gynecological history on the bone mineral content and muscle cross-sectional area. J Musculoskelet Neuronal Interact 6:195–200

Takada M, Engelke K, Hagiwara S, Grampp S, Genant HK (1996) Accuracy and precision study in vitro for peripheral quantitative computed tomography. Osteoporos Int 6:207–212

Tucci JR, Tonino RP, Emkey RD, Peverly CA, Kher U, Santora AC 2nd (1996) Effect of three years of oral alendronate treatment in postmenopausal women with osteoporosis. Am J Med 101:488–501

Ulrich D, Rietbergen BV, Laib A, Ruegsegger P (1999) The ability of three-dimensional structural indices to reflect mechanical aspects of trabecular bone. Bone 25:55–60

Wachter NJ, Augat P, Mentzel M, Sarkar MR, Krischak GD, Kinzl L, Claes LE (2001) Predictive value of bone mineral density and morphology determined by peripheral quantitative computed tomography for cancellous bone strength of the proximal femur. Bone 28:133–139

Wang Q, Alen M, Nicholson P, Lyytikainen A, Suuriniemi M, Helkala E, Suominen H, Cheng S (2005) Growth patterns at distal radius and tibial shaft in pubertal girls: a 2-year longitudinal study. J Bone Miner Res 20:954–961

Webb S (1998) The mathematics of image formation and image processing. In: Webb S (ed) The physics of medical imaging. Institute of Physics Publishing, London, pp 534–566

Wu C, Hans D, He Y, Fan B, Njeh CF, Augat P, Richards J, Genant HK (2000) Prediction of bone strength of distal forearm using radius bone mineral density and phalangeal speed of sound. Bone 26:529–533

Zanchetta JR, Bogado CE, Ferretti JL, Wang O, Wilson MG, Sato M, Gaich GA, Dalsky GP, Myers SL (2003) Effects of teriparatide [recombinant human parathyroid hormone (1–34)] on cortical bone in postmenopausal women with osteoporosis. J Bone Miner Res 18:539–543

Quantitative Ultrasound

Reinhard Barkmann

CONTENTS

11.1
Introduction

Measurement methods using ultrasound waves have been successfully employed in materials testing as well as medical diagnosis for a long time. Unlike medical ultrasonography, quantitative ultrasound (QUS) methods are not primarily used to obtain images from the inner human body but to measure quantitative variables by which to assess tissue properties. QUS devices are less expensive and smaller than axial dual-energy X-ray absorptiometry (DXA) or quantitative computed tomography (QCT) devices and do not require the use of ionizing radiation. These advantages explain the motivation for using QUS devices for the assessment of osteoporosis, assuming that the performance is comparable. However, QUS is not just a cheap surrogate for measurement of bone mineral density (BMD). Ultrasound propagation is complex and affected by other properties of materials, as X-rays are. Ultrasound waves are affected not only by the amount of material but also by its elasticity and structure. For this reason, QUS might be able to yield additional information about bone fragility.

At present, QUS devices are mostly used for the prediction of osteoporotic fracture risk. The ability to estimate the probability of future fractures has been established in the case of a number of QUS approaches. However, other fields of interest beyond the assessment of primary osteoporosis are also being investigated, such as rheumatoid arthritis, the impact of steroids or haemodialysis, and disorders of growth and puberty in children. The situation is complicated by the introduction of different QUS methods and a variety of more or less different commercial devices.

This chapter will give an overview of the principles of existing methods of QUS, without attempting to give a profound physical explanation of the observed associations between ultrasound propagation and the material properties of bone. Computational methods simulating the propagation of acoustic waves are useful in giving an impression of the nature of the interaction between ultrasound and bone in the different approaches. Within the different methods, the existence of various variables such as speed of sound and broadband ultrasound attenuation has to be taken into account, as well as the impact of different technological solutions (e.g. waterbath/gel coupling, positioning, variable calculation). The status of validation varies: naturally, new devices based on modern technology have yet to prove their worth compared with the older devices. Whatever the technology, however, adequate quality control has to be carried out regularly and the

R. Barkmann, PhD
Medizinische Physik, Klinik für Diagnostische Radiologie,
Universitätsklinikum Schleswig-Holstein Campus Kiel,
Michaelisstrasse 9, 24105 Kiel, Germany

user must be aware of limitations and sources of error. With these issues kept in mind, and handled responsibly, QUS devices could play an important role in the diagnosis of osteoporosis. Because of the complex nature of ultrasound propagation, further development of new methods and devices can be expected. More sophisticated analysis of the received signals may even open up opportunities for estimating other aspects of bone quality in addition to density.

11.2
Basics of Ultrasound Transmission through Bone

Sound waves are mechanical waves, which, unlike X-ray radiation, need a medium for propagation. For example, air transports the sound waves of human speech, and ocean water serves as transport medium for the communication of whales. Sound waves in the frequency range above 20 kHz are denoted as ultrasound. The velocity of the propagation of the ultrasonic wave depends on the nature of the medium, lowest in gases such as air, highest in solids. In between is the range for liquids and biological soft tissue. The velocity in bone covers a wide range, in compact bone more similar to the velocity in solids and in cancellous bone more similar to the velocity in soft tissue, at least in high porous bone due to the high marrow content.

QUS methods are parametrical and are in general not used for the reconstruction of an image (Laugier et al. 1994). This means that the interaction of bone and the ultrasound wave is analysed in order to obtain quantitative variables which are associated with properties of the skeletal site such as density, structure or strength. Even imaging devices do not use the image for diagnostic purposes but to find an anatomically correct positioning of the region of interest. Apart from investigational approaches, all devices comprise at least one sender and one receiver separated from each other. Given the strong attenuation of high-frequency ultrasound in (especially trabecular) bone, the frequency range is limited to typically 0.1–2 MHz (Evans and Tavakoli 1990; Langton et al. 1984).

Unlike X-ray-based measurements of bone density (DXA, QCT), QUS offers a variety of variables which, in different ways, are affected not only by the amount of material but also its elasticity and structure. Commonly used are variables of ultrasound velocity and attenuation. Velocity of the ultrasound wave, usually called speed of sound (SOS), is calculated as ratio of transducer distance and time-of-flight of the ultrasound wave between the transducers. Mostly, it is a mixture of velocities in bone, overlying soft tissue and, in some devices, water. Speed of sound in bone is primarily affected by density and elasticity (Katz and Meunier 1987). The attenuation of the wave additionally depends on scattering on inhomogeneities and absorption in the medium (Njeh et al. 1999b). In cancellous bone, attenuation increases strongly with frequency. The best performance in osteoporosis measurements shows the (approximately linear) slope of attenuation with increasing frequency, called broadband ultrasound attenuation (BUA). Unfortunately, the theoretically very well-known associations between material variables and ultrasound variables are complicated in an inhomogeneous material like bone. This is true not only for cancellous bone but also for compact bone, which mechanically and acoustically is anisotropic (Katz and Meunier 1987).

Until today no theoretical approach is able to describe ultrasound propagation through cancellous bone exactly and predict the measured variables correctly. Methods simulating ultrasound propagation through bone are more successful. Using software for the simulation of ultrasound propagation (Wave2000 pro, CyberLogic Inc., NY, NY, USA), we will depict the propagation of the ultrasound wave through bone, which might help to elucidate the "black box" called ultrasound in bone (Barkmann et al. 2000a).

11.3
Technology of QUS Approaches

Three different methods are used today in commercially available devices: transverse transmission in cancellous bone, transverse transmission in cortical bone, and axial transmission in cortical bone (Barkmann et al. 1999; Glüer 1997). These methods, together with the specific interactions between QUS and bone, will be described in this section.

11.3.1
Transverse Transmission of Cancellous Bone

Transverse transmission in cancellous bone (including transmission through a thin cortical shell) is the most common approach. Following the introduction by LANGTON et al. in 1984 of a method of measuring ultrasound transmission through the human calcaneus, a variety of devices have now been developed. All these machines measure the calcaneus, but the technology varies with regard to the coupling of the ultrasound wave into the body and the selection of the region to be measured. The basic principle is depicted in Figure 11.1.

Several variations of this technique have been developed. These include:

● The use of gel as a coupling medium instead of water, making water reservoirs unnecessary. This method requires different techniques to ensure proper coupling into the skin. One solution is to use transducers with variable separation which are pressed against the skin, usually with the help of rubber pads (Cuba Clinical, McCue; Sahara, Hologic, Bedford, MA, USA). Another approach uses a small water reservoir with the transducers immersed and a diaphragm between the water and the skin. The gel-covered diaphragm is pressed against the skin by increasing water pressure (Achilles Express, Lunar/GE, Madison, WI, USA).

● Scanning transducers with the creation of an image instead of using fixed transducers. From the image topography, a region of interest (ROI) can be calculated automatically (Fig. 11.2) (UBIS5000, Diagnostic Medical Systems, Pérois, France; DTU-one, Osteometer/OSI, Hawthorne, CA, USA). In this way errors due to variable positioning caused by different foot sizes can be avoided. A different approach is used by another device (QUS-2, Metra/Quidel, San Diego, CA, USA), which does not create an image but automatically detects the back and the bottom edges of the bone and calculates the optimal position for the measurement inside the calcaneus.

● Focused rather than nonfocused transducers. Focused transducers are used to increase lateral resolution, enhancing the quality of an image. These transducers are only used in the two imaging devices.

● Use of an array of ultrasound transducers for the assessment of an image. Instead of a single transducer, an array is implemented as receiver (InSight, Lunar/GE). By integrating over an area

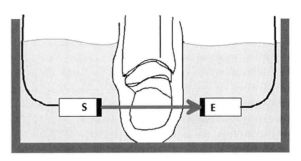

Fig. 11.1. Principle of transverse transmission in the calcaneus. The foot and the transducers are immersed in a water bath. The *arrow* marks the direction of penetration from the transmitter *T* to the receiver *R*. Water is used to ensure proper coupling of the acoustic wave into the skin

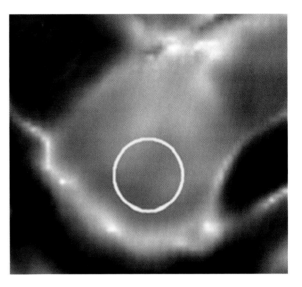

Fig. 11.2. Acoustic image of the calcaneus as created by the UBIS5000. The *circle* marks the automatically assessed region of interest

identical with the surface of the receiving transducer in the former devices (Achilles+, Achilles Express, Lunar/GE), similar results can be obtained. The whole area of the array is used to depict an image of the calcaneus, which is used to check for correct positioning (Fig. 11.3).

Because high frequencies are subject to strong damping in cancellous bone, the usual sonographic range above 2 MHz cannot be used. A typical range in calcaneus measurements is 0.2–0.8 MHz. SOS and BUA are the usual variables employed, as are combinations of SOS and BUA (stiffness index, quantitative ultrasound index [QUI]). The SOS (unit: m/s) is not only the velocity of ultrasound propagation

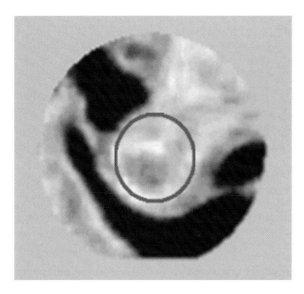

Fig. 11.3. Image of the heel bone as assessed by the InSight device using transducer arrays. The *circle* marks the measured region

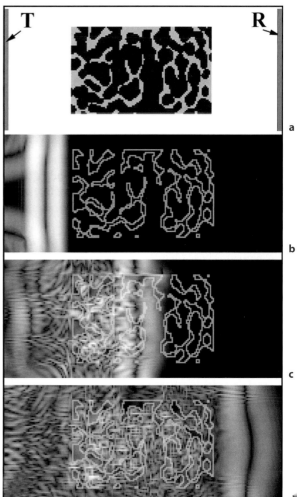

Fig. 11.4a–d. Transmission of an ultrasound wave through trabecular bone (simulation). **a** Image of trabecular bone specimen used for the simulation. The ultrasound wave starts from the transmitter (*T*) and moves towards the receiver (*R*). **b** The wave propagating through soft tissue. One oscillation is depicted as two grey stripes. **c** The wave interacts with the trabecular bone. Parts of the wave always travel through solid trabecular material at a higher velocity and enter marrow again. **d** The resulting wave propagated faster, is attenuated and has a greater bandwidth

in bone, but is also affected by the velocities in the overlying soft tissue and coupling medium. In addition, different techniques are in use, preventing direct comparison of SOS values from different devices. This is not necessarily a disadvantage, however, the impact of the various techniques and sources of error on the sensitivity of the method in detecting and following up osteoporotic changes has to be taken into account. Ultrasound waves of different frequencies are attenuated in cancellous bone to different extents. Attenuation always increases with frequency, at first in a linear fashion. The slope of the attenuation curve vs frequency represents BUA (unit: dB/MHz). BUA is lower in osteoporotic bone than in healthy bone. Bone material covers only 10%–20% of the volume of the cancellous part of the calcaneus. Bone marrow alone would cause only a slight dependence of attenuation on frequency, and hence a low BUA. An increase in bone mass causes distortion of the ultrasound propagation and greater attenuation of higher frequencies, and hence a higher BUA. Figure 11.4 depicts the change of an ultrasound wave during transmission through cancellous bone.

SOS and BUA are affected by properties of the soft tissue layers (BARKMANN and GLÜER 1999). The most important sources of error are temperature and a possible presence of oedema. Due to the fat content, SOS depends negatively on foot temperature. Therefore, SOS measurements should not be taken on patients with very cold feet. The impact on BUA is

less pronounced and positive. Therefore, combined variables (stiffness, QUI) might offer a higher precision due to a partial compensation of the temperature impact. The ability to recognize osteoporotic bone, however, is not necessarily improved. The effect of oedema, which effects SOS and BUA in the same direction, cannot be compensated.

Many studies have investigated the relationships between QUS variables and bone properties of the calcaneus. Since ultrasound propagation is affected not only by density, the impact of trabecular structure and elastic modulus as well as associations with breaking strength have been investigated. In this context, it should be remembered that different definitions of density exist. Density of the solid bone material such as trabeculae and cortical shell is the mass of the material divided by its volume. This only covers the solid bone material, not bone/marrow distributions. Apparent density is the mass of a complete bone volume divided by the volume itself, thus taking into account both bone and marrow. This variable depends not only on bone density, which is nearly constant, but also on the ratio between bone volume and marrow volume in cancellous bone. BMD, as measured by DXA, is not a true volumetric density but a planar variable, where the mass of the bone is divided by the covered area. This variable also depends on bone width. BMD as well as QUS variables strongly depend on the region measured inside the calcaneus, and correlations between QUS and DXA are usually moderate. However, when measured at exactly the same region, correlations increase substantially up to 0.9 (CHAPPARD et al. 1997). Unlike DXA, QUS strongly depends on the degree of alignment of the trabecular structure. SOS and BUA, measured in proximodistal direction differ significantly from these variables measured in mediolateral and anteroposterior direction (STRELITZKI et al. 1997). However, in vivo measurements are taken only in the mediolateral direction, where BMD and structural variables are strongly correlated; only minor contributions of the structure to the relationship between QUS and BMD could be found (NICHOLSON et al. 2001). In a recent study by NICHOLSON and BOUXSEIN (NICHOLSON and BOUXSEIN 2000), elastic modulus of trabecular bone cylinders from human calcaneus bones was substantially reduced by compressing the specimens beyond the reversible region. Despite these strong decreases in elasticity, no changes in QUS variables appeared, indicating that the strong relationship between ultrasound velocity and elastic modulus in a homogenous solid material does not exist in a composite material such as in the calcaneus (solid bone/marrow). Taking these results into account, it is most likely that QUS on the calcaneus mostly reflects its density as measured by DXA.

The transformation of the ultrasound wave during propagation through trabecular bone can be seen in Figure 11.4 in a simulation using a rectangular piece of cancellous bone (Fig. 11.4a). An ultrasound wave propagates from the left to the right side. Three stages of the propagation of one oscillation are depicted, the undisturbed wave (Fig. 11.4b), the wave inside the bone (Fig. 11.4c) and the wave after transmission through bone (Fig. 11.4d). After transmission, the wave has travelled faster than in marrow alone (increased SOS) and the wavelength has increased. The increased wavelength is equivalent with a spectral shift to lower frequencies or a stronger attenuation of higher frequencies. BUA, which is defined as the increase of attenuation with frequency, therefore, is increased after transmission through bone. In general, SOS and BUA increase with the amount of penetrated trabecular bone material.

11.3.2
Transverse Transmission of Cortical Bone

Only one device (DBMSonic Bone Profiler, Igea, Carpi, Italy) uses this method and only the proximal finger phalanges II–V are measured. Using a hand-held caliper, two transducers, one acting as a transmitter and one as a receiver, are positioned on opposite sites of the metaphysis of the phalanges (WUSTER et al. 2000). Measurement site is depicted in Figure 11.5.

The standard variable is amplitude-dependent-speed of sound (AD-SoS). This is calculated as the ratio between transducer separation and the time of flight of the ultrasound wave. Time of flight is measured as the time interval between the starting time of the signal (A in Fig. 11.6) and the time when the signal received reaches a constant trigger level (B). In an impaired bone, the AD-SoS is lower, but the amplitude is also decreased. In this case, the trigger level is reached at a later point in time, leading to a further decrease of the AD-SoS. Therefore, this variable depends on the amplitude of the signal received, combining the effects of the decreases in velocity

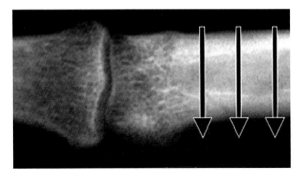

Fig. 11.5. Region of ultrasound propagation through the phalanx

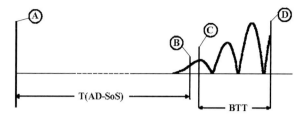

Fig. 11.6. Typical shape of the signal received as detected by the DBMSonic Bone Profiler, depicted as amplitude versus time. *A* Time when transmitted signal started. *B* Time for the calculation of AD-SOS. *C* Time for the calculation of bone transmission time (*BTT*). *D* Time when a wave through pure soft tissue would have arrived, assuming a soft tissue velocity of 1,570 m/s. The signal is cut off at this time because the main information on bone status is contained in the part of the signal which arrived before this time

and amplitude in impaired bone. However, in some applications this combination might be a disadvantage, e.g. in measurements in children, where the amplitude does not change during growth and the inclusion of the amplitude only gives room for an increase in the precision error. Similar to calcaneus measurements AD-SoS combines velocities in bone and in soft tissue. Therefore, the thickness of the soft tissue is a source of error and changes in thickness effect the precision of the method. Both dependencies, on amplitude and soft tissue thickness, are overcome through a recently introduced variable, the bone transmission time (BTT) (formerly called time frame) (MAULONI et al. 2000; WUSTER et al. 2000). BTT is calculated as the difference in time when the first peak of the signal received reaches its maximum (C) and the time that would be measured if no bone but only soft tissue was present between the transducers (D). BTT only depends on bone properties; it would be equal to zero if no bone was present.

BARKMANN et al. (2000a) compared ultrasound variables in vivo with bone geometry, as assessed using magnetic resonance imaging. Associations were also tested using phantoms and the simulation of ultrasound propagation. Two significant correlations were found: between ultrasound velocity and the cortical cross-sectional area, and between the amplitude of the signal received and the cross-sectional area of the medullary canal. Bone width was only a minor confounder. The velocity parameter used was not identical with AD-SoS but correlated strongly with BTT. During ageing or impairment, cortical area typically decreases and the medullary canal area increases, so SOS and amplitude also decrease. The combined AD-SoS variable is affected

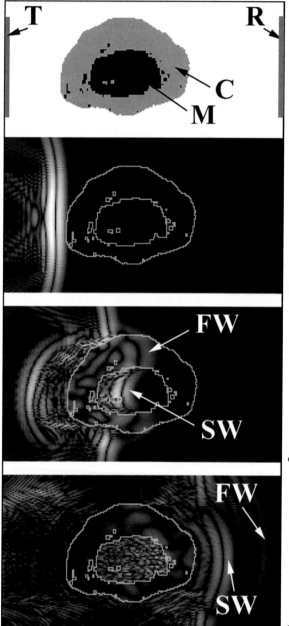

Fig. 11.7a–d. Propagation of ultrasound waves through the finger phalanx consisting of compact bone (*C*) and the medullary canal (*M*) containing bone marrow. **a** Cross-sectional image of a finger phalanx containing cortex (*C*) and medullary canal (*M*) as well as the transducers (transmitter *T* and receiver *R*). **b** Ultrasound wave as transmitted from the transmitter to the left before entering the bone. **c** Split wave consisting of the first wave (*FW*) propagating through the cortex and second wave (*SW*) penetrating the medullary canal. **d** Re-emitted parts of the wave before detection by the receiver

by these decreases in the same direction, combining both effects. Besides cortical area cortical density and porosity are also determinants of QUS variables (BARKMANN et al. 2000; SAKATA et al. 2004).

In a simulation, the propagation of different waves through cortex and the medullary canal can be seen distinctly (Fig. 11.7). The wave, transmitted from a transmitter to the left, is split into two parts, a first wave (FW) propagating through compact bone and a second wave (SW) propagating though the medullary canal. The first wave, which arrives earliest, is evaluated by the device. The second wave arrives later, typically later than the cut-off of the signal received.

11.3.3
Axial Transmission of Cortical Bone

This is another mode that is available in only one commercial device (Omnisense, Sunlight Ultrasound Technologies, Rehovot, Israel). Only one probe is used, comprising a variety of ultrasound transducers and measuring ultrasound propagation through a thin layer beneath the surface of the bone (BARKMANN et al. 2000b; HANS et al. 1999). Unlike with the other devices, the site to be examined has to be assessed from only one side, offering the potential to measure a variety of bones. Figure 11.8 depicts the principal arrangement of the transducers and the propagation of the ultrasound wave.

Ultrasound velocity is measured on the basis of transducer separation and the time of flight of the wave. This time is affected by properties of the overlying soft tissue. However, by using an array of transducers and by evaluating different pathways, the effect of the soft tissue can be mostly compensated and a pure velocity in bone can be calculated.

Depending on signal frequency and cortical thickness, different types of waves propagate through the bone (NICHOLSON et al. 2002). If cortical thickness is much larger than the wavelength (3–4 mm) no impact of thickness on the velocity of the lateral wave can be expected (NJEH et al. 1999c). The separate effect of cortical thickness and cortical BMD has been studied at the tibia. SOS correlated best with the outermost band of cortical BMD (PREVHRAL et al.2001), but both cortical thickness and cortical BMD contributed independently to SOS (SIEVÄNEN et al. 2001; PREVHRAL et al. 2001; NJEH et al.1999c). Theoretically, both cortical porosity and composition should affect SOS but this has not been studied in sufficient detail yet.

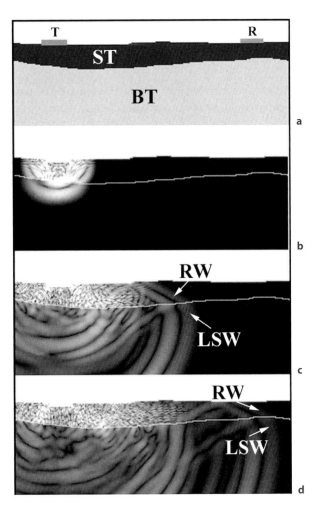

Fig. 11.8a–d. Axial transmission of an ultrasound wave through cortical bone. **a** Cross-sectional image of bone (*BT*), overlaying soft tissue (*ST*) and way of measured ultrasound wave (*white arrows*) also showing transmitter (*T*) and receiver (*R*). **b** Emitted wave penetrating into the bone. **c** Wave propagating parallel to the surface (*LSW*, lateral wave) and from this wave into soft-tissue re-emitted wave (*RW*). **d** Re-emitted wave, arriving at the receiver

11.3.4
Summary of Technological Approaches

The three QUS methods differ substantially and are used to assess different skeletal sites and different bone properties. For this reason, results obtained with one type of device do not necessarily reflect the performance to be expected with another approach. Even within the groups, differences exist. Devices that measure the calcaneus use different technological approaches in respect of imaging capabilities, water-coupling vs gel-based coupling, temperature control, signal processing, and so on. These aspects and potential differences among the QUS parameters need to be taken into account.

In recent years, we have gained knowledge on the associations between QUS parameters and bone properties. Ultrasound propagation through bone has been visualized, enabling sophisticated study of QUS interactions with bone. Although there are no 100% correlations between QUS parameters and bone properties, and the potential of a dedicated analysis of different parameters of ultrasound transmission has not been finally resolved, the bone variables which affect ultrasound propagation most can be identified. In the clinical range, both SOS and BUA (trabecular transverse transmission) mainly measure bone density of the calcaneus as assessed using DXA. In finger phalanges (cortical transverse transmission), AD-SOS correlates with relative cross-sectional area (BARKMANN et al. 2000a). However, the material density of the compact bone varies only within a very limited range, so relative cross-sectional area and density as measured using DXA are strongly correlated. For this reason, AD-SOS in adults can be regarded as mainly measuring cortical bone density as DXA does. SOS as measured in axial transmission mode is affected by the elasticity, apparent cortical density and (in bones with a small cortex) cortical thickness (NJEH et al. 1999c).

Despite these associations, different kinds of diseases might alter QUS parameters in another way than bone density. One example is shown in a study measuring the impact of Paget's disease on bone density and axial transmission of ultrasound (PANDE et al. 2000). A typical feature of this disease is an increase in bone mineral content but with deterioration in bone quality. The study showed that bone density as measured using DXA was increased in the affected tibia but SOS was decreased, indicating an association with bone quality not measurable by DXA.

11.4
Clinical Applications for QUS

Currently we lack diagnostic criteria that would make QUS suitable for the diagnosis of osteoporosis. It has been demonstrated that the WHO criteria cannot simply be used with QUS. Different QUS approaches may show very different age-related declines. Consequently, the number of subjects who fall below the T-score threshold of –2.5 will vary and different percentages of subjects will be identified as osteoporotic, which is inconsistent with the notion of a constant percentage of subjects with osteoporosis. In addition, the limitation in measuring peripheral bones further restricts the use of QUS for diagnostic purposes. Correlations with the bone density of the main fracture sites in the spine and femur are modest and therefore their bone mass status cannot be assessed.

The main field of application for QUS is the estimation of fracture risk. Several studies show that QUS is well suited to the estimation of osteoporotic fracture risk. However, the differences between the methods must be taken into account, and it must also be remembered that different devices using the same approach may perform in different ways. To date, several prospective QUS studies have been published for transverse transmission measurements in the calcaneus and one for transverse transmission measurements of the finger phalanges. The two largest prospective studies, with sample sizes of 6,000–10,000 women, showed that QUS measurements at the calcaneus can be used to predict hip fracture risk in older women.

In the EPIDOS study (HANS et al. 1996), relative risks were similar for QUS (Lunar Achilles) and DXA (2.0 for BUA, 1.7 for SOS and 1.9 for femoral neck BMD). In the SOF-study (BAUER et al. 1997), BUA performed as well as BMD of the calcaneus (relative risks, 2.0; 2.2) but femoral neck performed better (relative risk, 2.6). However, the device used in this study is no longer available on the market. Using the same device, hazard ratios of 1.8–2.3 were found for spine BMD, femoral neck BMD and BUA for osteoporotic fractures. In a smaller study, a relative risk of 1.5 was found for the prediction of vertebral fractures and 1.9 for the prediction of non-spine fractures (HUANG et al. 1998). Extrapolating data from the EPIDOS study, HANS and coworkers calculated that the prediction of hip fractures remained significant up to 7.5 years for the stiffness variable of the Achilles (10 years for femoral neck BMD) (HANS et al. 2004). For transverse transmission at the phalanges, one smaller study has been conducted showing a relative risk of 1.5 for the prediction of non-spine fractures.

Prospective studies are the ideal tool for documenting the ability of a device to estimate fracture risk. However, they take several years and require a large number of participants. With reservations, adequate proof is provided if (1) the device under investigation yields results that correlate highly with results obtained using a validated device and (2) several independent cross-sectional studies document its ability to discriminate between fractures and non-fractures. In a large Swiss study, Ge-Lunar Achilles + and Hologic Sahara performed equally well (KRIEG et al. 2003) in discriminating between women with and without non-vertebral fractures and better than the Igea DBMSonic 1200. In a population-based European multicenter study, the calcaneus QUS-devices Achilles + (GE-Lunar), DTU-one (Osteometer/OSI), QUS-2 (Metra/Quidel) and UBIS 5000 (DMS) performed equally well and as well as central DXA in discriminating between women with and without vertebral fractures (GLÜER et al. 2004). SOS performed slightly better than BUA, and AD-SoS measurements at the finger phalanges (Igea DBMSonic Bone Profiler) were comparable with BUA measurements at the calcaneus. Similar results for discrimination of patients with multiple vertebral fractures have been reported by HARTL et al. (2002). For axial transmission measurements, odds ratios were somewhat lower than for BMD in the same subject group (KNAPP 2001).

Quantitative ultrasound measurements, especially at the calcaneus, appear to perform similarly to central DXA measurements for the prediction of prevalent and incident fractures. Similar results have been found with several devices, perhaps with slight differences for different variables. For hip fracture discrimination, QUS might be slightly worse compared with DXA at the femur, but QUS might be advantageous in the prediction of all types of fractures. Combinations of different QUS variables do not seem to provide any benefit. Some issues still must be clarified before these results can be reproduced in a clinical setting. Quality control procedures have to be defined, for example, there is a lack of anthropometric phantoms, and results obtained on different devices have to be standardized (GLÜER et al. 1997). In the future, it will be important to calculate absolute 5- or 10-year risks for fracture for standardized QUS-results or specific for single devices and variables (KANIS et al. 2005). Once these data are available, a fracture risk assessment comparable to DXA should be possible, at least when performed with the methodologic rigor required.

11.5
Perspectives

Given the positive results of the prospective studies for the assessment of fracture risk and the positive results of many cross-sectional studies, QUS methods have the potential for widespread use. The main field of application is in the assessment of fracture risk, where validated QUS devices may have a part to play alongside existing risk factors. Once data are available on therapy response in patients with low QUS values, a decision for treatment might become feasible based on clinical risk factors and QUS measurements without the need for DXA. Monitoring treatment with QUS, though not recommended today, may become possible once the sources of error can be better controlled, the quality of repetitive measurements can be guaranteed, and once we know more about the associations between treatment-induced changes in bone and changes in QUS parameters. Recently conducted studies have shown promising results. For example, changes comparable to central DXA were measured for QUS at finger phalanges with alendronate and estradiol therapy (INGLE 2005) and for QUS at the calcaneus with alendronate therapy (GONNELLI 2002). The lack of ionizing radiation makes QUS an interesting tool for the assessment of juvenile growth disorders, and reference data for children have been published for transverse transmission methods in the calcaneus and the finger phalanges (BARKMANN et al. 2001; BARONCELLI et al. 2001; VAN DEN BERGH et al. 2000; Drozdzowska et al. 2005).

Ultrasound propagation is affected by bone structure and composition. At the calcaneus, however, structure and BMD are highly correlated and no separate assessment of microstructure can be performed in clinical practice yet. At cortical measurement sites, the prospects of obtaining more detailed information are better, because of the smaller impact of bone marrow composition. Several bone properties have been identified as having an impact on ultrasound velocity in cortical bone such as lamellar microstructure (HASEGAWA et al. 1995), acoustical impedance (RAUM et al. 2005) and porosity (RAUM et al. 2005; SAKATA et al. 2004). Further technological refinements are required – specifically the definition of multiple QUS variables tailored to reflect specific aspects of bone composition – in order to use QUS for the assessment of specific treatment effects or for the differentiation of different bone disorders. Corresponding research is being conducted for transverse transmission methods (BARKMANN et al. 2000b; SAKATA et al. 2004) and axial transmission methods (NICHOLSON et al. 2002; MOILANEN et al. 2004; TATARINOV et al. 2005).

References

Barkmann R, Glüer CC (1999) Error sources in quantitative ultrasound measurement. In: Njeh CF, Hans D, Fuerst T, Glüer CC and Genant HK (eds) Quantitative ultrasound: assessment of osteoporosis and bone status. Martin Dunitz, London, pp 101–108

Barkmann R, Scheffzyk R (2000) Extended measurement procedures of transverse quantitative ultrasound techniques for an improved assessment of cortical structure of the phalanges. Osteoporosis Int 11:S3

Barkmann R, Glüer CC, Heller M (1999) Methoden der in vivo-Ultraschallmesstechnik am Skelett: Grundlagen und technische Realisierung. J Miner Stoffwechs 6:22–27

Barkmann R, Lüsse S, Stampa B et al (2000a) Assessment of the geometry of human finger phalanges using Quantitative Ultrasound in vivo. Osteoporos Int 11:745–755

Barkmann R, Kantorovich E, Singal C et al (2000b) A new method for quantitative ultrasound measurements at multiple skeletal sites: first results of precision and fracture discrimination. J Clin Densitometry 3:1–7

Barkmann R, Rohrschneider W, Vierling M et al (2002) German pediatric reference data for quantitative transverse transmission ultrasound of finger phalanges. Osteoporos Int 13:55–61

Baroncelli GI, Federico G, Bertelloni S et al (2001) Bone quality assessment by quantitative ultrasound of proximal phalanxes of the hand in healthy subjects aged 3–21 years. Pediatr Res 49:713–718

Bauer DC, Glüer CC, Cauley JA et al (1997) Broadband ultrasound attenuation predicts fractures strongly and independently of densitometry in older women: a prospective study. Arch Intern Med 157:629–634

Chappard C, Laugier P, Fournier B et al (1997) Assessment of the relationship between broadband ultrasound attenuation and bone mineral density at the calcaneus using BUA imaging and DXA. Osteoporos Int 7:316–322

Drozdzowska B, Pluskiewicz W, Halaba C et al (2005) Quantitative ultrasound at the hand phalanges in 2850 females aged 7 to 77 yr: a cross-sectional study. J Clin Densitom 8:216–221

Evans JA, Tavakoli MB (1990) Ultrasonic attenuation and velocity in bone. Phys Med Biol 35:1387–1396

Gluer CC (1997) Quantitative ultrasound techniques for the assessment of osteoporosis: expert agreement on current status. The International Quantitative Ultrasound Consensus Group. J Bone Miner Res 12:1280–1288

Gluer CC, Eastell R, Reed DM et al (2004) Association of five quantitative ultrasound devices and bone densitometry with osteoporotic vertebral fractures in a population-based sample: the OPUS Study. J Bone Miner Res 19:782–793

Gonnelli S, Cepollaro C (2002) The use of ultrasound in the assessment of bone status J Endocrinol Invest 25:389–397

Gonnelli S, Cepollaro C, Pondrelli C et al (1996) Ultrasound parameters in osteoporotic patients treated with salmon calcitonin: a longitudinal study. Osteoporos Int 6:303–307

Gonnelli S, Montagnani A, Cepollaro C et al (2000) Quantitative ultrasound and bone mineral density in patients with primary hyperparathyroidism before and after surgical treatment. Osteoporos Int 11:255–260

Hans D, Dargent-Molina P, Schoott AM et al (1996) Ultrasonographic heel measurements to predict hip fracture in elderly women: the EPIDOS prospective study. Lancet 348:511–514

Hans D, Srivastav SK, Singal C et al (1999) Does combining the results from multiple bone sites measured by a new quantitative ultrasound device improve discrimination of hip fracture? J Bone Miner Res 14:644–651

Hans D, Schott AM, Duboeuf F et al (2004) Does follow-up duration influence the ultrasound and DXA prediction of hip fracture? The EPIDOS prospective study Bone 35:357–363

Hartl F, Tyndall A, Kraenzlin M et al (2002) Discriminatory ability of quantitative ultrasound parameters and bone mineral density in a population-based sample of post-menopausal women with vertebral fractures: results of the Basel Osteoporosis Study, J Bone Miner Res 17:321–330

Hasegawa K, Turner CH, Recker RR et al (1995) Elastic properties of osteoporotic bone measured by scanning acoustic properties. Bone 16:85–90

Huang C, Ross PD, Yates AJ et al (1998) Prediction of fracture risk by radiographic absorptiometry and quantitative ultrasound: a prospective study. Calcif Tissue Int 63:380–384

Ingle BM, Hay SM, Bottjer HM et al (1999a) Changes in bone mass and bone turnover following ankle fracture. Osteoporos Int 10:408–415

Ingle BM, Hay SM, Bottjer HM et al (1999b) Changes in bone mass and bone turnover following distal forearm fracture. Osteoporos Int 10:399–407

Ingle BM, Machado AB, Pereda CA et al (2005) Monitoring alendronate and estradiol therapy with quantitative ultrasound and bone mineral density J Clin Densitom 8:278–286

Kanis J, Glüer CC (2000) An update on the diagnosis and assessment of osteoporosis with densitometry. Osteoporosis Int 11:192–202

Kanis JA, Johnell O, Oden A et al (2005) Ten-year probabilities of clinical vertebral fractures according to phalangeal quantitative ultrasonography, Osteoporos Int 16:1065–1070

Katz J, Meunier A (1987) The elastic anisotropy of bone. J Biomechanics 20:1063–1070

Knapp KM, Blake GM, Spector D et al (2001) Multisite quantitative ultrasound: precision, age and menopause- related changes, fracture discrimination, and T-score equivalence with dual-energy X-ray absorptiometry, Osteoporo Int 12:456–464

Krieg MA, Jacquet AF, Bremgartner M et al (1999) Effect of supplementation with vitamin D3 and calcium on quantitative ultrasound of bone in elderly institutionalized women: a longitudinal study. Osteoporos Int 9:483–488

Krieg M, Cornuz J, Ruffieux C et al (2003) Comparison of three bone ultrasounds for the discrimination of subjects with and without osteoporotic fractures among 7562 elderly women. J Bone Miner Res 18:1261–1266

Langton CM, Palmer SB, Porter RW (1984) The measurement of broadband ultrasound attenuation in cancellous bone. Eng Med 13:89–91

Laugier P, Giat P, Berger G (1994) Broadband ultrasonic attenuation imaging: a new imaging technique of the os calcis. Calcif Tiss Int 54:83–86

Mauloni M, Rovati LC et al (2000) Monitoring bone effect of transdermal hormone replacement therapy by ultrasound investigation at the phalanx: a four-year follow-up study. Menopause 7:402–412

Mele R, Masci G, Ventura V et al (1997) Three-year longitudinal study with quantitative ultrasound at the hand phalanx in a female population. Osteoporos Int 7:550–557

Moilanen P, Kilappa V, Nicholson PH et al (2004) Thickness sensitivity of ultrasound velocity in long bone phantoms. Ultrasound Med Biol 30:1571–1521

Nicholson PH, Bouxsein ML (2000) Quantitative ultrasound does not reflect mechanically induced damage in human cancellous bone.[In Process Citation]. J Bone Miner Res 15:2467–72

Nicholson PH, Muller R, Cheng XG et al (2001) Quantitative ultrasound and trabecular architecture in the human calcaneus. J Bone Miner Res 16:1886–1892

Nicholson PH, Moilanen P, Karkkainen T et al (2002) Guided ultrasonic waves in long bones: modelling, experiment and in vivo application. Physiol Meas 23:755–768

Njeh CF, Boivin CM, Gough A et al (1999a) Evaluation of finger ultrasound in the assessment of bone status with application of rheumatoid arthritis. Osteoporos Int 9:82–90

Njeh CF, Hans D, Fuerst T et al (1999b) Quantitative ultrasound: assessment of osteoporosis and bone status. Martin Dunitz, London

Njeh CF, Hans D, Wu C et al (1999c) An in vitro investigation of the dependence on sample thickness of the speed of sound along the specimen. Med Eng Phys 21:651–659

Njeh CF, Saeed I, Grigorian M et al (2001) Assessment of bone status using speed of sound at multiple sites. J Ultrasound Med 20:1219–1228

Pande KC, Bernard J, McCloskey EV et al (2000) Ultrasound velocity and dual-energy X-ray absorptiometry in normal and pagetic bone. Bone 26:525–528

Prevrhal S, Fuerst T, Fan B et al (2001) Quantitative ultrasound of the tibia depends on both cortical density and thickness. Osteoporos Int 12:28–34

Raum K, Leguerney I, Chandelier F et al (2005) Bone microstructure and elastic tissue properties are reflected in QUS axial transmission measurements Ultrasound Med Biol 31:1225–1235

Roben P, Barkmann R,Ullrich S et al (2001) Assessment of phalangeal bone loss in patients with rheumatoid arthritis by quantitative ultrasound. Ann Rheum Dis 60:670–677

Rosenthall L, Caminis J, Tenehouse A (1999) Calcaneal ultrasonometry: response to treatment in comparison with dual X-ray absorptiometry measurements of the lumbar spine and femur. Calcif Tissue Int 64:200–204

Sakata S, Barkmann R, Lochmuller EM et al (2004) Assessing bone status beyond BMD: evaluation of bone geometry and porosity by quantitative ultrasound of human finger phalanges. J Bone Miner Res 19:924–930

Sievänen H, Cheng S, Ollikainen S et al (2001) Ultrasound velocity and cortical bone characteristics in vivo. Osteoporos Int 12:399–405

Strelitzki R, Nicholson PHF, Evans JA (1997) Low-frequency ultrasound velocity measurements in human calcaneal trabecular bone. Physiol Meas 18:119–127

Tatarinov A, Sarvazyan N, Sarvazyan A (2005) Use of multiple acoustic wave modes for assessment of long bones: model study, Ultrasonics 43:672–680

van den Bergh JP, Noordam C, Ozyilmaz A et al (2000) Calcaneal ultrasound imaging in healthy children and adolescents: relation of the ultrasound variables BUA and SOS to age, body weight, height, foot dimensions and pubertal stage. Osteoporos Int 11:967–976

Wuster C, Albanese C, De Aloysio D et al (2000) Phalangeal osteosonogrammetry study: age-related changes, diagnostic sensitivity, and discrimination power. The Phalangeal Osteosonogrammetry Study Group [In Process Citation]. J Bone Miner Res 15:1603–1614

Magnetic Resonance Imaging

Thomas M. Link

CONTENTS

patients without osteoporotic fractures. Thus, several new emerging techniques have been aimed at quantifying trabecular bone structure in addition to BMD. In recent years a number of studies have been performed that applied magnetic resonance imaging (MRI) to the study of trabecular bone and bone quality. Two MRI techniques have been most thoroughly studied in osteoporosis:
- High-resolution MRI (HR-MRI)
- T2* decay characteristics

Currently high-resolution techniques are increasingly used to directly quantify trabecular bone architecture with computer-based structure analysis software. This technique requires high-field scanners with fast gradients and surface coils with a high signal-to-noise ratio. T2* decay characteristics measure field inhomogeneities caused by susceptibility differences at the marrow–bone boundaries and thus quantify the amount of mineralized elements, providing information about both bone density as well as bone structure. The latter technique, however, is currently less frequently used.

12.1 Introduction

Although bone mineral density (BMD) is one of the most important contributing factors to bone strength and fracture risk, studies have shown that changes in bone quality and structure independent of BMD influence both bone strength and propensity to fracture. The influence of these other factors may partially explain the observed overlap in bone mineral measurements between patients with and

T. M. Link, MD
Department of Radiology, University of California San Francisco, 400 Parnassus Avenue, A367, Box 0628, San Francisco, CA 94143, USA

12.2 High-Resolution MRI

Average trabecular diameter ranges from 0.05 to 0.2 mm depending on anatomic site and location within the bone. Modern high-field (1.5- and 3-T) clinical scanners with fast gradients and optimized coil design provide spatial resolutions of down to 0.15 mm in plane and slice thicknesses as low as 0.3 mm; these spatial resolutions have been obtained in vitro in bone specimens and in vivo in the phalanges, the distal radius, and the calcaneus (KUEHN et al. 1997; LINK et al. 1998a; MAJUMDAR et al. 1999; WEHRLI et al. 2001a). Using HR-MRI, however, a number of imaging problems inherent to MRI and technical parameters have to be considered. Due to susceptibility effects between bone and bone marrow, trabeculae may appear thicker in gradient echo images than in spin echo images. Variation of the TE also changes trabecular dimensions; for this reason MAJUMDAR et al. (1995) recommended as small a TE as possible (TE < 10 ms). In addition, TR and bandwidth may also have a substantial impact on spatial resolution. In order to obtain images that are comparable, the imaging parameters have to be standardized.

Previous studies used gradient echo and spin-echo sequences to visualize trabecular bone architecture. The advantage of gradient echo sequences is a faster acquisition time but more artifacts, while spin-echo sequences require longer acquisition time and have lower signal-to-noise-ratio yet less artifacts (MAJUMDAR et al. 1996, 1999; WEHRLI et al. 2001a; LINK et al. 2002b). In particular the amplification of the trabecular dimensions is more pronounced in the gradient echo images (LINK et al. 2003a). Representative trabecular bone images obtained with gradient echo and spin-echo sequences are shown in Figure 12.1.

In deriving quantitative parameters from images one of the primary factors affecting the quantitative measures is accurate segmentation of the bone and bone marrow components. As the image resolution is degraded, the segmentation of the bone and marrow phases becomes complicated due to partial volume averaging effects. The observed density profile at the trabecular bone edge has a transition region between marrow and bone. When the image resolution is comparable to trabecular dimensions the size of this transition zone is not negligible. As a result, the intensity histogram in a region comprising trabecular bone and bone marrow may not be bimodal as one would expect in a two-phase model where pixels consist of a single component. In image processing there is no established technique for measuring the accuracy of any segmentation scheme. Every thresholding scheme has some associated subjectivity that may either be operator-dependent or dependent on the automated criteria specified in an algorithm. Several techniques may be applied when segmenting high-resolution images into bone and bone marrow. Intensity-derived thresholding schemes based on the histogram of signal intensities and internal calibration techniques

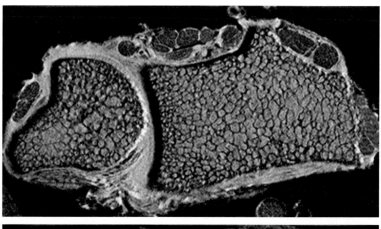

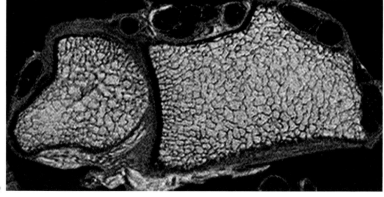

Fig. 12.1a,b. High resolution MR images of the distal radius obtained with a gradient echo (**a**) and spin-echo (**b**) sequence obtained at 1.5 T. Note increased susceptibility artefacts in (**a**) with thicker appearing trabeculae

(MAJUMDAR et al. 1996, 1997; OUYANG et al. 1997) have been used, but because these are obtained from a single value, an apparent thickening of trabeculae or a loss of thinner trabeculae within the same image may result. An adaptive or local thresholding algorithm based on an edge detection schema may result in the detection of the heterogeneity of bone marrow in the trabecular spaces and thus inaccurately classify marrow components as bone. Bayesian estimation techniques, the relative merits and resolution dependence of which remain to be evaluated, have also been proposed (WU et al. 1993). After the images have been segmented into two phases, they may be used to calculate morphological parameters derived from the standard histomorphometry of bone structure such as trabecular bone area fraction (BV/TV), trabecular width (Tb.Th), trabecular number (Tb.N), and trabecular spacing or separation (Tb.Sp) using run length analysis methods or more complex structure measures such as fractal dimension.

An important factor that affects the absolute quantification of trabecular bone area fraction, trabecular width, and spacing is the spatial resolution of the image, which, if it is comparable to the dimensions of the structure to be measured, can lead to errors in the estimated dimensions. It is evident that when the image resolution is equivalent to trabecular dimensions, the accuracy with which the dimensions of trabecular structure can be measured is prone to error, regardless of the segmentation scheme. For example, if the image resolution is 0.1 mm, and the trabecular thickness is of the order of 0.1 mm, an error of one pixel may potentially be reflected as a 100% error in the estimated trabecular width. Similarly a trabecula that is 0.05–0.1 mm thick will be detected as a 0.1-mm structure. The errors in measuring trabecular spacing will be less pronounced, because the marrow spaces are wider than the individual trabeculae. Thus, since the standard histomorphometry measures derived from MR images reflect an average given the limited spatial resolution, they are denoted as "apparent" measures: the apparent (app.) BV/TV, app. Tb.Th, app. Tb.N, and app. Tb.Sp.

12.2.1
Validation of the Technique

In vitro HIPP et al. showed that structure parameters obtained from MR images at 8.6 T with a spatial resolution of 0.092 mm were highly correlated to

the true histomorphological measures determined in optical images: (for BV/TV $R^2 = 0.81$, for Tb.N $R^2 = 0.53$, and for Tb.Sp $R^2 = 0.73$) (HIPP et al. 1996). Using lower spatial resolutions which may also be applied in vivo (0.156×0.156×0.3 mm), MAJUMDAR et al. showed that, compared to true histomorphological measures, partial volume effects in the MR images result in an overestimation of trabecular bone area fraction and trabecular width (approximately three-fold) as well as an underestimation of trabecular spacing (approximately 1.6-fold) (MAJUMDAR et al. 1996). LINK et al. (2003b) compared trabecular bone structure parameters in distal radius specimens assessed with clinical HR-MRI at 1.5 T with those determined in specimen sections (Fig. 12.2). The authors found significant correlations between MRI-derived structure parameters and those derived from macropathological sections, with r values of up to 0.75 ($p < 0.01$). The highest correlations were found for app. BV/TV and Tb.Sp.

12.2.2
Clinical Application

A disadvantage of HR-MRI in vivo are relatively long acquisition times of up to 6–15 min. In addition, fast gradients are required together with dedicated coils with a small field of view and a high signal-to-noise ratio (SNR). Due to these requirements and to motion artifacts in the axial skeleton, the use of HR-MRI is at present limited to peripheral sites such as the calcaneus and the distal radius.

However, application of newer MR techniques to imaging of the proximal femur is work in progress.

Previous studies in the calcaneus and distal radius have shown that structure analysis of high resolution MR images gives additional information to BMD in differentiating patients with and without osteoporotic fractures; some of the studies found even better performance than BMD for the structure parameters (LINK et al. 1998a, 2002b; WEHRLI et al. 1998, 2001a). Figures 12.3 and 12.4 illustrate differences in structure between patients with osteoporotic fractures and normal age-matched controls.

It has also been shown that MRI-based structure analysis techniques were useful in evaluating pre- and post-cardiac-transplant patients with and without osteoporotic spine fractures (LINK et al. 2000). The purpose of this study was to use HR-MRI to analyze the trabecular bone structure of the calcaneus in patients before and after cardiac transplan-

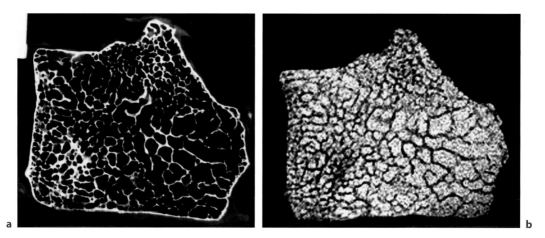

Fig. 12.2a,b. Corresponding contact radiograph of specimen macro-section (**a**) and high-resolution MR image (slice thickness 0.9 mm) (**b**) of a distal radius specimen, showing the similarities in the depiction of trabecular bone architecture. [Images from LINK et al. (2003b)]

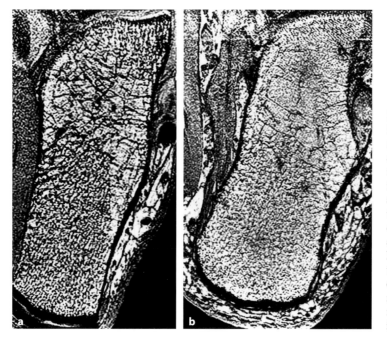

Fig. 12.3a,b. Axial high-resolution MR images of the calcaneus of two age-matched postmenopausal female subjects. **a** Trabecular bone structure of a postmenopausal patient with no osteoporotic fractures. **b** Trabecular bone structure of a patient with an osteoporotic fracture of the right hip. The images clearly depict the differences between the two subjects in the appearance of the "density" of the trabecular network. The marrow spaces between the trabeculae appear widest in the image of the fracture patient. Moreover, both the number of the trabeculae and their thickness are lower in the fracture patient than in the age-matched normal subject

tation and to compare this technique with BMD in predicting therapy-induced bone loss and vertebral spine fracture status. Significant differences were found between patients before and after cardiac transplantation in regard to both structure measures and BMD. In 36% (16/44) of the post-cardiac transplant patients vertebral fractures were found. While structure measures showed significant differences between patients with and without vertebral fractures (Fig. 12.5), differences were nonsignificant for BMD. ROC analysis also showed a higher

diagnostic performance for structure measures in differentiating patients with and without vertebral fractures. Correlation between some of the structure measures and the time after cardiac transplantation was moderately significant, but for BMD the correlation was nonsignificant.

Additional studies were performed in patients with renal failure and renal transplantation (LINK et al. 2002a) as well as patients on chronic hemodialysis (WEHRLI et al. 2004). The results of these studies indicated that structural measures obtained

with fracture

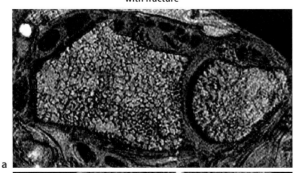

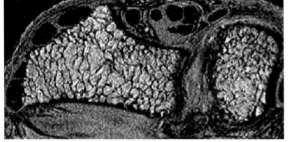

b

without fracture

Fig. 12.4a,b. High-resolution MR images in the axial plane through the distal radius in (**a**) a postmenopausal subject without and (**b**) one with an osteoporotic hip fracture. Qualitative differences in the trabecular structure between both subjects are clearly visualized. [Images from MAJUMDAR et al. (1999)]

from HR-MR images may be used to characterize fracture incidence in kidney transplant patients and that micro-MRI may have potential to characterize the structural implications of metabolic bone disease, potentially providing a noninvasive tool for the evaluation of therapies for renal osteodystrophy.

12.2.3
Longitudinal Studies

In vivo precision errors of 2%–6% were calculated for MRI-based structure measurements, which are in the same range as the precision error of quantitative CT of the spine (OUYANG et al. 1997; NEWITT et al. 2002). As yet only a small number of longitudinal studies analyzing the impact of anti-osteoporotic drugs on trabecular bone architecture have been performed (VAN RIETBERGEN et al. 2002; POTHU- AUD et al. 2004). RIETBERGEN et al. analyzed the effects of idoxifene on trabecular bone in HR-MR images of the calcaneus at baseline and after 1 year of treatment. Mechanical parameters of a trabecular volume of interest in the calcaneus were calculated using micro-finite element analysis. Although there

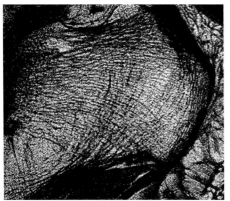

a

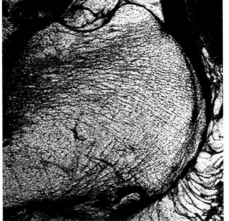

b

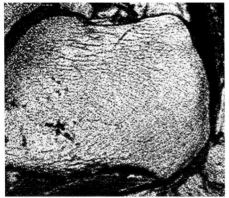

c

Fig. 12.5a–c. Sagittal high-resolution T1-weighted spin-echo MR images of the calcaneus in (**a**) a 40-year-old healthy male, (**b**) a 56-year-old patient 16 months after cardiac transplantation with no fractures, and (**c**) a 65-year-old patient 14 months after cardiac transplantation with three vertebral fractures. The trabecular structure is most dense in (**a**), with narrow trabecular separation, whereas in (**b**) the trabecular structure is sparser and the trabeculae are thin. In (**c**) the trabecular structure is basically gone and the individual trabeculae appear very thin

were no significant differences between the mean changes in the treated groups and the placebo group, there were significant changes from baseline within groups after 1 year of treatment. This study was the first demonstration that longitudinal changes in bone mechanical properties due to trabecular micro-architectural changes may be quantified in long-term clinical studies. It was concluded that the application of these techniques may increase the clinical significance for pharmaceutical trials.

12.3
New Technical Developments

With the advent of 3 T MRI imaging of trabecular bone is getting more feasible. The higher field strength increases signal-to-noise-ratios two-fold compared to standard 1.5-T MRI, thus imaging time may be reduced and/or spatial resolution may be increased for high resolution imaging of trabecular bone. A previous study in calcaneus cadaver specimens showed that using MicroCT as a standard of reference trabecular bone was significantly ($p< 0.05$) better visualized at 3 T than at 1.5 T (Phan et al. 2005). Correlations of true bone structure measurements with those determined in high resolution MRI for BV/TV and Tb.Sp were r = 0.68–0.72 at 1.5 T versus $r = 0.87$ at 3 T. Figure 12.6 visualizes differences in the depiction of the structure at 1.5 T

and 3 T. However, in addition to a better depiction of the bone structure it should also be noted that trabeculae appear more amplified at 3 T, meaning that trabeculae are 2-fold thicker at 3T while they are only 1.6-fold thicker at 1.5 T as compared to the dimensions obtained with MicroCT. This amplification is due to increased susceptibility effects at the higher field strength. Current developments in the field also aim at imaging more central regions of the skeleton. Since osteoporotic fractures at the proximal femur are particularly detrimental for individual patients imaging at this site would be particularly important. In a preliminary study comparing the trabecular bone architecture at 1.5 T and 3 T in six healthy volunteers Krug et al. (2005) found that the bone structure of the proximal femur is substantially better depicted at 3 T. However, the spatial resolution of the images limited the application of 3D structural analysis, making the assessment more akin to 2D textural measures, which may be correlated to histomorphometric measures but are not identical measures (Fig. 12.7). Still, this feasibility study established the potential of MRI as a means of imaging proximal femur structure, but improvements in technique and spatial resolution enhancements are warranted.

In addition to the new 3-T MR scanners the first 7-T whole body MR scanners are now also available and researchers are starting to explore the potential of these machines. Future research will be dedicated to pushing the limits of trabecular bone imaging using this equipment.

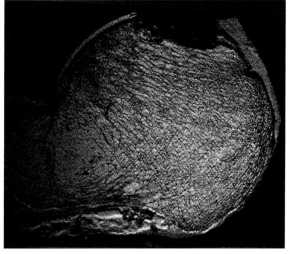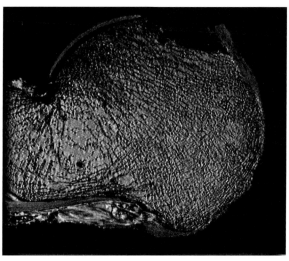

a   b

Fig. 12.6a,b. Sagittal MR images of calcaneus specimens obtained at 1.5 T (**a**) and 3T (**b**). Note enhanced visualization of the trabecular bone architecture at 3 T with better delineation of trabeculae, but also thicker appearing trabeculae due to increased susceptibility artefacts

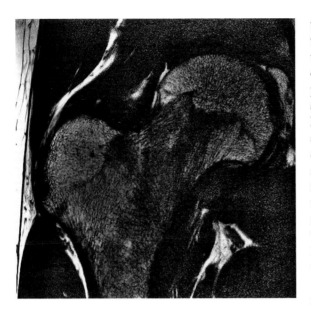

Fig. 12.7. Coronal MR image of the right hip joint obtained at 3 T with trabecular structure clearly visualized at the trochanteric region, but less well visualized at the femoral head and neck. [Images from KRUG et al. (2005)]

12.4
Structure Parameters

A number of structure measures to analyze trabecular bone architecture are currently available and research focuses on developing and optimizing these measures to better predict biomechanical strength in vitro and fracture risk in vivo. Below we described some of the standard parameters and newer parameters that have shown potential in diagnosing osteoporosis.

12.4.1
Morphological Parameters Based on Bone Histomorphometry

The standard structure measures that are currently used are based on bone histomorphometry and require binarization of MR images. Thresholding techniques with high reproducibility are used to obtain these datasets. Intensity-derived thresholding techniques based on the histogram of signal intensities and internal calibration techniques have been applied previously (MAJUMDAR et al. 1996, 1997; OUYANG et al. 1997). From these binarized datasets morphological parameters are calculated. The total number of bright pixels contributing to

the bone phase in the binarized image relative to the total number of pixels in the region of interest is used to compute apparent BV/TV. The total number of black and white pixel edges that cross a set of parallel rays at a given angle θ through the image are counted, then a measure of the mean intercept length is computed as the ratio between the total area of the bright pixels and half the number of edges. The mean value of the intercept length for all angles provides the width of the bright pixels and is defined as app. Tb.Th. From these measurements two other morphological parameters are determined: app. Tb.N = number of bright pixels/app. Tb.Th and app. Tb.Sp = (1/app. Tb.N)–app. Tb.Th. Morphological 2D and 3D measures are currently used to quantify trabecular bone architecture.

In addition to these standard measures, the connectivity of the trabecular network as determined from the Euler number or the complexity of the network as determined from extensions of fractal-based box-counting techniques may also be used to characterize trabecular bone structure from MR images. These latter measures, however, have not been shown to be particularly useful in MR images (LINK et al. 2000).

12.4.2
Digital Topological Analysis (DTA)

The use of DTA to analyze trabecular bone architecture has been previously described by two groups (GOMBERG et al. 2000, 2001, 2003, 2004; WEHRLI et al. 2001b). This technique makes use of data obtained from a skeletonization process that converts trabecular struts into curves and trabecular plates into surfaces. Using digital topological analysis (DTA), the topological class of each voxel in the VOI can be determined by look-up tables as previously described by WEHRLI et al. (2002). Topological classes are surfaces, curves, and their mutual junctions and whether the voxel is situated in the interior or edge of a structure. Dividing the total number of voxels in each class by the VOI produces topological class densities such as surface, curve, or junction densities that are thus, by default, normalized to bone size. Two composite parameters can be computed that characterize overall network integrity: the surface-to-curve ratio (SCR) and topological erosion index (TEI). The various normalized topological class densities are surface interiors (S), curve interiors (C), surface edges (SE), curve edges (CE), surface–surface junctions (SS), and curve–curve junctions (CC). Profile elements (PE) are a special class of curves that consists of two voxel-wide surfaces that represent an intermediate structural type between surfaces and curves in the plate to rod bone loss etiology. The surface-to-curve ratio is a measure of the ratio of plates to rods in the analysis volume. The topological erosion index is defined as the ratio of the sum of all topological parameters expected to increase with trabecular bone erosion (C, CC, CE, SE, and PE) to the sum of all those expected to decrease with erosion (S and SS). These measurements have been previously used with good results to distinguish subjects with vertebral fractures and unfractured controls (WEHRLI et al. 2001a) and in differentiating eugonadal from hypogonadal men (BENITO et al. 2003).

12.4.3
3D Scaling Index Methods (SIM)

The scaling index method is a tool for estimating the local scaling properties of point distributions in higher dimensions. By analyzing these scaling properties it is possible to differentiate between different structural elements in a point distribution (e.g. rod-like, plate-like structures). Considering the three-dimensional tomographic image data as a point distribution one can apply the SIM, which gives a decomposition of the image according its structural elements. In a previous in vitro study it has been demonstrated that the complex 3D SIM is well suited for the description of trabecular bone structure and the prediction of biomechanical strength (BOEHM et al. 2003). This methodology has also been applied with good results to in vivo data differentiating postmenopausal females with and without osteoporotic vertebral fractures (MUELLER et al. 2002).

12.5
Other MR Based Techniques

12.5.1
T2* Decay Characteristics

As shown by the studies of DAVIS et al. (1986), FORD and WEHRLI (1991), FORD et al. (1993), WEHRLI et al. (1989, 1991, 1995), and MAJUMDAR (1991), the marrow relaxation time T2* may be used to study

the density and quality of the trabecular bone network. This method uses standard MRI techniques and can be used in the wrist, calcaneus, spine, and femur. The technical background of this technique may be explained by differences in magnetic susceptibility at the interface of bone trabeculae and marrow, which result in spatial inhomogeneities in the magnetic field. These inhomogeneities result in dephasing of the transverse magnetization, which leads to a decrease in the marrow T2* values. The decrease in T2* and its decay characteristics provide information about the density and structure of the surrounding trabecular network.

Figure 12.8a shows a coronal gradient-echo MR image through the left proximal femur of a postmenopausal normal patient with an echo time of 40 ms. With increasing echo time the signal in the proximal femur decreases. The white box indicates the region of interest used to analyze the femur neck. The graph shown in Fig. 12.8b shows the exponential decrease in signal intensity with increasing echo time. Compared to the dotted curve the lower black curve, with a faster T2* decay, corresponds to denser bone with more pronounced susceptibility effects between bone marrow and trabeculae. Thus a patient with osteoporotic bone would have a curve located above the dotted curve with a much slower T2* decay.

The significant correlation coefficients between T2* values and BMD of the femur and spine found by LINK et al. (1998b) and FUNKE et al. (1994) show similarities between the two measures. GRAMPP et al. (1996) obtained similar results in the distal radius, showing that approximately 50% of the variability in 1/T2* could be attributed to the trabecular BMD. Thus, additional factors must account for the other 50% of the variability, including those related to trabecular architecture and direction and connectivity of the trabecular network.

Several studies (WEHRLI et al. 1991; FUNKE et al. 1994; GRAMPP et al. 1996) showed that T2* increases with age. In the proximal femur LINK et al. (1998b) showed that correlations between T2* and age were even stronger than correlations between BMD and age. These finding are supported by results in the distal radius (GRAMPP et al. 1996); T2* compared to BMD determined by dual-energy X-ray absorptiometry (DXA) and peripheral quantitative CT was the most sensitive parameter by which to predict age-related changes in this study. While the authors did not find significant differences in the distal radius between T2* in healthy subjects and that in osteo-

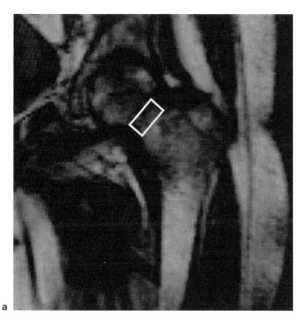

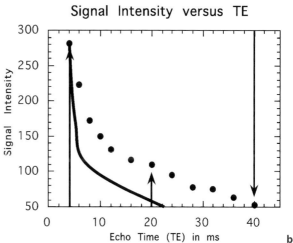

Signal Intensity versus TE

a

b

Fig. 12.8. a Coronal gradient echo MR image through the left proximal femur of a postmenopausal normal patient with an echo time of 40 ms. The *box* indicates the region of interest used to analyze the femoral neck. The graph (**b**) shows the exponential decrease in signal intensity with increasing echo time. Compared to the *dotted curve*, the lower *black curve*, with a faster T2* decay, corresponds to denser bone with more pronounced susceptibility effects between bone marrow and trabeculae. [Images from LINK et al. (1998)]

porotic postmenopausal patients with spine fractures, the results of LINK et al. showed that healthy subjects and osteoporotic postmenopausal patients with hip fractures could be distinguished using T2* measurements of the proximal femur. As yet, however, it is not clear whether the T2* characteristics provide additional information to that provided by BMD in the prediction of fracture risk. Currently research in this arena is limited and application of this technique to clinical practice appears unlikely.

12.5.2
Bone Marrow Perfusion

A new approach to evaluate osteoporosis and potentially fracture risk is dynamic MR imaging of the bone marrow, as it is known that viability of the bone marrow contributes to healthy bone status and reduced fracture risk. A small number of studies has been performed to investigate blood perfusion of vertebral bodies (CHEN et al. 2001; SHIH et al. 2004a,b). CHEN et al. (2001) examined non-fractured, normal-appearing vertebral bodies and studied bone perfusion with regard to age and sex. Rate of vertebral bone marrow perfusion revealed a significant decrease in subjects older than 50 years.

Women demonstrated a higher marrow perfusion rate than men younger than 50 years and a more marked decrease than men older than 50 years (CHEN et al. 2001). In another study lumbar spine bone marrow perfusion was prospectively assessed with dynamic magnetic resonance (MR) imaging and perfusion was correlated with bone mineral density (BMD) in female subjects (SHIH et al. 2004b). A significant positive correlation was found for BMD with peak enhancement ratio of lumbar vertebrae among all subjects ($r = 0.63$, $p < .001$), all postmenopausal women ($r = 0.50$, $p < .001$), and postmenopausal women without hormone replacement therapy ($r = 0.61, p < .001$). Both BMD and peak enhancement ratio were inversely correlated with age. The authors concluded bone marrow perfusion may be able to detect a vascular component in the pathogenesis of osteoporosis (SHIH et al. 2004a,b).

12.6
Conclusion and Future Perspectives

The advances in MRI combined with image processing techniques have potential in vitro and in vivo applications in the study of trabecular bone architecture and its relationship to bone biomechanics, in assessing osteoporosis, and in fracture risk prediction. The noninvasive, 3D nature of MRI together with its ability to predict trabecular bone structure characteristics makes it particularly useful for in vivo studies. However, hardware and software improvements are still needed. At this stage HR-MRI of trabecular bone architecture is used as a research tool to study patient populations in clinical trials and in this setting it has established a role as a measure of bone quality versus bone mass, which is assessed with DXA and QCT. T2* measurements currently have no relevant role clinically, while, as shown in relatively recent studies, bone marrow perfusion as obtained from dynamic MRI may provide new insights in the pathophysiology of osteoporosis.

References

Benito M, Gomberg B, Wehrli FW, Weening RH, Zemel B, Wright AC, Song HK, Cucchiara A, Snyder PJ (2003) Deterioration of trabecular architecture in hypogonadal men. J Clin Endocrinol Metab 88:1497–1502

Boehm H, Raeth C, Newitt D, Majumdar S, Link T (2003) Local 3D scaling properties -- a new structure parameter for the analysis of trabecular bone in high resolution MRI: comparison with BMD in the prediction of biomechanical strength in vitro. Invest Radiol 38:269–280

Chen WT, Shih TT, Chen RC, Lo SY, Chou CT, Lee JM, Tu HY (2001) Vertebral bone marrow perfusion evaluated with dynamic contrast-enhanced MR imaging: significance of aging and sex. Radiology 220:213–218

Davis CA, Genant HK, Dunham JS (1986) The effects of bone on proton NMR relaxation times of surrounding liquids. Invest Radiol 21:472–477

Ford J, Wehrli F (1991) In vivo quantitative characterization of trabecular bone by NMR interferometry and localized proton spectroscopy. Magn Res Med 17:543–551

Ford J, Wehrli F, Chung H (1993) Magnetic field distribution in models of trabecular bone. Magn Res Med 30:373–379

Funke M, Bruhn H, Vosshenrich R, Rudolph O, Grabbe E (1994) Bestimmung der T2*-Relaxationszeit zur Charakterisierung des trabekulären Knochens. Fortschr Roentgenstr 161:58–63

Gomberg BR, Saha PK, Song HK, Hwang SN, Wehrli FW (2000) Topological analysis of trabecular bone MR images. IEEE Trans Med Imaging 19:166–174

Gomberg BR, Saha PK, Song HK, Hwang SN, Wehrli FW (2001) Three-dimensional digital topological analysis of trabecular bone. Adv Exp Med Biol 496:57–65

Gomberg BR, Saha PK, Wehrli FW (2003) Topology-based orientation analysis of trabecular bone networks. Med Phys 30:158–168

Gomberg BR, Wehrli FW, Vasilic B, Weening RH, Saha PK, Song HK, Wright AC (2004) Reproducibility and error sources of micro-MRI-based trabecular bone structural parameters of the distal radius and tibia. Bone 35:266–276

Grampp S, Majumdar S, Jergas M, Newitt D, Lang P, Genant H (1996) Distal radius: in vivo assessment with quantitative MR imaging, peripheral quantitative CT and dual X-ray absorptiometry. Radiology 198:213–218

Hipp J, Jansujwicz A, Simmons C, Snyder B (1996) Trabecular Bone Morphology from Micro-Magnetic Resonance Imaging. J Bone Miner Res 11:286–292

Krug R, Banerjee S, Han ET, Newitt DC, Link TM, Majumdar S (2005) Feasibility of in vivo structural analysis of high-resolution magnetic resonance images of the proximal femur. Osteoporos Int 16:1307–1314

Kuehn B, Stampa B, Heller M, Glueer C (1997) In vivo assessment of trabecular bone structure of the human phalanges using high resolution magnetic resonance imaging. Osteoporos Int 7:291

Link TM, Majumdar S, Augat P, Lin J, Newitt D, Lu Y, Lane N, Genant H (1998a) In vivo high resolution MRI of the calcaneus: differences in trabecular structure in osteoporosis patients. J Bone Miner Res 13:1175–1182

Link TM, Majumdar S, Augat P, Lin J, Newitt D, Lu Y, Lane N, Genant H (1998b) MRI T2* decay characteristics of the proximal femur for assessment of osteoporosis and fracture discrimination. Radiology 209:531–536

Link TM, Lotter A, Beyer F, Christiansen S, Newitt D, Lu Y, Schmid C, Majumdar S (2000) Post-cardiac transplantation changes in calcaneal trabecular bone structure: a magnetic resonance imaging study. Radiology 217:855–862

Link TM, Saborowski S, Kisters K, Kempkes M, Kosch M, Newitt D, Lu Y, Waldt S, Majumdar S (2002a) Changes in calcaneal trabecular bone structure assessed with high resolution MRI in patients with kidney transplantation. Osteoporos Int 13:119–129

Link TM, Vieth V, Matheis J, Newitt D, Lu Y, Rummeny E, Majumdar S (2002b) Bone structure of the distal radius and the calcaneus versus BMD of the spine and proximal femur in the prediction of osteoporotic spine fractures. Eur Radiol 12:401–408

Link TM, Ross C, Nägele E, Bauer J, Kuhn V, Eckstein F (2003a) Spinecho or gradient echo sequences for high resolution MRI of trabecular bone – which sequence performs better in the assessment of osteoporosis and the prediction of bone structure? RSNA. Scientific Meeting Program, p 572

Link TM, Vieth V, Stehling C, Lotter A, Beer A, Newitt D, Majumdar S (2003b) High resolution MRI versus multislice spiral CT -- which technique depicts the trabecular bone structure best? Eur Radiol 13:663–671

Majumdar S (1991) Quantitative study of the susceptibility difference between trabecular bone and bone marrow: computer simulations. Magn Reson Med 22:101–110

Majumdar S, Newitt D, Jergas M, Gies A, Chiu E, Osman D, Keltner J, Keyak J, Genant H (1995) Evaluation of technical factors affecting the quantification of trabecular bone structure using magnetic resonance imaging. Bone 17:417–430

Majumdar S, Newitt D, Mathur A, Osman D, Gies A, Chiu E, Lotz J, Kinney J, Genant H (1996) Magnetic resonance imaging of trabecular bone structure in the distal radius: relationship with X-ray tomographic microscopy and biomechanics. Osteoporos Int 6:376–385

Majumdar S, Newitt D, Kothari M, Link T, Augat P, Lin J, Lang T, Genant H (1997) Measuring 3D trabecular structure and anisotropy using magnetic resonance. Osteoporos Int 7:272

Majumdar S, Link T, Augat P, Lin J, Newitt D, Lane N, Genant H (1999) Trabecular bone architecture in the distal radius using MR imaging in subjects with fractures of the proximal femur. Osteoporos Int 10:231–239

Mueller D, Link T, Bauer J, Morfill G, Rummeny E, Raeth C (2002) A newly developed 3D-based scaling index algorithm to optimize structure analysis of trabecular bone in patients with and without osteoporotic spine fractures. Radiology 225(p):603

Newitt DC, van Rietbergen B, Majumdar S (2002) Processing and analysis of in vivo high-resolution MR images of trabecular bone for longitudinal studies: reproducibility of structural measures and micro-finite element analysis derived mechanical properties. Osteoporos Int 13:278–287

Ouyang X, Selby K, Lang P, Majumdar S, Genant H (1997) High resolution MR imaging of the calcaneus: age-related changes in trabecular structure and comparison with DXA measurements. Calcif Tissue Int 60:139–147

Phan C, Matsuura M, Bauer J, Dunn TC, Newitt D, Lochmuller EM, Eckstein F, Majumdar S, Link TM (2006) Trabecular bone structure of the calcaneus: comparison of high resolution MR imaging at 3.0 and 1.5 Tesla using microCT as a standard of reference. Radiology 239:488–496

Pothuaud L, Newitt DC, Lu Y, MacDonald B, Majumdar S (2004) In vivo application of 3D-line skeleton graph analysis (LSGA) technique with high-resolution magnetic resonance imaging of trabecular bone structure. Osteoporos Int 15:411–419

Shih TT, Chang CJ, Tseng WY, Hsiao JK, Shen LC, Liu TW, Yang PC (2004a) Effect of calcium channel blockers on vertebral bone marrow perfusion of the lumbar spine. Radiology 231:24–30

Shih TT, Liu HC, Chang CJ, Wei SY, Shen LC, Yang PC (2004b) Correlation of MR lumbar spine bone marrow perfusion with bone mineral density in female subjects. Radiology 233:121–128

van Rietbergen B, Majumdar S, Newitt D, MacDonald B (2002) High-resolution MRI and micro-FE for the evaluation of changes in bone mechanical properties during longitudinal clinical trials: application to calcaneal bone in postmenopausal women after one year of idoxifene treatment. Clin Biomech (Bristol, Avon) 17:81–88

Wehrli FW, Ford JC, Gusnard DA, Listerud J (1989) The inhomogeneity of magnetic susceptibility in vertebral body bone marrow. Proceedings of the 8th Annual Meeting SMRM I:217

Wehrli F, Ford J, Attie M, Kressel H, Kaplan F (1991) Trabecular structure: preliminary application of MR interferometry. Radiology 179:615–621

Wehrli F, Ford J, Haddad J (1995) Osteoporosis: clinical assessment with quantitative MR imaging in diagnosis. Radiology 196:631–641

Wehrli F, Hwang S, Ma J, Song H, Ford J, Haddad J (1998) Cancellous bone volume and structure in the forearm: noninvasive assessment with MR microimaging and image processing. Radiology 206:347–357

Wehrli F, Gomberg B, Saha P, Song H, Hwang S, Snyder P (2001a) Digital topological analysis of in vivo magnetic resonance microimages of trabecular bone reveals structural implications of osteoporosis. J Bone Miner Res 16:1520–1531

Wehrli FW, Gomberg BR, Saha PK, Song HK, Hwang SN, Snyder PJ (2001b) Digital topological analysis of in vivo magnetic resonance microimages of trabecular bone reveals structural implications of osteoporosis. J Bone Miner Res 16:1520–1531

Wehrli FW, Saha PK, Gomberg BR, Song HK, Snyder PJ, Benito M, Wright A, Weening R (2002) Role of magnetic resonance for assessing structure and function of trabecular bone. Top Magn Reson Imaging 13:335–355

Wehrli FW, Leonard MB, Saha PK, Gomberg BR (2004) Quantitative high-resolution magnetic resonance imaging reveals structural implications of renal osteodystrophy on trabecular and cortical bone. J Magn Reson Imaging 20:83–89

Wu Z, Chung H, Wehrli F (1993) Sub voxel tissue classification in NMR microscopic images of trabecular bone. Proceedings of the SMRM, New York, p 451

Structure Analysis Using High-Resolution Imaging Techniques

Thomas M. Link

CONTENTS

13.1 Introduction

According to the NIH consensus development panel in 2001 bone strength in the setting of osteoporosis is determined by bone mass and bone quality (NIH CONSENSUS DEVELOPMENT PANEL ON OSTEOPOROSIS PREVENTION 2001). Important components of bone quality are bone micro- and macrostructure. Currently there is substantial interest in better measuring bone quality and pharmaceutical companies are interested in using these measures as biomarkers in drug trials.

T. M. LINK, MD
Department of Radiology, University of California San Francisco, 400 Parnassus Avenue, A367, Box 0628, San Francisco, CA 94143, USA

The most widely used diagnostic techniques in osteoporosis are bone mass measurements such as bone mineral densitometry with either dual X-ray absorptiometry (DXA) or quantitative computed tomography (QCT). Bone mass has been shown to be a good predictor of fracture risk in osteoporosis. However, studies have indicated that the bone mass alone may be of limited value in determining the strength of cancellous bone, and that the trabecular bone architecture is another important factor in assessing bone strength and fracture risk (VESTERBY et al. 1991; WALLACH et al. 1992; DALSTRA et al. 1993; WIGDEROWITZ et al. 2000). So far, diagnostic techniques focusing on the noninvasive analysis of bone structure are considerably less developed and standardized. In recent years a number of researchers have worked on the analysis of high-resolution images of trabecular bone to characterize the trabecular architecture using a number of either 2D or 3D structural analysis techniques.

Several imaging techniques have been described for examining trabecular bone structure, e.g., conventional, projectional radiography, high-resolution computed tomography (CT), and high-resolution magnetic resonance imaging (MRI). Imaging and structural analysis protocols have been adapted to the different imaging modalities. Table 13.1 gives an overview of the studies using the different imaging techniques as well as the structural analysis algorithms.

13.2 High-Resolution Imaging Techniques

To analyze trabecular bone structure, high-resolution imaging is mandatory. Imaging techniques have been used at different skeletal sites: (1) conventional radiography at the calcaneus, the distal radius, the phalanges, the spine, and the femur

Table 12.1. High-resolution imaging techniques and structural analysis algorithms used for the characterization of trabecular bone in osteoporosis

Imaging technique	Textural/structural analysis technique
Conventional radiography	
In vitro:	
Femur, spine, and calcaneus specimens (LESPESSAILLES et al. 1998a,b; MILLARD et al. 1998; OUYANG et al. 1998)	Morphological parameters, fractal dimension
Spine specimens (LINK et al. 1997b; VEENLAND et al. 1997)	Morphological parameters, fractal dimension. Digital skeletons, mathematical filter techniques («white top hat»), co-occurrence matrices
In vivo:	
Lumbar spine (CALIGIURI et al. 1993, 1994)	Fast Fourier transform, fractal dimension
Metacarpals and phalanges (GERAETS et al. 1990; VEENLAND et al. 1994)	Digital skeletons, mathematical filter techniques ("white top hat"), co-occurrence matrices
Distal radius (GERAETS et al. 1990; WIGDEROWITZ et al. 2000)	Morphological parameters, digital skeletons, neural networks
Calcaneus (BENHAMOU et al. 1993; POTHUAUD et al. 1998)	Fractal dimension
High-resolution CT	
In vitro:	
Spine, calcaneus, distal radius, femur and iliac bone specimens (ITO et al. 1998; LINK et al. 1998d, 2003a; PATEL et al. 2005; RUEGSEGGER et al. 1996; WALDT et al. 1999; ISSEVER et al. 2002)	Fractal dimension, 2D and 3D parameters analogous to standard bone histomorphometry
In vivo:	
Lumbar spine (CHEVALIER et al. 1992; ITO et al. 1995, 2005; MUNDINGER et al. 1993) and distal radius (MULLER et al. 1996)	Digital skeletons, "run length" method, fractal dimension, 2D and 3D parameters analogous to histomorphometry
High-resolution MRI	
In vitro:	
Femur, calcaneus, distal radius and spine specimens (HIPP et al. 1996; LINK et al. 1998d, 2003a; LINK et al. 2003b; MAJUMDAR, 1999; VIETH 2001; ISSEVER 2002)	2D and 3D parameters analogous to histomorphometry, fractal dimension, digital skeletons, autocorrelation functions
In vivo:	
Distal radius (MAJUMDAR et al. 1999; LINK et al. 2002b; WEHRLI et al. 1998, 2001)	Morphological parameters, fractal dimension and digital skeletons, autocorrelation, tubularity, digital topological analysis
Distal tibia (WEHRLI et al. 2004)	
Calcaneus (LINK et al. 2002a,b)	
(LINK et al. 1998a)	

(GERAETS et al. 1990; BENHAMOU et al. 1993, 1994; CALIGIURI et al. 1994; LINK et al. 1997b; VEENLAND et al. 1997; LESPESSAILLES et al. 1998a,b; MILLARD et al. 1998; OUYANG et al. 1998); (2) high-resolution CT at the spine (LAVAL-JEANTET et al. 1989; ITO et al. 1995; MEIER et al. 1995; GORDON et al. 1998; LINK et al. 1998b; CORTET et al. 1999, 2000a,b, 2002); and (3) high-resolution MRI at the calcaneus, the distal radius, the distal tibia and the proximal femur (CHUNG et al. 1995; MAJUMDAR and GENANT 1995; MAJUMDAR et al. 1999; GENANT et al. 1996; HIPP et al. 1996; LINK et al. 1998a, 1999; NEWITT et al. 2002b; GOMBERG et al. 2004; POTHUAUD et al. 2004).

13.2.1
Conventional Radiography

Conventional radiography has a spatial resolution of up to 0.04 mm, which may be obtained at peripheral skeletal sites but not in the axial skeleton; the diameter of bone trabeculae ranges from approximately 0.05 to 0.2 mm. However, radiography delivers projection images of the trabecular architecture. These images may reflect bone structure accurately at peripheral sites such as the calcaneus, the distal radius, and to some extent the proximal femur. Figure 13.1 shows two images of the calcaneus one

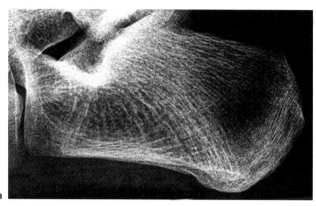 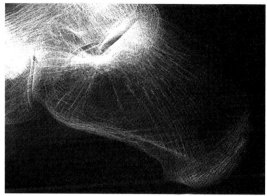

Fig. 13.1a,b. Lateral calcaneus radiographs obtained in a young, healthy female volunteer (**a**) and a postmenopausal patient with osteoporotic fractures (**b**). The differences in the bone structure are clearly visualized

with normal and one with scarce trabecular bone structure in a patient with osteoporotic spine fractures.

13.2.1.1
In Vitro Studies

A number of in vitro studies have been performed correlating the biomechanical strength of bone specimens with the textural parameters derived from radiographs of the same specimens. OUYANG et al. (1998) analyzed cubic specimens of human vertebrae that were cut along three orthogonal anatomical orientations. Contact radiographs of the bone cubes along all three orientations were obtained. The specimens were tested in compression along three orthogonal orientations of the cube and the corresponding elastic moduli were calculated. Quantitative computed tomography (QCT) was used to obtain a measure of trabecular bone mineral density (BMD). A specialized digital image processing procedure was designed to assess trabecular bone structure. Global gray level thresholding and local thresholding algorithms were used to extract the trabecular bone network. Apparent trabecular bone fraction (ABV/TV), mean intercept length (I.Th), mean intercept separation (I.Sp), and number of nodes (N.Nd) were measured from the extracted trabecular network. The fractal dimension of the trabecular bone texture was also measured using a box counting algorithm. Paired t-test showed that the mean value of each texture parameter (except ABV/TV) and elastic modulus along the superoinferior orientation was significantly different ($p < 0.05$) from those along the mediolateral and anteropos-

terior orientations. Trabecular textural parameters correlated significantly with BMD and elastic modulus. These parameters also reflected the anisotropy of trabecular structure.

LIN et al. (1999) analyzed conventional radiographs of human proximal femoral specimens with fractal analysis to quantify trabecular texture patterns and used these measures in conjunction with BMD to predict bone strength. Radiographs were obtained from 59 human femoral specimens. The radiographs were analyzed using three different fractal geometry-based techniques, namely, semivariance, surface area, and Fourier analysis. Maximum compressive strength (MCS) and shear stress (MSS) were determined with a materials testing machine; BMD was measured using QCT. MCS and MSS both correlated significantly with BMD (MCS: $R = 0.49$–0.54, MSS: $R = 0.69$–0.72). Fractal dimension also correlated significantly with both biomechanical properties (MCS: $R = 0.49$–0.56, MSS: $R = 0.47$–0.54). Using multivariate regressional analysis, the fractal dimension in addition to BMD improved correlations with biomechanical properties (MCS: $R_{adj} = 0.66$–0.72, MSS: $R_{adj} = 0.77$–0.83). The authors concluded that both BMD and fractal dimension showed statistically significant correlation with bone strength and that the fractal dimensions provided additional information beyond BMD in correlating with biomechanical properties.

In another study WIGDEROWITZ et al. (2000) studied the trabecular bone structure of radius specimens using computerized spectral analysis of their radiographic images and tested the specimens to failure under compression. Multilayered perceptron neural networks were used to integrate the various image parameters reflecting the periodicity and the spatial distribution of the trabeculae and to predict the mechanical strength of the specimens. The correlation between each of the isolated image parameters and bone strength was generally significant, but weak. The values of mechanical parameters predicted by neural networks, however, had a very high correlation with those observed, namely r = 0.91 for the load at fracture and r = 0.93 for the ultimate stress. Both these correlations were superior to those obtained with dual-energy X-ray absorptiometry and with the cross-sectional area from CT scans: r = 0.87 and r = 0.49, respectively.

13.2.1.2
In Vivo Studies

In an in vivo study POTHUAUD et al. (1998) used morphological textural parameters to analyze radiographs of the calcaneus in 39 postmenopausal patients with and 39 age-matched women without osteoporotic vertebral fractures. Significant differences were found between patients with osteoporotic spine fracture and age-matched controls, and receiver operating characteristic (ROC) analysis showed higher diagnostic performance in differentiating fracture and nonfracture patients for textural measures than for BMD of the proximal femur (DXA).

In vivo analysis of the spine, however, may be more complex, since the variability of image quality due to reduced exposure dose and differences in patients' sizes and weights has to be taken into account. On the other hand, some authors obtained relatively good results in differentiating patients with and without osteoporotic fractures using lumbar spine radiographs compared to BMD (CALIGIURI et al. 1993; ISHIDA et al. 1993; CALIGIURI et al. 1994). The use of conventional radiographs for textural analysis requires standardized film-screen combinations and exposure parameters; the use of a calibration phantom may improve the standardization and reproducibility of textural analysis (CHEN et al. 1994; VEENLAND et al. 1996a,b).

13.2.2
High-Resolution Computed Tomography

Unlike conventional radiography, CT is a tomographic technique, which may also be used to obtain 3D images of trabecular bone architecture. Using high-resolution CT (HR-CT), in vivo an in-plane spatial resolution of down to 0.4 mm and a slice thickness of 1 mm are obtained with clinical scanners; thus trabecular architecture is subjected to partial volume effects and individual trabeculae are not depicted. With the advent of multislice spiral CT (MSCT) spatial resolution increased both in plane (spatial resolution down to 0.25 mm) and concerning slice thickness (down to 0.5 mm); however, still with this technique partial volume effects are substantial. On the other hand it has been found that the pseudotrabecular structure depicted by these images correlates with biomechanical measures of bone strength and the trabecular architecture (LINK et al. 1998c; WALDT et al. 1999; ISSEVER et al. 2002; LINK et al. 2003a).

In addition, micro-CT systems are now available with isotropic spatial resolutions of 0.028–0.25 mm. Most of these systems can only be used in vitro for small tissue samples or small animals (RUEGSEGGER et al. 1996; LAIB et al. 2000; ENGELKE et al. 2001). A new scanner has been made recently available for in vivo applications in humans for the peripheral skeleton (distal radius and tibia) with an isotropic spatial resolution of approximately 80 μm. Figure 13.2 shows 3D images obtained from micro-CT and MSCT datasets that were harvested from donors with and without osteoporotic vertebral fractures. The differences in structure are clearly visualized but also note differences in spatial resolution between micro-CT and MSCT (Fig. 13.2a–d).

13.2.2.1
In Vitro Studies

A number of in vitro studies have been performed correlating texture measures obtained from CT studies with biomechanical measures of bone strength and validating CT measures. In an early experimental study LINK et al. (1997a) obtained HR-CT images of trabecular bone cubes with a slice thickness of 1 mm and used four different groups of textural analysis techniques: morphological parameters analogous to bone histomorphometry, digital skeletons, fractal dimension, and co-occurrence matrices. These authors also analyzed different image postprocessing algorithms (global and local thresholding techniques) and different exposure doses. In addition, QCT was performed and elastic modulus was determined biomechanically. R^2 between elastic modulus and BMD was 0.78 ($p < 0.01$). R^2 for elastic modulus versus most of the textural measures was

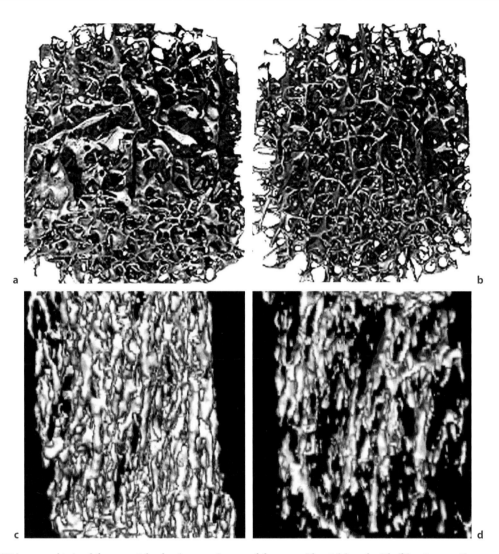

Fig. 13.2a–d. Micro-CT images obtained from vertebral spine specimens of donors without (**a**) and with (**b**) osteoporotic spine fractures. While structure appears more plate-like in (**a**), it is more rod-like in (**b**). Corresponding multislice CT images of the same specimens are shown in (**c**) and (**d**), limitations in depiction of structure are evident, but differences in structure between non-fractured and fractured subject are still well appreciated

also significant. Textural measures in addition to measures of BMD in a multivariate regression model significantly increased R^2 up to 0.87. The textural measures that obtained the best results were three morphological parameters (apparent bone fraction, trabecular separation, and thickness), as well as two of the co-occurrence matrices (energy and mean). The authors concluded that combining texture measures with BMD improved the prediction of biomechanical strength significantly.

WALDT et al. (1999) examined fresh vertebral motion segments and obtained correlations between textural measures and maximum compressive strength of the specimens that were superior to those between BMD and strength (WALDT et al. 1999). The best results were found for fractal dimension determined using a box-counting algorithm, a texture measure of complexity. A similar study in vertebral specimens was performed by BAUER et al. (2004). These authors compared texture measures obtained from single and multi-slice spiral CT (SSCT and MSCT) and found higher correlations between biomechanical strength and texture measures calculated in MSCT images compared to correlations found for texture measures determined in SSCT images and for BMD determined with standard QCT. Figure 13.3 shows images of the same vertebral specimen that was scanned with SSCT and

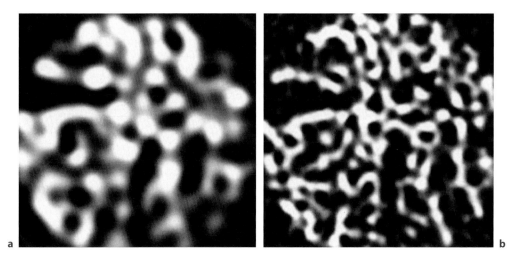

a   b

Fig. 13.3a,b. Single slice (**a**) and multislice (**b**) spiral CT image of the same bone specimen show differences in spatial resolution between the two techniques with better visualization of the structure using multislice CT

MSCT. Structure as visualized with MSCT was validated in the proximal femur and the distal radius with Micro-CT and contact radiographs obtained from specimen sections (ISSEVER et al. 2002; LINK et al. 2003a). Correlations between MSCT texture measures and true structure measures were highly significant but mildly lower than those found for high resolution MR structure measurements. Figure 13.4 depicts an MSCT image of the distal radius and a contact radiograph of the corresponding specimen section; similarities in structure are visualized but also limitations in spatial resolution, which make the CT image appear blurry.

PATEL et al. (2005) showed in a cadaver study that structural parameters of trabecular bone as obtained from high-resolution MSCT images of the calcaneus can be used to differentiate between donors with and without osteoporotic vertebral fractures (Fig. 13.5). Theoretically the previously described techniques are all applicable to in vivo examinations.

The use of micro-CT systems, that obtain substantially higher spatial resolution, however, will be restricted to in vitro studies or limited clinical applications at the distal radius and the distal tibia. Micro-CT is currently considered as a nondestructive gold standard measure to assess cancellous bone and its structural properties. This technique may be useful for analysis of bone biopsy specimens. MicroCT can characterize 3D structure of various animal models, and the longitudinal changes in 3D bone microarchitectural integrity that deteriorates in the transmenopausal period, is preserved with

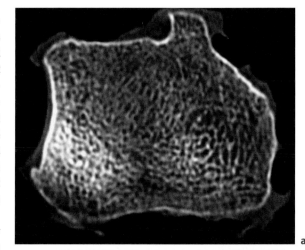

a

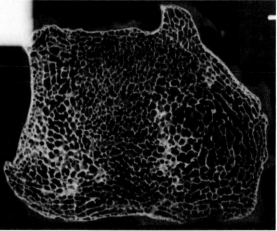

b

Fig. 13.4a,b. Distal radius high resolution multislice CT image (**a**) and corresponding contact radiograph of a specimen section (**b**). Trabeculae appear more coarse in (**a**) yet similarities in structure are clearly visualized

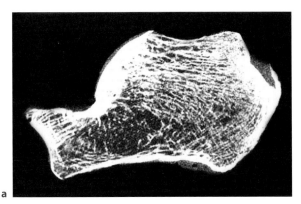

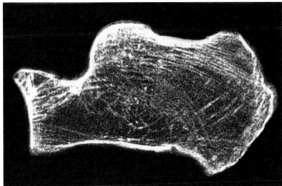

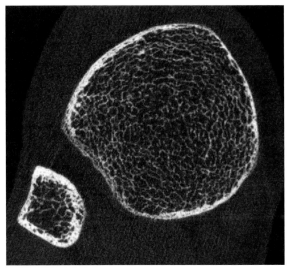

Fig. 13.6. High resolution CT image of the distal tibia obtained in a volunteer with a new in vivo micro-CT scanner for distal radius and tibia. (Image courtesy of Bruno Koller, PhD, Scanco Medical Systems, Zurich, Switzerland)

Fig. 13.5a,b. High resolution multislice CT images of whole calcaneus cadaver specimens obtained from a donor without (a) and with (b) osteoporotic vertebral fractures

HRT, and is improved with PTH treatment in postmenopausal women (JIANG et al. 2005). With spatial resolutions of 28 μm isotropic it is also possible to visualize microfractures and microcallus formations. The incidence and prevalence of microcallus appears of great importance in the context of damage accumulation and repair mechanisms in trabecular bone and thus in understanding the pathophysiology of osteoporosis.

13.2.2.2
In Vivo Studies

Most of the older clinical studies using single slice spiral CT data showed that structural measures obtained either similar or lower results than BMD in differentiating between patients with and those without osteoporotic fractures (CHEVALIER et al. 1992; MUNDINGER et al. 1993; ITO et al. 1995). Combining both measures showed better correlations than either structural measures or BMD alone in one of these studies (MUNDINGER et al. 1993). The somewhat disappointing results of these studies may

be explained by relatively low spatial resolution of these images, textural parameters and thresholding techniques, which may not have been optimal for CT imaging, and 2D analysis of the images. An interesting finding in the study of ITO et al. (1995) was that structural parameters, although they performed worse than BMD in all patients, performed better in the older patients (70- to 79-year-olds) (ITO et al. 1995). An initial study investigating vertebral bone structure with multislice CT, however, has shown promising results in differentiating patients with and without fractures (ITO et al. 2005). Structure parameters determined with this technique obtained better results in differentiating postmenopausal patients with and without vertebral fractures than BMD.

In vivo micro-CT systems for the distal radius and the distal tibia are now also available with spatial resolutions of down to 0.08 mm and optimized 3D structural analysis, which will assess the trabecular architecture more precisely (Fig. 13.6). Initial studies investigating this device are currently work in progress.

13.2.3
High-Resolution MRI

High-resolution MRI techniques are described in detail in Chap. 11. With improved hardware and software, as well as the high spatial resolutions obtained in vivo, MRI is a promising new technique for the analysis of trabecular bone architecture. The lack of radiation exposure makes this technique particularly attractive for clinical studies. Figure 13.7 shows a 3D visualization of a high resolution MRI dataset of a trabecular bone cube.

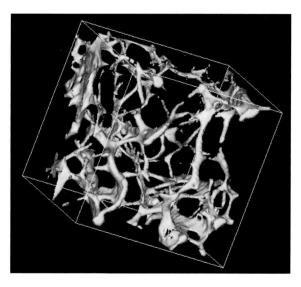

Fig. 13.7. 3D MR image obtained from a human cadaver spine bone cube (size, $12 \times 12 \times 12$ mm) at a spatial resolution of $0.117 \times 0.156 \times 0.3$ mm

13.3
Structure Analysis Techniques

A number of structure analysis techniques have been used for the assessment of trabecular bone architecture in high resolution radiological images; some of these have been described in more detail in the previous chapter. Most commonly used are morphological parameters based on standard histomorphometry (PARFITT et al. 1987; PARFITT 1988) including trabecular thickness, separation and number. Fractal measures calculated using different algorithms have also been used (MAJUMDAR et al. 1993; BENHAMOU et al. 1994; VEENLAND et al. 1996a,b; LESPESSAILLES et al. 1998b; LINK et al. 1998b, 1999; WALDT et al. 1999), other techniques used include mathematical filter techniques as well as co-occurrence matrices (VEENLAND et al. 1994, 1997; LINK et al. 1997a). Another technique which currently receives substantial attention is microfinite element modelling of trabecular bone images to determine biomechanical surrogate measures (NEWITT et al. 2002a). A detailed description of these parameters, however, is beyond the scope of this chapter.

13.4
Conclusion and Future Developments

The analysis of bone structure in addition to bone mass is an exciting new field in the diagnosis of osteoporotic bone. In vitro studies show that with high-resolution tomographic techniques trabecular architecture can be depicted and bone strength may be determined. It has also been shown that osteoporotic and nonosteoporotic individuals may be distinguished using these techniques. Best results, however, were obtained combining structural mea-

sures with BMD. Future developments include optimization of imaging hardware and improvement of 3D analysis techniques for high-resolution tomographic datasets. Using the advanced available hardware clinical studies are also required.

References

Bauer JS, Issever AS, Fischbeck M, Burghardt A, Eckstein F, Rummeny EJ, Majumdar S, Link TM (2004) Mehrschicht-CT zur Strukturanalyse des trabekulären Knochens -- Vergleich mit Mikro-CT und biomechanischer Festigkeit. Rofo 176:709–718

Benhamou C, Lespessailes E, Touliere D, Jacquet G, Harba R, Jennane R (1993) Fractal evaluation of trabecular bone microarchitecture: comparative study of calcaneus and ultradistal radius. J Bone Miner Res 8:263

Benhamou C, Lespessailles E, Jacquet G, Harba R, Jennane R, Loussot T, Tourliere D, Ohley W (1994) Fractal organization of trabecular bone images on calcaneus radiographs. J Bone Miner Res 9:1909–1918

Caligiuri P, Giger M, Favus M, Jia H, Doi K, Dixon L (1993) Computerized radiographic analysis of osteoporosis: preliminary evaluation. Radiology 186:471–474

Caligiuri P, Giger ML, Favus M (1994) Multifractal radiographic analysis of osteoporosis. Med Phys 21:503–508

Chen J, Zheng B, Chang Y, Shaw C, Towers J, Gur D (1994) Fractal analysis of trabecular patterns in projection radiographs. An assessment. Invest Radiol 29:624–629

Chevalier F, Laval-Jeantet A, Laval-Jeantet M, Bergot C (1992) CT image analysis of the vertebral trabecular network in vivo. Calcif Tissue Int 51:8–13

Chung HW, Wehrli FW, Williams JL,Wehrli SL (1995) Three dimensional nuclear magnetic resonance micro-imaging of trabecular bone. J Bone Miner Res 10:1452–1461

Cortet B, Dubois P, Boutry N, Bourel P, Cotten A, Marchandise X (1999) Image analysis of the distal radius trabecular network using computed tomography. Osteoporos Int 9:410–419

Cortet B, Boutry N, Dubois P, Bourel P, Cotten A, Marchandise X (2000a) In vivo comparison between computed tomography and magnetic resonance image analysis of the distal radius in the assessment of osteoporosis. J Clin Densitometry 3:15–26

Cortet B, Dubois P, Boutry N, Varlet E, Cotten A, Marchandise X (2000b) Does high-resolution computed tomography image analysis of the distal radius provide information independent of bone mass? J Clin Densitometry 3:339–351

Cortet B, Dubois P, Boutry N, Palos G, Cotten A, Marchandise X (2002) Computed tomography image analysis of the calcaneus in male osteoporosis. Osteoporos Int 13:33–41

Dalstra M, Huiskes R, Odgaard A (1993) Mechanical and textural properties of pelvic trabecular bone. J Biomech 27:375–389

Engelke K, Suss C, Kalender W (2001) Stereolithographic models simulating trabecular bone and their characterization by thin-slice- and micro-CT. Eur Radiol 11:2026–2040

Genant H, Engelke K, Fuerst T, Glueer C, Grampp S, Harris S, Jergas M, Lang T, Lu Y, Majumdar S, Mathur A, Takada M (1996) Noninvasive assessment of bone mineral and structure: state of the art. J Bone Miner Res 11:707–730

Geraets W, van der Stelt P, Netelenbos C, Elders P (1990) A new method for automatic recognition of the radiographic trabecular pattern. J Bone Miner Res 5:227–232

Gomberg BR, Wehrli FW, Vasilic B, Weening RH, Saha PK, Song HK, Wright AC (2004) Reproducibility and error sources of micro-MRI-based trabecular bone structural parameters of the distal radius and tibia. Bone 35:266–276

Gordon C, Lang T, Augat P, Genant H (1998) Image-based assessment of spinal structure bone from high-resolution CT images. Osteoporos Int 8:317–325

Hipp J, Jansujwicz A, Simmons C, Snyder B (1996) Trabecular bone morphology from micro-magnetic resonance imaging. J Bone Miner Res 11:286–292

Ishida T, Kazuya Y, Takigawa A, Kariya K, Itoh H (1993) Trabecular pattern analysis using fractal dimension. Jpn J Appl Phys 32:1867–1871

Issever AS, Vieth V, Lotter A, Meier N, Laib A, Newitt D, Majumdar S, Link TM (2002) Local differences in the trabecular bone structure of the proximal femur depicted with high-spatial-resolution MR imaging and multisection CT. Acad Radiol 9:1395–1406

Ito M, Ohki M, Hayashi K, Yamada M, Uetani M, Nakamura T (1995) Trabecular texture analysis of CT images in the relationship with spinal fracture. Radiology 194:55–59

Ito M, Nakamura T, Matsumoto T, Tsurusaki K,Hayashi K (1998) Analysis of trabecular microarchitecture of human iliac bone using microcomputed tomography in patients with hip arthrosis with or without vertebral fracture. Bone 23:163–169

Ito M, Ikeda K, Nishiguchi M, Shindo H, Uetani M, Hosoi T, Orimo H (2005) Multi-detector row CT imaging of vertebral microstructure for evaluation of fracture risk. J Bone Miner Res 20:128–1836

Jiang Y, Zhao J, Liao EY, Dai RC, Wu XP, Genant HK (2005) Application of micro-CT assessment of 3-D bone microstructure in preclinical and clinical studies. J Bone Miner Metab 23[Suppl]:122–131

Laib A, Barou O, Vico L, Lafage-Proust M, Alexandre C, Rugsegger P (2000) 3D micro-computed tomography of trabecular and cortical bone architecture with application to a rat model of immobilisation osteoporosis. Med Biol Eng Comput 38:326–332

Laval-Jeantet A, Chevalier F, Pellot C, Bergot C (1989) CT imaging and the quest for information on the vertebral structure. Seventh International Workshop on Bone Densitometry, p 11

Lespessailles E, Jullien A, Eynard E, Harba R, Jacquet G, Ildefonse J, Ohley W, Benhamou C (1998a) Biomechanical properties of human os calcanei: relationships with bone density and fractal evaluation of bone microarchitecture. J Biomech 31:817–824

Lespessailles E, Roux J, Benhamou C, Arlot M, Eynard E, Harba R, Padonou C, Meunier P (1998b) Fractal analysis of bone texture on os calcis radiographs compared with trabecular microarchitecture analyzed by histomorphometry. Calcif Tissue Int 63:121–125

Lin J, Grampp S, Link T, Kothari M, Newitt D, Felsenberg D, Majumdar S (1999) Fractal analysis of proximal femur radiographs: correlation with biomechanical properties and bone mineral density. Osteoporos Int 9:516–524

Link TM, Majumdar S, Augat P, Lin J, Newitt D, Genant H (1997a) Trabecular bone structure using texture analysis of high resolution MR images versus biomechanically determined bone strength in an experimental model. Osteoporosis Int 7:289

Link TM, Majumdar S, Konermann W, Meier N, Lin JC, Newitt D, Ouyang X, Peters PE, Genant HK (1997b) Texture analysis of direct magnification radiographs: correlation with bone mineral density and biomechanical properties. Academic Radiology 4:167–176

Link TM, Majumdar S, Augat P, Lin J, Newitt D, Lu Y, Lane N, Genant H (1998a) In vivo high resolution MRI of the calcaneus: differences in trabecular structure in osteoporosis patients. J Bone Miner Res 13:1175–1182

Link TM, Majumdar S, Lin J, Augat P, Gould R, Newitt D, Ouyang X, Lang T, Mathur A, Genant H (1998b) Assessment of trabecular structure using high-resolution CT images and texture analysis. J Comput Assist Tomogr 22:15–24

Link TM, Majumdar S, Lin J, Augat P, Gould R, Newitt D, Ouyang X, Lang T, Mathur A, Genant H (1998c) Assessment of trabecular structure using high-resolution CT images and texture analysis. J Comput Assist Tomo 22:15–24

Link TM, Majumdar S, Lin J, Newitt D, Augat P, Ouyang X, Mathur A, Genant H (1998d) A comparative study of trabecular bone properties in the spine and femur using high resolution MRI and CT. J Bone Miner Res 13:122–132

Link TM, Majumdar S, Grampp S, Guglielmi G, van Kuijk C, Imhof I, Glueer C, Adams J (1999) Imaging of trabecular bone structure in osteoporosis. Eur Radiol 9:1781–1788

Link TM, Saborowski S, Kisters K, Kempkes M, Kosch M, Newitt D, Lu Y, Waldt S, Majumdar S (2002a) Changes in calcaneal trabecular bone structure assessed with high resolution MRI in patients with kidney transplantation. Osteoporos Int 13:119–129

Link TM, Vieth V, Matheis J, Newitt D, Lu Y, Rummeny E, Majumdar S (2002b) Bone structure of the distal radius and the calcaneus versus BMD of the spine and proximal femur in the prediction of osteoporotic spine fractures. Eur Radiol 12:401–408

Link TM, Vieth V, Stehling C, Lotter A, Beer A, Newitt D, Majumdar S (2003a) High resolution MRI versus Multislice spiral CT -- which technique depicts the trabecular bone structure best? Eur Radiol 13:663–671

Link TM, Vieth V, Langenberg R, Meier N, Lotter A, Newitt D, Majumdar S (2003b) Structure analysis of high resolution magnetic resonance imaging of the proximal femur: in vitro correlation with biomechanical strength and BMD. Calcif Tissue Int 72:156–165

Majumdar S, Genant H (1995) Magnetic resonance imaging in osteoporosis. Eur J Radiol. 20:193–197

Majumdar S, Link T, Augat P, Lin J, Newitt D, Lane N, Genant H (1999) Trabecular bone architecture in the distal radius using MR imaging in subjects with fractures of the proximal femur. Osteoporos Int 10:231–239

Majumdar S, Weinstein R, Prasad R (1993) The fractal dimension of trabecular bone: a measure of trabecular structure. Calcif Tissue Int 52:168

Meier N, Link T, Fiebich M, Bick U, Lenzen H, Peters P (1995) Digital bone structure analysis from computer tomographs of the human lumbar spine. CAR 1995, conference proceedings, Berlin, Springer

Millard J, Augat P, Link T, Kothari M, Newitt D, Genant H, Majumdar S (1998) Power spectral analysis of trabecular bone structure from radiographs: correlation with bone mineral density and biomechanics. Calcif Tissue Int 63:482–489

Muller R, Hildebrand T, Hauselmann H, Ruegsegger P (1996) In vivo reproducibility of three-dimensional structural properties of noninvasive bone biopsies using 3D-pQCT. J Bone Miner Res 11:1745–1750

Mundinger A, Wiesmeier B, Dinkel E, Helwig A, Beck A, Schulte-Moenting J (1993) Quantitative image analysis of vertebral body architecture-improved diagnosis in osteoporosis based on high-resolution computed tomography. Osteoporos Int 3:138–147

Newitt DC, Majumdar S, van Rietbergen B, von Ingersleben G, Harris ST, Genant HK, Chesnut C, Garnero P, MacDonald B (2002a) In vivo assessment of architecture and micro-finite element analysis derived indices of mechanical properties of trabecular bone in the radius. Osteoporos Int 13:6–17

Newitt DC, van Rietbergen B, Majumdar S (2002b) Processing and analysis of in vivo high-resolution MR images of trabecular bone for longitudinal studies: reproducibility of structural measures and micro-finite element analysis derived mechanical properties. Osteoporos Int 13:278–287

NIH Consensus Development Panel on Osteoporosis Prevention, Diagnosis, and Therapy (2001) Osteoporosis prevention, diagnosis, and therapy. JAMA 285:785–795

Ouyang X, Majumdar S, Link T, Lu Y, Augat P, Lin J, Newitt D, Genant H (1998) Morphometric texture analysis of spinal trabecular bone structure assessed using orthogonal radiographic projections. Medical Physics 25:2037–2045

Parfitt M (1988) Bone histomorphometry: standardization of nomenclature, symbols and units. Summary of a proposed system. Bone and Mineral 4:1–5

Parfitt M, Drezner M, Glorieux F, Kanis J, Malluche H, Meunier P, Ott S, Recker R (1987) Bone histomorphometry: standardization of nomenclature, symbols and units.

Report of the ASBMR histomorphometry nomenclature committee. J Bone Miner Res 2:595–610

Patel PV, Prevrhal S, Bauer JS, Phan C, Eckstein F, Lochmuller EM, Majumdar S, Link TM (2005) Trabecular bone structure obtained from multislice spiral computed tomography of the calcaneus predicts osteoporotic vertebral deformities. J Comput Assist Tomogr 29:246–253

Pothuaud L, Lespessailles E, Harba R, Jennane R, Royant V, Eynard E, Benhamou C (1998) Fractal analysis of trabecular bone texture on radiographs: discriminant value in post menopausal osteoporosis. Osteoporos Int 8:618–625

Pothuaud L, Newitt DC, Lu Y, MacDonald B, Majumdar S (2004) In vivo application of 3D-line skeleton graph analysis (LSGA) technique with high-resolution magnetic resonance imaging of trabecular bone structure. Osteoporos Int 15:411–419

Ruegsegger P, Koller B, Muller R (1996) A microtomographic system for the nondestructive evaluation of bone architecture. Calcif Tissue Int 58:24–29

Veenland J, Grashuis J, Mer van der F, Beckers A, Gelsema E (1996a) Estimation of fractal dimension in radiographs. Med Phys 23:585–594

Veenland J, Link T, Konermann W, Meier N, Grashuis J, Gelsema E (1996b) Comparison of two fractal dimension estimation methods in predicting fracture risk in vertebrae. Osteoporosis Int 6, S1:146

Veenland J, Link T, Konermann W, Meier N, Grashuis J, Gelsema E (1997) Unraveling the role of structure and density in determining vertebral bone strength. Calcif Tissue Int 61:474–479

Veenland JF, Grashuis JL, Gelsema ES, Beckers ALD, van Kujik C (1994) Texture analysis of trabecular bone in radiographs to detect osteoporosis. Symposium for Computer Assisted Radiology, pp 77–82

Vesterby A, Mosekilde L, Gundersen HJ, Melsen F, Mosekilde L, Holme K, Sorensen S (1991) Biologically meaningful determinants of the in vitro strength of lumbar vertebrae. Bone 12:219–224

Waldt S, Meier N, Renger B, Lenzen H, Fiebich M, Rummeny E, Link T (1999) Strukturanalyse hochauflösender Computertomogramme als ergänzendes Verfahren in der Osteoporosediagnostik: in vitro Untersuchungen an Wirbelsäulensegmenten. Rofo 171:136–142

Wallach S, Feinblatt J, Avioli L (1992) The bone quality problem. Calcif Tissue Int 51:169–172

Wehrli F, Hwang S, Ma J, Song H, Ford J, Haddad J (1998) Cancellous bone volume and structure in the forearm: noninvasive assessment with MR microimaging and image processing. Radiology 206:347–357

Wehrli FW, Gomberg BR, Saha PK, Song HK, Hwang SN, Snyder PJ (2001) Digital topological analysis of in vivo magnetic resonance microimages of trabecular bone reveals structural implications of osteoporosis. J Bone Miner Res 16:1520–1531

Wehrli FW, Leonard MB, Saha PK, Gomberg BR (2004) Quantitative high-resolution magnetic resonance imaging reveals structural implications of renal osteodystrophy on trabecular and cortical bone. J Magn Reson Imaging 20:83–89

Wigderowitz C, Paterson C, Dashti H, McGurty D, Rowley D (2000) Prediction of bone strength from cancellous structure of the distal radius: can we improve on DXA? Osteoporos Int 11:840–846

Densitometry in Clinical Practice

STEPHAN GRAMPP

CONTENTS

14.1 Introduction

The focus of radiological efforts are early diagnosis of the bone mineral status, identification of patients at risk and accurate prediction of treatment outcome. The most commonly used methods are dual-energy X-ray absorptiometry (DXA) and quantitative computed tomography (QCT), which together with conventional radiographs constitute the basic diagnostic modalities. All of these have been described in detail in previous chapters. Additionally, clinical risk factors such as low body weight, previous fractures, etc., shall be taken into account. Data acquired from an individual patient are generally compared to data from an age-, sex-, and ethnicity-matched control population. Those are routinely provided in the software of the diagnostic equipment. The bone mass measurement predicts a patient's future risk of fracture, and osteoporosis can be diagnosed even in the absence of prevalent fractures. Which measurement sites are most appropriate for the purpose may vary depending on the specific characteristics of the individual patient. The basic and supplementary techniques employed in any given clinical case should be based on knowledge of their strengths and limitations.

Osteoporosis is defined as a decrease in bone mass accompanied by structural and architectonic changes leading to a decrease in bone strength and ultimately to an increase in fracture propensity. The most important information the clinician seeks from the radiologist relates to this last. Bone strength itself depends on several factors such as bone mineral density, bone structure and size, elastic modulus, bone marrow and the ability to heal microfractures. Mass density and elastic modulus are highly correlated and are both influenced by trabecular configuration, biomechanical properties and fatigue damage. Both measures reflect the biomechanical properties of trabecular bone (ASHMAN and RHO 1988; CEDER et al. 1981; GLÜER 1997; GREENFIELD et al. 1975; JERGAS et al. 1995b). Bone mineral density (BMD) as defined by radiological techniques is in this context the most important determinant of bone fragility and fracture risk (CUMMINGS et al. 1993, 1995; GENANT et al. 1996; MILLER et al. 1996). The incidence of fractures has increased in the last few decades due to the increased life expectancy in industrial countries (BOYCE and VESSEY 1985). Early diagnosis of osteoporosis and assessment of treatment efficacy are therefore of great clinical and scientific interest. Bones which predominantly consist of trabecular structures are generally the preferred measuring sites for the assessment of BMD (ADAMS 1997; GENANT et al. 1996; GLÜER et al. 1996; GRAMPP et al. 1997a; GUGLIELMI et al. 1995, 1997; LINK et al. 1998). This is based on the fact that trabecular bone responds to metabolic stimuli about eight times as fast as does cortical bone, accordingly changes in bone mass are first detectable in these regions. In

S. GRAMPP, MD
Univ. Dozent, Dr. Grampp and Dr. Henk OEG, Röntgenordination, Lenaustrasse 23, 2000 Stockerau, Austria

addition, the incidence of fractures is greater in bones with larger trabecular parts (e.g., vertebral bodies, femoral neck, and distal radius) (FROST 1964; JONES et al. 1987). As described in detail in previous chapters, it is now possible to evaluate by various means the appendicular or axial skeleton or both, as well as the trabecular bone or cortical bone envelopes, with a high degree of accuracy and precision, and a modest capacity for determining bone strength and predicting fracture risk (GENANT et al. 1996; ADAMS 1997; GUGLIELMI et al. 1997). In general the more measurements performed the more complex and accurate the information about the skeletal status of an individual.

14.2
Diagnosis and Prediction of Treatment Outcome

At the beginning of a diagnostic work-up, in almost all cases, conventional X-rays are performed (GRAMPP et al. 1997b). Bone density measurements are always compared to those from age-, sex-, and ethnicity-matched controls, since bone density decreases with age, and differences exist between sexes and races. A normative database, such as is given by all manufacturers in the software of their systems, is mandatory for the interpretation of BMD (Fig. 14.1). Usually the estimated bone density is given as a T-score and a Z-score. The T-score refers to the peak bone mass of young normal adults and is calculated similarly to the Z-score. The Z-score shows the patient's results as the deviation from the mean of age-matched controls divided by the standard deviation of this mean, which is an indication of biological variability. These scores are instrumental in predicting the fracture risk of patients. One of the basic principles is that prevention of osteoporotic fractures will reduce morbidity as well as mortality in the population and therefore reduces costs for the health system. For adequate prevention, patients who have a high fracture risk but have not yet suffered a fracture need to be identified. There are several clinical reasons for this. Firstly, asymptomatic individuals with decreased bone mass are at higher risk of fracture than are normal individuals. Secondly, it frequently happens that reasons for low bone mass in individuals are identified, that are not due to ageing, which in most cases is accompanied

by an inactive lifestyle. If patients with a low bone mass are identified and receive appropriate therapy, further bone loss and further increase of fracture risk can be avoided (LINDSAY and TOHME 1990; ROSS et al. 1991, 1993; WATTS et al. 1990). If these individuals are not identified, the bone loss will continue without restriction and intervention.

The same is not true of children in exactly the same terms. In children assessment of BMD and BMC may only be helpful in selected cases such as patients with a malnutrition syndrome or anorexia nervosa, or those undergoing treatment for tumors and other malignant diseases (GORDON 2000; HARKE 1999; RESCH et al. 2000; SEEMAN et al. 2000). Using a T-score for patients below the age of 18–20 years is not helpful. Here the use of the Z-score to compare an individual measurement to the age-matched population is the method of choice. Some manufac-

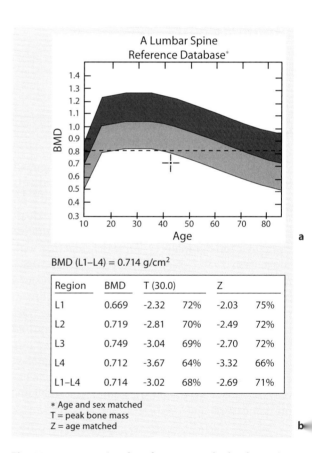

BMD (L1–L4) = 0.714 g/cm²

Region	BMD	T (30.0)		Z	
L1	0.669	-2.32	72%	-2.03	75%
L2	0.719	-2.81	70%	-2.49	72%
L3	0.749	-3.04	69%	-2.70	72%
L4	0.712	-3.67	64%	-3.32	66%
L1–L4	0.714	-3.02	68%	-2.69	71%

* Age and sex matched
T = peak bone mass
Z = age matched

b

Fig. 14.1. a Normative data for BMD at the lumbar spine (L1–L4; PA) in a female population. Age is represented on the *x*-axis, BMD on the *y*-axis. Peak bone mass is reached in the third decade; from this point on the BMD decreases with age. **b** The BMD (in g/cm²) of the individual measurement together with T and Z scores. A datapoint for the patient's individual measurement is given

turers give normative values for ages from birth on in their default databases (Fig. 14.2). As regards the interpretation, value and practicability of measurement techniques, I should like to mention the "Consensus of an international panel on the clinical utility of bone mass measurements in the detection of low bone mass in the adult population" by MILLER et al., published in 1996. This consensus reflects most facets of present state-of the-art diagnostic procedures and can be applied and interpreted for general practice.

The measurement of bone mass is an indicator of the future fracture risk of the individual patient. Densitometry is the only direct and objective method for accurate assessment of bone mass and estimation of the fracture risk. It is quite unlikely that treatment will be initiated without a baseline measurement. The decision about appropriate treatment should be made on the basis not only of the radiographic findings, but also the measurement site, the patient's age and the fracture risk assessment.

In general a diagnosis can be reached by bone mass measurement, even without prevalent fractures. The basic concept is that there is a relationship between BMD and fracture risk which can be used to quantify the risk in an individual. Fracture risk increases about 1.5–2.5 times with every standard deviation decrease in T-score (difference from peak bone mass) (CUMMINGS et al. 1993; HUI et al. 1988; Ross et al. 1991, 1993). A T-score of –1 doubles the fracture risk; a T-score of –2 increases the risk four times, and a T-score of –3 increases the risk eight times.

The World Health Organisation (WHO) defined the presence of osteoporosis for Caucasian women who have not suffered a fracture (KANIS 1994). These women are regarded as osteoporotic if they have a T-score more than 2.5 SD below the peak bone mass. A total of 95% of individuals who will have a fracture are below this threshold. On the other hand, it is also important to identify individuals who have not yet experienced such a severe decrease in bone mass, but whose risk of fracture is nevertheless elevated. For this group of individuals the WHO uses the term osteopenic. Their measured values correspond with T-scores between –1.0 and –2.5. These values may not, in all cases, warrant instant intervention; however, these individuals should at least be monitored thereafter.

The diagnosis according to the WHO criteria should be made by a measurement of the lumbar spine and/or at the hip, because the two sites are

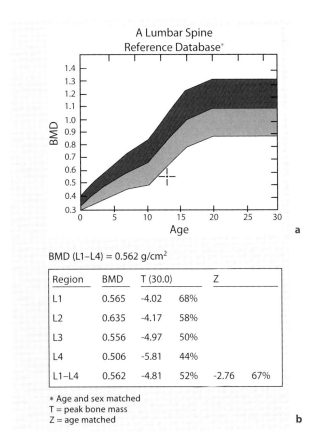

BMD (L1–L4) = 0.562 g/cm²

Region	BMD	T (30.0)		Z	
L1	0.565	-4.02	68%		
L2	0.635	-4.17	58%		
L3	0.556	-4.97	50%		
L4	0.506	-5.81	44%		
L1–L4	0.562	-4.81	52%	-2.76	67%

* Age and sex matched
T = peak bone mass
Z = age matched

Fig. 14.2. a Normative data for the BMD at the lumbar spine (L1–L4; PA) in girls. Age is represented on the x-axis, BMD on the y-axis. **b** The BMD (in g/cm²) of the individual measurement together with T and Z scores. A datapoint for the patient's individual measurement is given as in adults

where most osteoporotic fractures occur. As mentioned above, the T-score levels are recommended for women only. However, until conclusive data are available for men, these levels are most commonly applied for them as well (GRAMPP et al. 1999b, 2001; KRESTAN et al. 2001).

The assessment of bone mass is a major factor in patient management. There are a number of clinical standard situations where knowledge of bone mass and fracture risk determine the clinical management. These are:

- In women over the age of 50 who have an additional risk factor for osteoporosis
- In women over the age of 65 (even without having an additional risk factor for osteoporosis)
- In patients with diseases that carry a high bone loss rate
- In long-term treatment with drugs that cause a high bone loss rate (e.g. corticosteroids)

- In cases of oestrogen deficiency
- In cases where low bone density is suspected on conventional radiographs
- In cases of primary hyperparathyroidism
- After the occurrence of a vertebral, femoral or radial fracture or any other fracture without appropriate trauma

Follow-up exams are necessary for the assessment of these conditions and the effect of therapeutic interventions.

The measurement site and method should be selected according to the patient's individual case. Bone density measurements are frequently performed to quantify bone loss seen on conventional radiographs. In such cases the suspected part of the skeleton should be measured if possible. Most fractures occur at the lumbar spine or the proximal femur, and therefore these sites are recommended as basic examination locations (MELTON et al. 1992). Since fractures of the femur do carry the most serious consequences in terms of mortality and morbidity, this particular site is regarded as clinically the most important (ALFFRAM 1964; CEDER et al. 1981; THOMAS and STEVEN 1974; WALLACE 1983). In elderly patients (< 65 years) measurements of the lumbar spine by DXA are frequently falsified by degenerative changes to a significant amount (ITO et al. 1993; RAND et al. 1997; YU et al. 1995). The correct diagnosis can be obtained by performing the measurement with QCT of the spine or by using the DXA measurement at the proximal femur.

The basic purpose of all measurements is to obtain knowledge about the fracture risk of an individual. For an assessment of global skeletal fracture risk, all techniques and sites (distal radius, calcaneus, spine, proximal femur) have comparable statistical significance (HUI et al. 1988; Ross et al. 1991; SEELEY et al. 1990). The specific risk at a specific site, however, is best estimated by measuring at that site. If measurements at the spine or femur reveal an increased fracture risk, a diagnosis has already been established and further measurements may not be necessary.

14.3
Choice of Technique

In clinical practice, the choice of any technique depends on its limitations and advantages.

In numerous studies the highest diagnostic sensitivity was found for QCT of the lumbar spine, regarded by many researchers as the diagnostic gold standard (GRAMPP et al. 1996, 1997a, 2001a; GUGLIELMI et al. 1994; PACIFICI et al. 1990; REINBOLD et al. 1986; VAN BERKUM et al. 1989; YU et al. 1995). Measurements at peripheral sites generally show the highest sensitivity for fracture risk estimation at those specific sites (CUMMINGS et al. 1993; GLÜER et al. 1996).

The choice of technique must be based on the information desired and the anatomic and pathological conditions of the case. Relevant criteria are the radiological appearance and the patient's history (previous fracture, Sudeck's dystrophy, degenerative changes).

The decision about the measurement site and method is the focus of the radiological effort. Currently, DXA is clinically the most relevant method because it is associated with short measurement times, reasonable costs, and low radiation exposure. After an initial spinal radiograph, DXA of the lumbar spine (in all patients up to the age of 65 with no significant degenerative changes of the spine) and/or the hip (in patients over the age of 65 or in whom significant degenerative changes at the spine are present) should be performed. For special applications, or if a CT scanner is available (which in many institutions it is not), QCT of the lumbar spine may be performed as the primary examination (GRAMPP et al. 2001a).

In addition to the basic quantitative measurements at the spine and hip, there are a number of methods for quantification of the skeletal status of peripheral bones (GENANT et al. 1996). These may currently be regarded as additional techniques. The single measurement of a peripheral bone such as phalanx, calcaneus or radius should not be used to make the basis for a decision about the treatment of an individual.

In recent years numerous publications have dealt with the subject of finding the most accurate, cheap, reliable and convenient method for the diagnosis of osteoporosis and estimation of fracture risk (GENANT et al. 1996; GRAMPP et al. 1997a, 1999b). Quantitative ultrasound measurements – usually at the calcaneus – have been at the center of the scientific discussion. This method may not be useful as the sole measurement for assessment of the skeletal status of an individual (GRAMPP et al. 1999b; KRESTAN et al. 2001), but recent publications indicate that quantitative ultrasound of the calcaneus can quite successfully be used as a screening or pre-screening method and will be used in clinical practice (GRAMPP et al. 2001b). Patients identified with this method should then be measured or imaged using one of the "basic techniques" described next.

Basic techniques for the diagnosis of osteoporosis include:

- QCT of the lumbar spine (GRAMPP et al. 1997a; GUGLIELMI et al. 1997)
- DXA of the lumbar spine and proximal femur (GUGLIELMI et al. 1994; JERGAS et al. 1995a)
- Conventional radiographs (GRAMPP et al. 1997b)

Supplementary methods which may be used for special applications or follow-up (i.e. not for primary diagnosis, but which provide additional information about the skeletal status) include:

- Peripheral CT of the radius and other sites (GRAMPP et al. 1995; GUGLIELMI et al. 1997)
- DXA of the radius and whole body (HERD et al. 1993; MAZESS et al. 1988; STEIGER et al. 1992)
- Quantitative ultrasound of the calcaneus, phalanges and other sites (GRAMPP et al. 1996, 2001b; GUGLIELMI et al. 1999; KRESTAN et al. 2001; RESCH et al. 1990)
- Magnetic resonance imaging of trabecular structure (LINK et al. 1999)
- Vertebral DXA morphometry (SMYTH et al. 1999)

In all instances appropriate follow-up intervals should be chosen. All modalities for bone mass assessment, used in clinical routine (DXA, QCT) have precision errors of approximately 1%–3% (GENANT et al. 1996). Depending on site and technique, average annual bone loss in healthy postmenopausal women is between 0.2% and 1.2% (GRAMPP et al. 1997a). These annual changes are quite small in comparison to the precision errors (GLÜER et al. 1994). For this reason, a difference between measurements of more than 2.8 times the precision error is regarded as real (VERHEJ et al. 1992). Therefore, the interval between follow-up measurements should be relatively long so that only real differences are diagnosed. Follow-up measurements should be performed at intervals of more than 2 years. An exception to this is the start of glucocorticoid therapy or organ transplantation, where changes of up to 15% per year have been observed. In such cases a follow-up measurement may be performed after 6 months.

The follow-up measurement is certainly an important tool for the physician in the management of the patient, because knowledge of the bone mass changes may influence patient compliance. From this point of view, more frequent measurements may be desired in some cases.

The ideal time for a baseline measurement is during or at the end of the menopause. For the initial assessment, examination of the lumbar spine and proximal femur seem advisable. If possible, additional sites such as the distal radius or calcaneus may be measured to complete the picture, since significant discrepancies occur between values measured at different sites (GRAMPP et al. 1996, 1997a). For follow-up measurements after an established diagnosis, measuring at just one site is sufficient in most cases.

The densitometric result report should be accompanied by a clinical interpretation. Quantitative data should always be accompanied by a specific diagnosis with description of the skeletal status, to ensure rapid flow of complex information between the radiologist and the referring physician (GRAMPP et al. 2001a).

The following information should be included:

- Measurement technique used (QCT, pQCT, DXA, QUS)
- Region investigated (lumbar spine, proximal femur)
- Direction of beam (PA, lateral, axial)
- Condition of measurement site (degenerative change, history of fracture)
- Absolute value, (with unit of measurement e.g. 1.049 g/cm^2)
- T-score (standard deviation)
- Z-score (standard deviation)
- Diagnosis with skeletal status (osteoporosis/osteopenia – WHO criteria) and comparison to age-matched data (Z-score)

14.4
Conclusion

There are a number of different possibilities for designing a diagnostic work-up of patients, depending on the target population and on the equipment available. On the basis of our experience, and in view of the scientific literature, at least one of the methods, referred to above as basic techniques, should be included in the diagnostic protocol. "Supplementary techniques" can be added depending on the individual case or the patient group and on what particular information about a skeletal site or bone compartment is desired.

We recognize that the T-score may be of limited value as a diagnostic criterion because in some instances (e.g. QCT of the spine, where the slope of the age-dependent normal values in the reference populations is especially steep) it may overestimate the pathological condition of an individual or diagnose all people of a certain comparatively young age as osteoporotic. Here, the supplementary use of the Z-score (e.g. for patients aged above 60 or 65 years) adds valuable information about the individual patient.

Diagnostic scores which take account of more influencing factors than age and BMD, such as "lifetime fracture risk" or others are currently the focus of intense ongoing scientific discussion. However, since there is no accepted consensus about their use and clinical value, I currently recommend continuing to use the T-score as the lowest common denominator accepted by the majority of international scientists.

References

Adams JE (1997) Single and dual X-ray absorptiometry. Eur Radiol 7:20–31

Alffram P (1964) An epidemiological study of cervical and trochanteric fractures of the femur in an urban population. Acta Orthop Scand [Suppl] 65:1–114

Ashman RB, Rho JY (1988) Elastic modulus of trabecular bone material. J Biomech 21:177–181

Boyce WJ, Vessey MP (1985) Rising incidence of fracture of the proximal femur. Lancet 175:150–151

Ceder L, Elmquist D, Svensson SE (1981) Cardiovascular and neurologic function in elderly patients sustaining a fracture of the neck or the femur. J Bone Joint Surg (Br) 63B:560–566

Choi K, Kuhn JL, Ciarelli MJ, Goldstein SA (1990) The elastic moduli of human subchondral, trabecular, and cortical bone tissue and the size-dependency of cortical bone modulus. J Biomech 23:1103–1113

Cummings SR, Black DM, Nevitt MC, Browner W, Cauley J, Ensrud K et al (1993) Bone density at various sites for prediction of hip fractures: the study of osteoporotic fractures. Lancet 341:72–75

Cummings SR, Nevitt MC, Browner WS, Stone K, Fox K, Ensrud K, et al (1995) Risk factors for hip fractures in white women. N Engl J Med 332:767–773

Frost HM (1964) Dynamics of bone remodelling. In: Frost H (ed) Bone biodynamics. Little Brown, Boston, pp 315–334

Genant HK, Engelke K, Fuerst T, Glüer CC, Grampp S, Harris ST et al (1996) Noninvasive assessment of bone mineral and structure: state of the art. J Bone Miner Res 11:707–730

Glüer CC (1997) Quantitative ultrasound techniques for the assessment of osteoporosis: expert agreement on current status. The international quantitative ultrasound consensus group. J Bone Miner Res 12:1280–1288

Glüer CC, Blunt B, Engelke K, Jergas M, Grampp S, Genant HK (1994) "Characteristic follow-up time" – a new concept for standardized characterization of a technique's ability to monitor longitudinal changes. Bone Miner 25 [Suppl 2]:S40

Glüer CC, Cummings SR, Bauer DC, Stone K, Pressman A, Mathur A et al (1996) Osteoporosis: association of recent fractures with quantitative US findings. Radiology 199:725–732

Gordon CM (2000) Bone density issues in the adolescent gynecology patient. J Pediatr Adolesc Gynecol 13:157–161

Grampp S, Lang P, Jergas M, Glüer CC, Mathur A, Engelke K, Genant HK (1995) Assessment of the skeletal status by peripheral quantitative computed tomography of the forearm: short-term precision in-vivo and comparison to dual X-ray absorptiometry. J Bone Miner Res 10:1566–1576

Grampp S, Jergas M, Lang P, Steiner E. Fuerst T, Glüer CC, Genant HK (1996) Quantitative CT assessment of the lumbar spine and radius in patients with osteoporosis. Am J Roentgenol l67:133–140

Grampp S, Genant HK, Mathur A, Lang P, Jergas M, Takada M et al (1997a) Comparisons of non-invasive bone mineral measurements in assessing age-related loss, fracture discrimination, and diagnostic classification. J Bone Miner Res 12:697–711

Grampp S, Steiner E, Imhof H (1997b) Radiological diagnosis of osteoporosis. Eur Radiol 7:11–19

Grampp S, Dobnig H, Willvonseder R (1999a) Empfehlung zur klinischen Anwendung und Relevanz der densitometrischen Verfahren. J Mineralstoffwechsel 6:19–21

Grampp S, Henk CB, Fuerst TP, Lu Y, Bader TR, Kainberger F., Imhof H (1999b) Diagnostic agreement of quantitative ultrasound of the calcaneus with dual X-ray absorptiometry of the spine and femur. Am J Roentgenol 173:329–334

Grampp S, Dobnig H, Willvonseder R, Leb G (2001a) Leitlinien zur Anwendung densitometrischer Verfahren. J Mineralstoffwechsel 8:50–51

Grampp S, Henk CB, Lu Y, Krestan C, Resch H, Kainberger, Youseffzadeh S, Imhof H (2001b) Cut-off levels for quantitative ultrasound of the calcaneus in the distinction of healthy and osteoporotic individuals. Radiology 220:400–405

Greenfield MA, Craven JD, Wishko DS, Huddleston AL, Friedman R, Stern R (1975) The modulus of elasticity of human cortical bone: an in-vivo measurement and its clinical implications. Radiology 115:163–166

Guglielmi G, Grimston SK, Fischer KC, Pacifici R (1994) Osteoporosis: diagnosis with lateral and posteroanterior dual X-ray absorptiometry compared with quantitative CT. Radiology 192:845–850

Guglielmi G, Glüer CC, Majumdar S, Blunt BA, Genant HK (1995) Current methods and advances in bone densitometry. Eur Radiol 5:129–139

Guglielmi G, Schneider P, Lang TF, Giannatempo GM, Cammisa M, Genant HK (1997) Quantitative computed tomography at the axial and peripheral skeleton. Eur Radiol 7:32–42

Guglielmi G, Cammisa M, De Serio A, Scillitani A, Chiodini I, Carnevale V et al (1999) Phalangeal US velocity discriminates between normal and vertebrally fractured subjects. Eur Radiol 9:1632–1637

Harke HT (1999) Pediatric bone densitometry: technical issues. Semin Muskuloskel Radiol 3:371–378

Herd RJM, Blake G.M, Parker JC, Ryan PJ, Fogelman I (1993) Total body studies in normal British women using dual energy X-ray absorptiometry. Br J Radiol 66:303–308

Hui SL, Slemenda CW, Johnston CC (1988) Age and bone mass as predictors of fracture in a prospective study. J Clin Invest 81:1804–1809

Ito M, Hayashi K, Yamada M, Uetani M, Nakamura T (1993) Relationship of osteophytes to bone mineral density and spinal fracture in men. Radiology 189:497–502

Jergas M, Breitenseher M, Glüer CC, Yu W, Genant HK (1995a) Estimates of volumetric bone density from projectional measurements improve the discriminatory capability of dual X-ray absorptiometry. J Bone Miner Res 10:1101–1110

Jergas MD, Majumdar S, Keyak JH, Lee IY, Newitt DC, Grampp S et al (1995b) Relationships between Young modulus of elasticity, ash density, and MRI derived effective transverse relaxation T2* in tibial specimens. J Comput Assist Tomogr 19:472–479

Jones CD, Laval-Jeantet AM, Laval-Jeantet MH, Genant HK (1987) Importance of measurement of spongious vertebral bone mineral density in the assessment of osteoporosis. Bone 8:201–206

Kanis JA (1994) Assessment of fracture risk and its application to screening for postmenopausal osteoporosis: synopsis of a WHO report. Osteoporos Int 4:368–381

Krestan C, Grampp S, Resch-Holeczke A, Henk CB, Imhof H, Resch H (2001) Diagnostic agreement of imaging ultrasonometry of the calcaneus with dual-energy X-ray absorptiometry of the spine and femur. Am J Roentgenol 177:213–216

Lindsay R, Tohme JF (1990) Estrogen treatment of patients with established postmenopausal osteoporosis. Obstet Gynecol 76:290–295

Link TM, Majumdar S, Augat P, Lin JC, Newitt D, Lane N, Genant HK (1998) Proximal femur: assessment for osteoporosis with T2* decay characteristics at MR imaging. Radiology 209:531–536

Link TM, Majumdar S, Grampp S, Guglielmi G, van Kuijk C, Imhof H, Glüer CC, Adams J (1999) Imaging of trabecular bone structure in osteoporosis. Eur Radiol 9:1781–1788

Mazess RB, Barden H, Ettinger M, Schultz E (1988) Bone density of the radius, spine, and proximal femur in osteoporosis. J Bone Miner Res 3:13–18

Melton LJ III, Chrischilles EA, Cooper C, Lane AW, Riggs BL (1992) Perspective. How many women have osteoporosis? J Bone Miner Res 7:1005–1010

Miller PD, Bonnick SL, Rosen CJ (1996) Consensus of an international panel on the clinical utility of bone mass measurements in the detection of low bone mass in the adult population. Calcif Tissue Int 58:207–214

Pacifici R, Rupich R. Griffin M, Chines A, Susman N, Avioli LV (1990) Dual energy radiography versus quantitative computer tomography for the diagnosis of osteoporosis. J Clin Endocrinol Metab 70:705–710

Rand T, Schneider B, Grampp S, Wunderbaldinger P, Migits H, Imhof H (1997) Influence of osteophytic size on bone mineral density measured with dual X-ray absorptiometry. Acta Radiol 37:210–213

Reinbold W, Genant HK, Reiser U, Harris S, Ettinger B (1986) Bone mineral content in early-postmenopausal and postmenopausal osteoporotic women: comparison of measurement method. Radiology 160:469–478

Resch II, Pietschmann P, Bernecker P, Krexner E, Willvonseder R (1990) Broadband ultrasound attenuation: a new diagnostic method in osteoporosis. Am J Radiol 155:825–828

Resch H, Nwerkla S, Grampp S, Resch A, Zapf S, Piringer S (2000) Ultrasound and X-ray based bone densitometry in patients with anorexia nervosa. Calcif Tissue Int 66:338–341

Ross PD, Davis JW, Epstein RS, Wasnich RD (1991) Preexisting fractures and bone mass predict vertebral fracture incidence in women. Ann Intern Med 114:919–923

Ross PD, Genant HK, Davis JW, Wasnich RD (1993) Predicting vertebral fracture incidence from prevalent fractures and bone density among non-black, osteoporotic women. Osteoporos Int 3:120–126

Seeley DG, Browner WS, Cummings SR, Genant HK (1990) Which fractures are associated with low appendicular bone mass in elderly women? Ann Intern Med 115:128

Seeman E, Karlsson MK, Duan Y (2000) On exposure to anorexia nervosa, the temporal variation in axial and appendicular skeletal development predisposes to site specific deficits in bone size and density: a cross sectional study. J Bone Miner Res 15:2259–2265

Smyth PP, Taylor CJ, Adams JE (1999) Vertebral shape: automatic measurement with active shape models. Radiology 211:571–578

Steiger P, Cummings SR, Black DM, Spencer NE, Genant HK (1992) Age-related decrements in bone mineral density in women over 65. J Bone Miner Res 7:625–632

Thomas TG, Steven RS (1974) Social effects of fractures of the neck of the femur. Br Med J 3:456–458

Van Berkum FN, Birkenhäger JC, Van Veen LC, Zeelenberg J, Birkenhäger-Frenkel DH, Trouerbach WT (1989) Noninvasive axial and peripheral assessment of bone mineral content: a comparison between osteoporotic women and normal subjects. J Bone Miner Res 4:679–685

Verhej LF, Blokland JA, Papapoulos SE, Zwinderman AH, Pauwels EKJ (1992) Optimization of follow-up measurements of bone mass. J Nucl Med 33:1406–1410

Wallace W (1983) The increasing incidence of fractures of the proximal femur: an orthopedic epidemic. Lancet 2:1413–1414

Watts NB, Harris ST, Genant HK, Wasnich RD, Miller PD, Jackson RD (1990) Intermittent cyclical etidronate treatment of postmenopausal osteoporosis. N Engl J Med 323:73–79

Yu W, Glüer CC, Grampp S, Jergas M, Fuerst T, Wu CY, Genant HK (1995) Spinal bone mineral assessment in postmenopausal women: a comparison between dual X-ray absorptiometry and quantitative computed tomography. Osteoporosis Int 5:433–439

Practical Cases

CHRISTIAN KRESTAN and HERWIG IMHOF

Case 1

A 68-year-old woman with postmenopausal osteo-porosis (menopause 21 years ago).

Studies

Radiographs: lumbar spine, lateral view; pelvis, (anteroposterior view, AP). Dual-energy X-ray absorptiometry (DXA): lumbar spine, PA (L1–L4); right proximal femur.

Findings

Spine. The lateral view radiograph shows multiple osteoporotic vertebral fractures (T12–L4), spondylosis deformans, and osteochondrosis (Fig. 15.1).

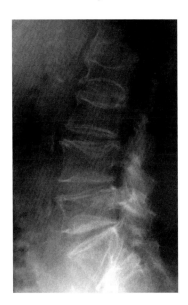

Fig. 15.1

C. Krestan, MD; H. Imhof, MD
Universitätsklinik für Radiodiagnostik, Waehringer Guertel 18–20, 1090 Vienna, Austria

Pelvis. In the AP radiograph of the pelvis (Fig. 15.2) the trabecular structure of the right proximal femur is moderately reduced and can be classified as a grade III on the Singh index (Singh et al. 1970). The left proximal femur has been replaced by a total hip prosthesis.

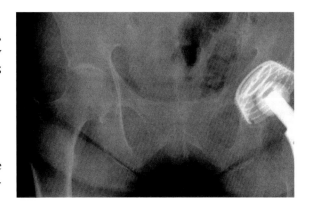

Fig. 15.2

Dual-Energy X-Ray Absorptiometry. Due to the multisegmental fractures of the lumbar spine, DXA (Fig. 15.3) gives falsely elevated numbers for bone mineral density (BMD) and therefore cannot be used. Quantitative CT (QCT) would not be appropriate as an alternate method because of the verte-

BMD (L1–L4) = 0.789 g/cm^2

Region	BMD	T (30.0)		Z	
L1	0.731	-1.76	79%	+0.02	100%
L2	0.784	-2.22	76%	-0.23	97%
L3	0.853	-2.10	79%	-0.01	100%
L4	0.779	-3.06	70%	-0.91	89%
L1–L4	0.789	-2.34	75%	-0.33	96%

T = peak bone mass
Z = age matched

Fig. 15.3

bral fractures. The DXA measurement of the right proximal femur (Fig. 15.4) cannot give meaningful numbers either, as the automatic software is unable to calculate the whole region of interest or identify the outline of the bone because of the severely reduced bone density.

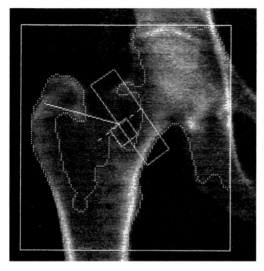

Fig. 15.4

Diagnosis

Manifest osteoporosis with multisegmental fractures of the lumbar spine which do not allow objective assessment of the bone mineral content or density by DXA or QCT.

Severe osteoporosis of the right proximal femur makes BMD measurement by DXA impossible. For this reason, quantification with standard methods is not possible in this case.

Case 2

A 56-year-old woman with a history of combined heart and lung transplant 3 months ago. Previous treatment with corticosteroids for several years.

Studies

Radiographs: lumbar spine, lateral view; pelvis AP. DXA: lumbar spine, PA (L1–L4); left proximal femur.

Findings

Spine. There are wedge-shaped vertebral bodies of the lower thoracic spine (T11–12). The trabecular structures of all vertebral bodies are markedly reduced and the cortical bone is thinned. Both findings are compatible with osteoporosis (SAVILLE 1967; GRAMPP et al. 1997) (Fig. 15.5).

Pelvis. There are moderate degenerative changes in both hip joints with joint space narrowing and moderate subcortical sclerosis. The trabecular structures in the proximal femur are reduced, equivalent to Singh index grade III (Fig. 15.6).

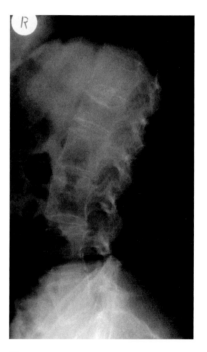

Fig. 15.5

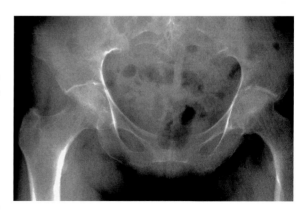

Fig. 15.6

Dual-Energy X-Ray Absorptiometry. The mean BMD of the lumbar spine is 0.508 g/cm², equivalent to a T score of –4.9 and a Z score of –3.73 (Fig. 15.7)

The mean BMD at the left femoral neck region is 0.543 g/cm² equivalent to a T score of –3.52 and a Z score of –2.13. (Fig. 15.8)

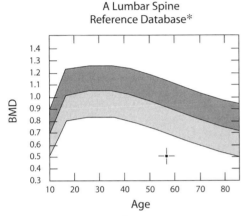

A Lumbar Spine
Reference Database*

BMD (L1–L4) = 0.508 g/cm²

Region	BMD	T (30.0)		Z	
L1	0.486	-4.00	52%	-2.97	60%
L2	0.528	-4.54	51%	-3.40	59%
L3	0.510	-5.22	47%	-4.02	54%
L4	0.505	-5.55	45%	-4.32	52%
L1–L4	0.508	-4.90	49%	-3.73	55%

* Age and sex matched
T = peak bone mass
Z = age matched

Fig. 15.7

BMD (Neck[L]) = 0.543 g/cm²

Region	BMD	T		Z	
Neck	0.543	-3.52 (22.0)	61%	-2.13	72%
Troch	0.481	-2.68 (30.0)	67%	-1.85	74%
Inter	0.786	-2.58 (29.0)	68%	-1.78	76%
TOTAL	0.632	-2.86 (28.0)	65%	-1.99	73%
Ward's	0.538	-2.34 (20.0)	68%	-0.21	96%

T = peak bone mass
Z = age matched

Fig. 15.8

Diagnosis

The conventional radiographs show manifest osteoporosis of the lower thoracic spine with vertebral deformities and radiological evidence of osteoporosis of the lumbar spine.

According to the WHO definition, the BMD of the lumbar spine and left femoral neck is in the osteoporotic range; with respect to age, both values are below the normal range.

Case 3

A 61-year-old woman with suspected osteoporosis.

Studies

Radiographs: lumbar spine, lateral and AP views; pelvis, AP view. DXA: lumbar spine, PA (L1–L4); left proximal femur

Findings

Spine. In the L3/L4 segment the AP view demonstrates a lateral vertebral gliding of approximately 1 cm (Fig. 15.9). The intervertebral space

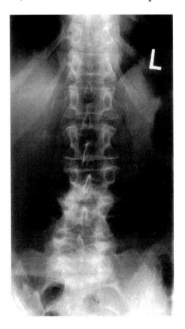

Fig. 15.9

L3–S1 is moderately narrowed. There are also some spondylotic reactions of the lumbar spine. L3/L4 shows marked subchondral sclerosis with sclerosis of L3, equivalent to hemispheric hyperostosis (Fig. 15.10).

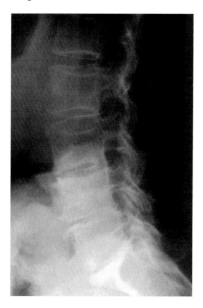

Fig. 15.10

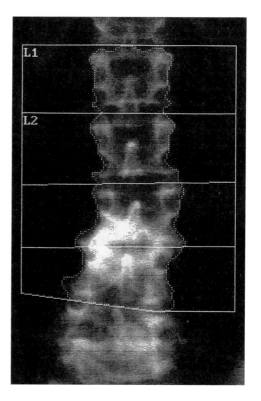

Pelvis. The AP view of the pelvis is normal (Fig. 15.11).

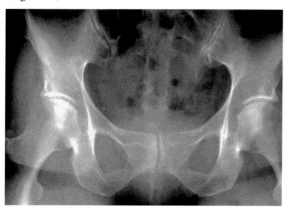

Fig. 15.11

Dual-Energy X-Ray Absorptiometry. Due to the lateral shift of L3/L4 and the sclerosis, both vertebrae have to be excluded from DXA. In L1/L2 the mean BMD is 0.669 g/cm², which reflects a T score of –2.82 and a Z score of –1.40 (Fig. 15.12). The BMD at the femoral neck is 0.647 g/cm² equivalent to a T score of –2.47 and a Z score of –0.76 (Fig. 15.13).

A Lumbar Spine
Reference Database*

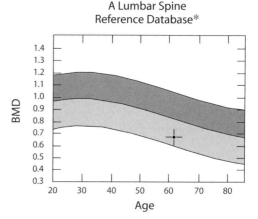

BMD (L1L2) = 0.669 g/cm²

Region	BMD	T (30.0)		Z	
L1	0.625	-2.73	68%	-1.39	80%
L2	0.710	-2.89	69%	-1.41	82%
N/A					
N/A					
L1L2	0.669	-2.82	68%	-1.40	81%

* Age and sex matched
T = peak bone mass
Z = age matched

Fig. 15.12

BMD (Neck[L]) = 0.647 g/cm^2

Region	BMD	T		Z	
Neck	0.647	-2.47 (22.0)	72%	-0.76	90%
Troch	0.632	-1.00 (30.0)	88%	+0.11	102%
Inter	0.903	-1.75 (29.0)	79%	-0.67	91%
TOTAL	0.770	-1.71 (28.0)	79%	-0.57	92%
Ward's	0.583	-1.93 (20.0)	73%	+0.58	112%

T = peak bone mass
Z = age matched

Fig. 15.13

Diagnosis

DXA of the lumbar spine shows osteoporotic values. L3 and L4 have to be excluded due to lateral vertebral shift and hemispheric hyperostosis of L3. According to the WHO definition, the BMD of the left femoral neck allows the diagnosis of osteopenia. With regard to age-adjusted values, both results are within the normal range.

Case 4

A 42-year-old man with a history of double lung transplant 12 months ago and high-dose steroid therapy. Lymphography 1 year ago.

Studies

Radiographs: lumbar and lower thoracic spine, AP and lateral views; pelvis, AP view. DXA: lumbar spine, PA (L1–L4); left proximal femur.

Findings

Spine. The lateral view shows a reduced lordosis of the lumbar spine; the vertebrae are of regular shape and height, but the trabecular structure appears markedly reduced (Fig. 15.14). There is residual contrast agent on the left side after lymphography (Fig. 15.15).

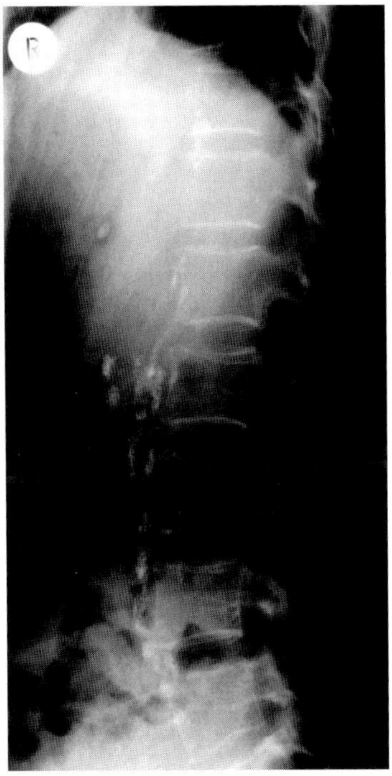

Fig. 15.14

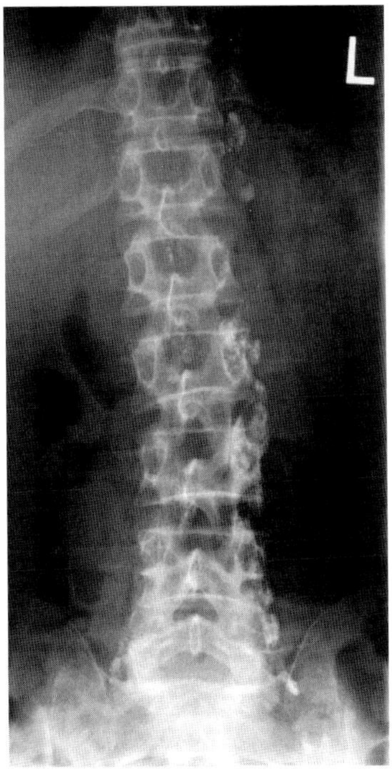

Fig. 15.15

Pelvis. The pelvic radiograph shows residual contrast agent overlying the right proximal femur (Fig. 15.16).

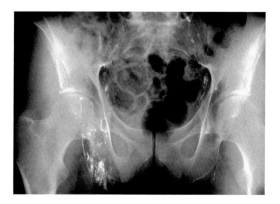

Fig. 15.16

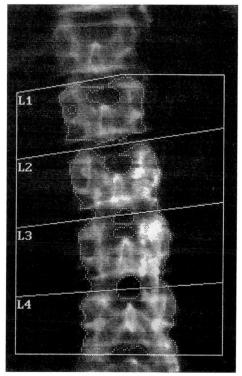

04.May.1998 09:23 [114 × 148]
Hologic QDR-4500A (S/N 45313)
Lumbar Spine V8.17a:3

BMD (L1–L4) = 0.894 g/cm^2

Region	BMD	T (30.0)		Z	
L1	0.689	-2.90	68%	-2.81	69%
L2	0.895	-1.81	82%	-1.72	83%
L3	1.007	-0.87	91%	-0.78	92%
L4	0.930	-1.95	81%	-1.86	82%
L1–L4	0.894	-1.79	82%	-1.64	83%

T = peak bone mass
Z = age matched

Fig. 15.17

Dual-Energy X-Ray Absorptiometry. The DXA of the lumbar spine (PA) cannot be used due to the residual contrast. The BMD value is 0.894 g/cm^2, equivalent to a T score of –1.79 and a Z score of –1.64 (Fig. 15.17).

The DXA of the left proximal femur gives a BMD of 0.044 g/m^2, corresponding to a T score of –4.9 and a Z score of –4.04 (Fig. 15.18).

k = 1.149 d0 = 52.8 (1.000H) 3.174

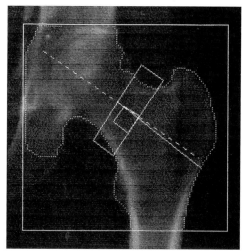

04.May.1998 09:27 [112 × 110]
Hologic QDR-4500A (S/N 45313)
Left Hip V8.17a:3

BMD (Neck[L]) = 0.440 g/cm^2

Region	BMD	T		Z	
Neck	0.440	-4.90	45%	-4.04	50%
Troch	0.424	-3.39	53%	-3.02	56%
Inter	0.733	-3.40	59%	-2.94	62%
TOTAL	0.568	-3.88	53%	-3.39	56%
Ward's	0.275	-4.64	33%	-3.47	40%

T = peak bone mass
Z = age matched

Fig. 15.18

Diagnosis

In the left femoral neck the value is in the osteoporotic range; in relation to the age-adjusted range it is well below normal.

The DXA value for the lumbar spine is not usable because of the residual overlying contrast agent.

Case 5

A 52-year-old man with a history of celiac disease.

Studies

Radiographs: lumbar spine, lateral view; pelvis, AP view. DXA: lumbar spine, PA (L1–L4); left proximal femur.

Findings

Spine. The conventional radiograph shows a wedge-shaped thoracic vertebral body (T12) with a 30% reduction in anterior height (Fig. 15.19). The trabecular structures are markedly reduced and column-like.The cortical borders are thinned.

Pelvis. The pelvic view shows normal cortical borders with moderate to severe reduction of the trabecular structures (Singh III–IV) (Fig. 15.20).

Dual-Energy X-Ray Absorptiometry. Lumbar spine (L1–L4) (Fig. 15.21): the BMD is 0.697 g/cm², equivalent to a T score of –3.59 and a Z score of –3.18. The region of interest at the femur (neck) has a BMD of 0.717 g/cm², equivalent to a T score of –2.38 and a Z score of –1.14. (Fig. 15.22).

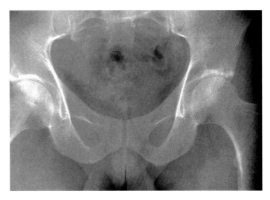

Fig. 15.20

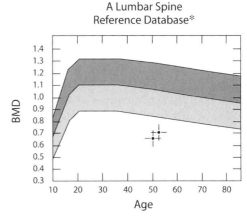

BMD (L1–L4) = 0.697 g/cm²

Region	BMD	T (30.0)		Z	
L1	0.611	-3.60	61%	-3.23	63%
L2	0.742	-3.20	68%	-2.80	71%
L3	0.727	-3.41	66%	-3.00	69%
L4	0.693	-4.11	61%	-3.69	63%
L1–L4	0.697	-3.59	64%	-3.18	67%

* Age and sex matched
T = peak bone mass
Z = age matched

Fig. 15.21

BMD (Neck[L]) = 0.717 g/cm²

Region	BMD	T (20.0)		Z	
Neck	0.717	-2.38	73%	-1.14	85%
Troch	0.590	-1.88	74%	-1.35	80%
Inter	0.865	-2.52	70%	-1.86	76%
TOTAL	0.758	-2.41	71%	-1.71	77%
Ward's	0.373	-3.82	45%	-2.13	59%

T = peak bone mass
Z = age matched

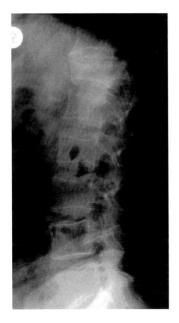

Fig. 15.19

Fig. 15.22

Diagnosis

Manifest osteoporosis, with values of the lumbar spine in the osteoporotic range (WHO) and also below normal age-adjusted values. The values in the femoral neck represent osteopenia and are slightly reduced in relation to age-adjusted values.

Case 6

A 49-year-old woman with suspected postmenopausal osteoporosis.

Studies

Radiographs: lumbar spine, lateral view; pelvis, AP. DXA: lumbar spine, PA (L1–L4); left proximal femur (neck).

Findings

Spine. No radiographic evidence of vertebral fractures or deformities, but the trabecular structures are markedly reduced (Fig. 15.23). There is little

osteophytic reaction at the sacrolumbar junction, with reduction of the intervertebral disk space L5–S1 and moderately increased subcortical sclerosis.

Pelvis. The cortical borders of the pelvis are regular, but the trabecular structures at the proximal femur are bilaterally reduced (Singh III) (Fig. 15.24).

Dual-Energy X-Ray Absorptiometry. Lumbar spine (Fig. 15.25): the BMD is 0.696 g/cm^2, equivalent to a T score of –3.19 and a Z score of –2.48.

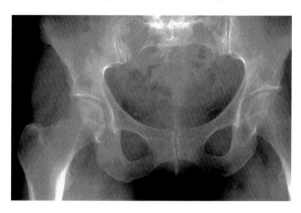

Fig. 15.24

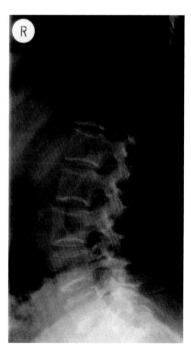

Fig. 15.23

A Lumbar Spine
Reference Database*

BMD (L1–L4) = 0.696 g/cm^2

Region	BMD	T (30.0)		Z	
L1	0.596	-2.99	64%	-2.37	70%
L2	0.643	-3.50	63%	-2.81	68%
L3	0.741	-3.12	68%	-2.39	74%
L4	0.759	-3.25	68%	-2.49	73%
L1–L4	0.696	-3.19	67%	-2.48	72%

* Age and sex matched
T = peak bone mass
Z = age matched

Fig. 15.25

At the femoral neck (Fig. 15.26) BMD is 0.569 g/cm^2, equivalent to a T score of –3.26 and a Z score of –2.3.

BMD (Neck[L]) = 0.569 g/cm^2

Region	BMD	T		Z	
Neck	0.569	-3.26 (22.0)	64%	-2.30	71%
Troch	0.582	-1.56 (30.0)	81%	-1.06	86%
Inter	0.989	-1.13 (29.0)	86%	-0.66	91%
TOTAL	0.788	-1.56 (28.0)	81%	-1.03	86%
Ward's	0.489	-2.79 (20.0)	61%	-1.17	79%

T = peak bone mass
Z = age matched

Fig. 15.26

Diagnosis

The radiographic appearance of the lumbar spine and femoral neck is compatible with osteopenia/osteoporosis.

According to the WHO definition, the DXA values at both sites are in the osteoporotic range and below the age-adjusted normal values.

Case 7

A 50-year-old man with osteoporosis.

Studies

Radiographs: lumbar spine, lateral view; pelvis, AP view. DXA: lumbar spine, PA (L1–L4); left proximal femur.

Findings

Spine. There is a loss of the lumbar lordosis and a 35% reduction of the height of the vertebral body of L1. The cortical bone is thinned, and the trabecular structures are columnar-like, representing grade 2 in Saville's classification (SAVILLE 1967) (Fig. 15.27).

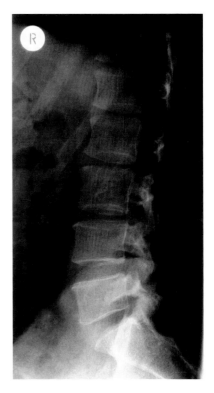

Fig. 15.27

Pelvis. There is no evidence of degenerative changes of the hip joint. The trabecular structures are moderately to severely reduced (Singh III–IV) (Fig. 15.28).

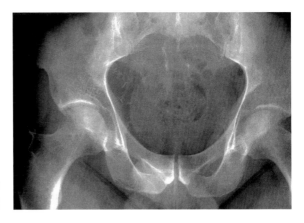

Fig. 15.28

Dual-Energy X-Ray Absorptiometry. The BMD at the lumbar spine is 0.775 g/cm^2, equivalent to a T score of –2.47 and a Z score of –1.38 (Fig. 15.29). The DXA of the femoral neck gives a BMD of 0.723 g/cm^2, equivalent to a T score of –1.72 and a Z score of –0.73 (Fig. 15.30).

A Lumbar Spine Reference Database*

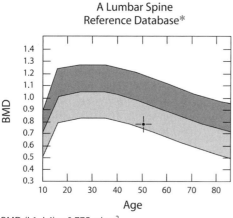

BMD (L1–L4) = 0.775 g/cm²

Region	BMD	T (30.0)		Z	
L1	0.742	-1.67	80%	-1.02	87%
L2	0.787	-2.19	77%	-1.47	83%
L3	0.847	-2.15	78%	-1.38	85%
L4	0.726	-3.54	65%	-2.75	71%
L1–L4	0.775	-2.47	74%	-1.73	80%

* Age and sex matched
T = peak bone mass
Z = age matched

Fig. 15.29

A Lumbar Spine Reference Database*

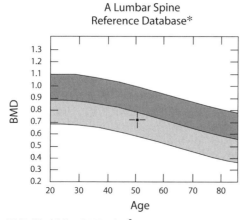

BMD (Neck[L]) = 0.723 g/cm²

Region	BMD	T		Z	
Neck	0.723	-1.72 (22.0)	81%	-0.73	91%
Troch	0.697	-0.28 (30.0)	97%	+0.25	103%
Inter	1.103	-0.32 (29.0)	96%	+0.18	102%
TOTAL	0.907	-0.57 (28.0)	93%	-0.02	100%
Ward's	0.618	-1.62 (20.0)	78%	+0.04	101%

* Age and sex matched
T = peak bone mass
Z = age matched

Fig. 15.30

Diagnosis

According to the WHO criteria, the BMD at the lumbar spine is on the border between osteopenia and osteoporosis. The BMD at the femoral neck is in the osteopenic range. BMD and conventional radiographs together allow the diagnosis of manifest osteoporosis.

Case 8

A 46-year-old woman with known Wilson's disease and suspected osteoporosis.

Studies

Radiographs: thoracic spine, lumbar spine (PA, lateral views); pelvis, AP view. DXA: lumbar spine, PA (L1–L4); left proximal femur.

Findings

Spine. The height and shape of the thoracic and lumbar vertebrae are normal, but there is reduced density of the trabecular structures (Fig. 15.31). The cortical borders are thinned with marked alteration at L1 and L4.

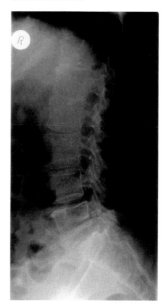

Fig. 15.31

Pelvis. There is a normal axis at both hip joints. The cortical borders of the pelvis and proximal femur are within normal limits, but the trabecular structures in both femurs are markedly reduced (Singh II) (Fig. 15.32).

Dual-Energy X-Ray Absorptiometry. The mean BMD at the lumbar spine is 0.739 g/cm², equivalent to a T score of –2.8 and a Z score of –2.29 (Fig. 15.33). In the left femoral neck the BMD is 0.678 g/cm², equivalent to a T score of –2.17 and a Z score of –1.41 (Fig. 15.34).

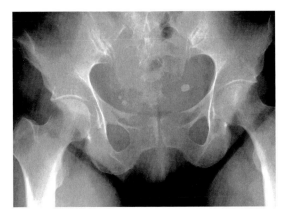

Fig. 15.32

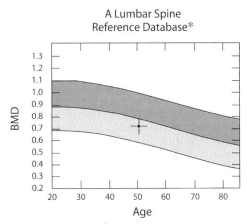

BMD (Neck[L]) = 0.678 g/cm²

Region	BMD	T		Z	
Neck	0.678	-2.17 (22.0)	76%	-1.41	83%
Troch	0.567	-1.72 (30.0)	79%	-1.37	82%
Inter	0.937	-1.50 (29.0)	82%	-1.16	85%
TOTAL	0.779	-1.63 (28.0)	80%	-1.24	84%
Ward's	0.494	-2.74 (20.0)	62%	-1.37	77%

* Age and sex matched
T = peak bone mass
Z = age matched

Fig. 15.34

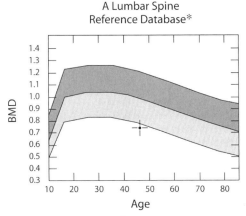

BMD (L1–L4) = 0.739 g/cm²

Region	BMD	T (30.0)		Z	
L1	0.567	-3.25	61%	-2.81	65%
L2	0.726	-2.75	71%	-2.25	75%
L3	0.764	-2.91	70%	-2.39	74%
L4	0.842	-2.49	75%	-1.95	80%
L1–L4	0.739	-2.80	71%	-2.29	75%

* Age and sex matched
T = peak bone mass
Z = age matched

Fig. 15.33

Diagnosis

The region of interest in the lumbar spine is in the osteoporotic range according to the WHO criteria; the BMD at the left femoral neck is in the osteopenic range. The value for the lumbar spine is below the age-adjusted normal range; for the femoral neck it is in the low normal region.

Case 9

A 25-year-old woman with a history of systemic lupus erythematosus.

Studies

Radiographs: lumbar spine, lateral view; pelvis, AP. DXA: lumbar spine, PA (L1–L4); left proximal femur.

Findings

Spine, Pelvis. Normal radiographic appearance of the lumbar spine and pelvis, with regular bone borders and regular bone architecture (Figs. 15.35, 15.36).

Dual-Energy X-Ray Absorptiometry. The DXA of the lumbar spine gives a BMD of 1.040 g/cm^2 (Fig. 15.37), equivalent to a T score of –0.06 and a Z score of 0. The BMD of the femoral neck (Fig. 15.38) is 0.923 g/cm^2, equivalent to a T score of 0.28 and a Z score of 0.29.

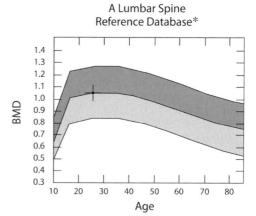

A Lumbar Spine
Reference Database*

BMD (L1–L4) = 1.040 g/cm^2

Region	BMD	T (30.0)		Z	
L1	0.966	+0.38	104%	+0.43	105%
L2	1.057	+0.26	103%	+0.32	104%
L3	1.082	-0.02	100%	+0.04	100%
L4	1.044	-0.65	94%	-0.59	94%
L1–L4	1.040	-0.06	99%	+0.00	100%

* Age and sex matched
T = peak bone mass
Z = age matched

Fig. 15.37

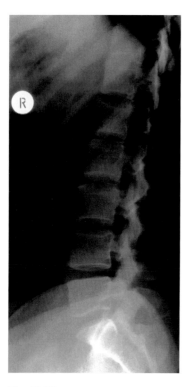

Fig. 15.35

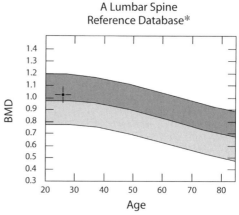

A Lumbar Spine
Reference Database*

BMD (Neck[L]) = 0.923 g/cm^2

Region	BMD	T		Z	
Neck	0.923	+0.28 (22.0)	103%	+0.29	103%
Troch	0.875	+1.71 (30.0)	121%	+1.75	122%
Inter	1.249	+0.73 (29.0)	109%	+0.74	109%
TOTAL	1.098	+1.03 (28.0)	113%	+1.03	113%
Ward's	1.024	+2.07 (20.0)	129%	+2.23	132%

* Age and sex matched
T = peak bone mass
Z = age matched

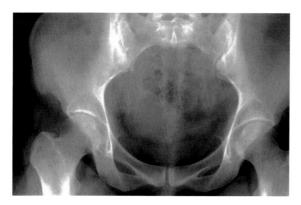

Fig. 15.36

Fig. 15.38

Diagnosis

Normal findings of the lumbar spine and femoral neck with normal bone densitometry values.

Case 10

A 13-year-old girl, height 147 cm, weight 48 kg, with a history of embryonal rhabdomyosarcoma. She underwent surgery 8 months ago, then postoperative radiochemotherapy.

Studies

DXA: lumbar spine, PA (L1–L4) (Fig. 15.39).

k = 1.143 d0 = 45.6 (1.000H) 6.626

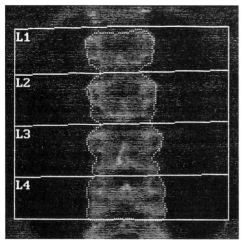

09.Aug.1999 08:04 [116 × 103]
Hologic QDR-4500A (S/N 45313)
Lumbar Spine V8.17a:3

Fig. 15.39

Findings

Dual-Energy X-Ray Absorptiometry. The mean BMD of the lumbar spine is 0.613 g/cm², equivalent to a T score of –3.95 and a Z score of –2.575 (Fig. 15.40).

Diagnosis

For the DXA of the lumbar spine in non-adults, a database exists covering the years from birth to adult

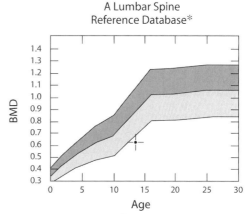

A Lumbar Spine
Reference Database*

BMD (L1–L4) = 0.613 g/cm²

Region	BMD	T (30.0)		Z	
L1	0.508	-3.79	55%		
L2	0.566	-4.20	55%		
L3	0.606	-4.35	56%		
L4	0.745	-3.37	67%		
L1–L4	0.613	-3.95	59%	-2.55	70%

* Age and sex matched
T = peak bone mass
Z = age matched

Fig. 15.40

age. In these cases only Z score assessment makes sense, as peak bone mass has not been reached yet.

The Z score is –2.55, which is below the normal age-adjusted bone mass.

Case 11

A 63-year-old woman with a history of dermatomyositis and suspected osteoporosis.

Studies

Radiographs: lumbar spine, lateral view; pelvis, AP view. DXA: lumbar spine, PA (L1–L4); left proximal femur.

Findings

Lumbar Spine. Residual barium in the small and large bowel is visible due to barium enema 10 days previously (Fig. 15.41). The lateral view of the lumbar spine shows a normal bone structure and a grade 1 anterolisthesis L5–S1 with spondylolysis.

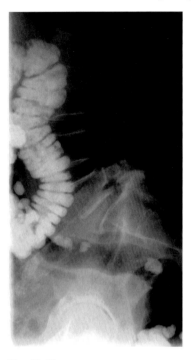

Fig. 15.41

Pelvis. The pelvic view radiograph shows overlying barium in the rectum (Fig. 15.42). The trabecular structure at the femoral neck is reduced (Singh grade IV). There is evidence of slight arthrosis of both hip joints as well as arthrosis of the sacroiliac joints with increased subcortical sclerosis.

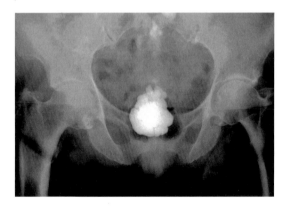

Fig. 15.42

Dual-Energy X-Ray Absorptiometry. The DXA of the lumbar spine cannot be used due to the overlying residual barium (Fig. 15.43).

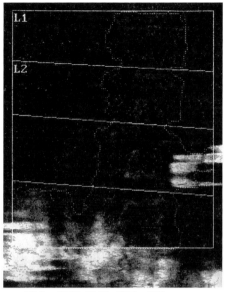

18.Aug.1999 09:46 [116 × 133]
Hologic QDR-4500A (S/N 45313)
Low Density Spine V8.17a:3

Fig. 15.43

k = 1.147 d0 = 48.2(1.000H) 5.743

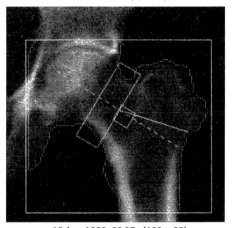

18.Aug.1999 09:37 [108 × 98]
Hologic QDR-4500A (S/N 45313)
Left Hip V8.17a:3

BMD (Neck[L]) = 0.793 g/cm^2

Region	BMD	T		Z	
Neck	0.793	-1.02 (22.0)	89%	+0.81	111%
Troch	0.704	-0.20 (30.0)	98%	+1.01	115%
Inter	1.145	-0.02 (29.0)	100%	+1.16	117%
TOTAL	0.952	-0.19 (28.0)	98%	+1.05	115%
Ward's	0.569	-2.06 (20.0)	71%	+0.58	113%

T = peak bone mass
Z = age matched

Fig. 15.44

There is no contrast agent overlying the proximal femur. The BMD of the left proximal femur (neck) is 0.793 g/cm², corresponding to a T score of –1.02 and a Z score of 0.81 (Fig. 15.44).

Diagnosis

The region of interest in the femoral neck gives a BMD which is on the border between normal and osteopenic values and normal age-adjusted values.

The DXA of the lumbar spine is unusable, as there is considerable residual contrast in the bowel overlying the bony structures.

Case 12

An 81-year-old woman with back pain and suspected osteoporosis.

Studies

Radiographs: lumbar spine: lateral view. DXA: lumbar spine, PA (L1–L4).

Findings

Spine. In the conventional radiograph of the lumbar spine the vertebral body of L1 shows a marked sclerotic internal structure with marked reduction of the vertebral height in the medial aspect (Figs. 15.45, 15.46) (DXA, PA).

There is also a considerable reduction of the intervertebral space, with spondylotic reactions in segments T12/L1 and L1/L2.

The spinous process of the lumbar spine shows significantly increased subchondral sclerosis (Baastrup's disease).

Dual-Energy X-Ray Absorptiometry. The DXA of vertebral body L1 shows a T score of +1.2 and a Z score of +3.61, equivalent to a pathologic BMD due to underlying Paget's disease (Fig. 15.47). The other vertebral bodies have a BMD between 0.843 g/cm² and 0.950 g/cm², equivalent to a T score between –1.15 and –2.48 and a Z score between 0.42 and 1.6.

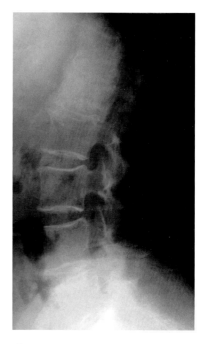

Fig. 15.45

k = 1.142 d0 = 43.7(1.000H) 7.727

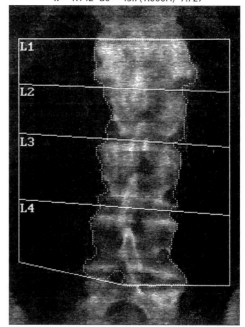

01.Apr.1999 10:04 [116 × 131]
Hologic QDR-4500A (S/N 45313)
Lumbar Spine V8.17a:3

Fig. 15.46

BMD (L1–L4) = 0.933 g/cm^2

Region	BMD	T (30.0)		Z	
L1	1.058	+1.21	114%	+3.61	160%
L2	0.902	-1.15	88%	+1.53	123%
L3	0.950	-1.22	88%	+1.60	123%
L4	0.843	-2.48	76%	+0.42	106%
L1–L4	0.933	-1.03	89%	+1.69	125%

T = peak bone mass
Z = age matched

Fig. 15.47

Diagnosis

Paget's disease of vertebral body L1. The other vertebral bodies have a T score between –1.15 and –2.48, which is in the osteopenic range by the WHO definition but above normal age-adjusted values (L1 must be excluded).

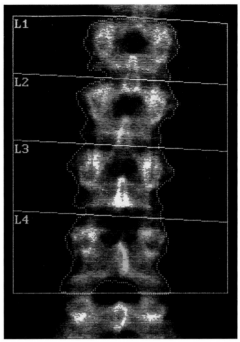

20.Aug.1999 09:42   [116 × 146]
Hologic QDR-4500A (S/N 45313)
Lumbar Spine V8.17a:3

Case 13

A 28-year-old man with a 4-year history of rheumatoid arthritis and low-dose steroid therapy.

Studies

DXA: lumbar spine, PA (L1–L4) (Fig. 15.48); left proximal femur (Fig. 15.49); right (Fig. 15.50) and left radii (Fig. 15.51).

Findings

DXA lumbar spine. The mean BMD is 1.251 g /cm^2, equivalent to a T score of 1.64 and a Z score of 1.46.

DXA Left Proximal Radius. The mean BMD in the femoral neck is 1.093 g/cm^2, equivalent to a T score of 1.04 and a Z score of 1.36.

DXA Left Radius. The BMD of the ultradistal region is 0.493 g/cm^2, equivalent to a T score of –0.29 and a Z score of –0.2.

A Lumbar Spine
Reference Database*

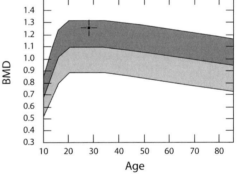

BMD (L1–L4) = 1.251 g/cm^2

Region	BMD	T (30.0)		Z	
L1	1.255	+2.25	125%	+2.25	125%
L2	1.318	+2.04	120%	+2.04	120%
L3	1.233	+1.18	112%	+1.18	112%
L4	1.210	+0.59	106%	+0.59	106%
L1–L4	1.251	+1.46	115%	+1.46	115%

∗ Age and sex matched
T = peak bone mass
Z = age matched

Fig. 15.48

BMD (Neck[L]) = 1.093 g/cm^2

Region	BMD	T (20.0)		Z	
Neck	1.093	+1.04	112%	+1.36	116%
Troch	0.900	+0.94	113%	+1.07	115%
Inter	1.282	+0.26	103%	+0.43	105%
TOTAL	1.167	+0.73	109%	+0.92	111%
Ward's	1.008	+1.46	121%	+1.90	129%

T = peak bone mass
Z = age matched

Fig. 15.49

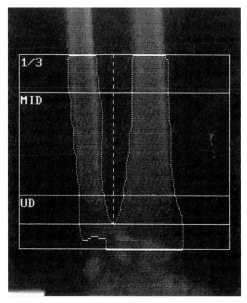

20.Aug.1999 09:59 [228 × 103]
Hologic QDR-4500A (S/N 45313)
Right Forearm V8.19a:3

BMD (Radius+Ulna[R] 1/3) = 0.799 g/cm^2

Region	BMD	T (20.0)		Z	
1/3	0.799	-0.48	97%	-0.42	97%
Mid	0.666	-0.52	96%	-0.48	96%
Ud	0.493	-0.29	97%	-0.20	98%
TOTAL	0.657	-0.41	97%	-0.35	97%

T = peak bone mass
Z = age matched

Fig. 15.50

BMD (Radius+Ulna[R] 1/3) = 0.807 g/cm^2

Region	BMD	T (20.0)		Z	
1/3	0.807	-0.34	98%	-0.28	98%
Mid	0.658	-0.68	95%	-0.64	95%
Ud	0.507	-0.04	100%	+0.05	101%
TOTAL	0.658	-0.40	97%	-0.34	97%

T = peak bone mass
Z = age matched

Fig. 15.51

DXA Right Radius. The BMD of the ultradistal region is 0.507 g/cm^2, equivalent to a T score of –0.04 and a Z score of 0.05.

Diagnosis

The BMD in all regions of interest is in the middle or slightly above the age-adjusted mean. According to the WHO definition, measurements at all sites represent normal values.

Case 14

A 41-year-old woman with a history of hysterectomy and ovariectomy.

Studies

Radiographs: lumbar spine, lateral view; pelvis, AP view. DXA: lumbar spine, PA (L1–L4); left proximal femur.

Findings

Spine. The radiograph of the lumbar spine shows normal height and shape of the vertebrae but severe loss of the trabecular structures with massive thinning of the cortical bone (Fig. 15.52).

Pelvis. The pelvis radiograph shows regular findings at the hip joints with moderate bone loss at the femoral neck (Singh III) (Fig. 15.53).

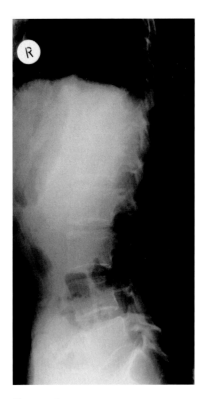

Fig. 15.52

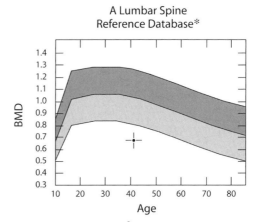

A Lumbar Spine
Reference Database*

BMD (L1–L4) = 0.664 g/cm²

Region	BMD	T (30.0)		Z	
L1	0.598	-2.97	65%	-2.73	67%
L2	0.686	-3.11	67%	-2.85	69%
L3	0.649	-3.95	60%	-3.67	62%
L4	0.708	-3.71	63%	-3.43	65%
L1–L4	0.664	-3.48	63%	-3.21	65%

* Age and sex matched
T = peak bone mass
Z = age matched

Fig. 15.54

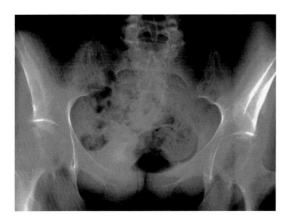

Fig. 15.53

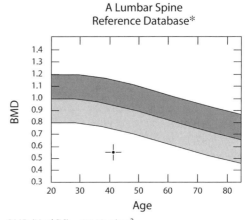

A Lumbar Spine
Reference Database*

BMD (Neck[L]) = 0.440 g/cm²

Region	BMD	T		Z	
Neck	0.440	-4.55 (22.0)	49%	-4.03	52%
Troch	0.381	-3.79 (30.0)	53%	-3.61	54%
Inter	0.609	-3.85 (29.0)	53%	-3.67	54%
TOTAL	0.500	-3.96 (28.0)	51%	-3.74	53%
Ward's	0.290	-4.60 (20.0)	36%	-3.57	43%

* Age and sex matched
T = peak bone mass
Z = age matched

Dual-Energy X-Ray Absorptiometry. The DXA of the lumbar spine gives a BMD of 0.664 g/cm², equivalent to a T score of –4.55 and a Z score of –3.21.(Fig. 15.54).

The DXA of the femoral neck gives a BMD of 0.440 g/cm², equivalent to a T score of –4.55 and a Z score of –4.03 (Fig. 15.55).

Fig. 15.55

Diagnosis

The radiographs support the diagnosis of osteopenia/osteoporosis with loss of bone architecture but without insufficiency fractures. Both sites (lumbar spine and femoral neck) have BMD values which are osteoporotic according to the WHO definition; the values are well below normal age-adjusted BMD values.

Case 15

A 58-year-old woman with postmenopausal osteoporosis and multiple vertebral fractures.

Studies

Radiographs: lumbar spine, lateral view; pelvis, AP view. DXA: lumbar spine, PA (L1–L4); DXA, left proximal femur.

Findings

Spine. The radiograph of the lumbar spine shows multiple vertebral fractures (T12, L1, L2, L4) (Fig. 15.56). There are moderate spondylotic reactions in the lumbar spine. The trabecular structures are severely reduced with thinning of the cortical bone. The spinous processes of the lumbar spine shows increased subcortical sclerosis (Baastrup's disease).

There is also moderate degenerative calcification of the aorta.

Pelvis. There is moderate reduction of the trabecular structures in both femoral necks (Singh grade III) (Fig. 15.57). The sacroiliac joints have degenerative changes such as subcortical sclerosis and spondylophytes.

Dual-Energy X-Ray Absorptiometry. Lumbar spine: due to the multiple fractures, calcification of the aorta, and the spondylotic reactions, the values will be falsely elevated and should not be used as a basis for BMD assessment (Fig. 15.58). Left proximal femur: the BMD at the femoral neck is 0.556 g/cm^2,

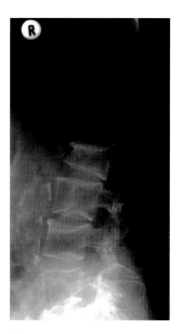

Fig. 15.56

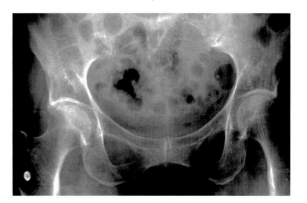

Fig. 15.57

equivalent to a T score of –3.38 and a Z score of –1.84 (Fig. 15.59).

Diagnosis

The bone architecture and the multiple vertebral fractures lead to the diagnosis of manifest osteoporosis. The DXA of the lumbar spine cannot be used because of the above-mentioned overlying calcifications of various regions. The BMD of the left femoral neck is in the osteoporotic range according to the WHO definition; the age-adjusted values are in the low normal range.

A Lumbar Spine
Reference Database*

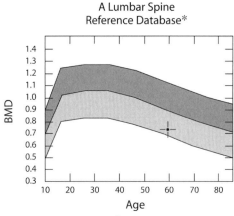

BMD (L1–L4) = 0.734 g/cm²

Region	BMD	T (30.0)		Z	
L1	0.652	-2.48	70%	-1.31	82%
L2	0.796	-2.11	77%	-0.81	90%
L3	0.701	-3.48	65%	-2.11	75%
L4	0.782	-3.04	70%	-1.62	81%
L1–L4	0.734	-2.85	70%	-1.52	81%

* Age and sex matched
T = peak bone mass
Z = age matched

Fig. 15.58

A Lumbar Spine
Reference Database*

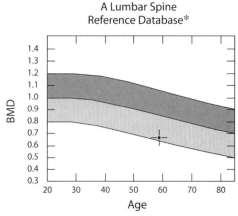

BMD (Neck[L]) = 0.556 g/cm²

Region	BMD	T		Z	
Neck	0.556	-3.38 (22.0)	62%	-1.84	75%
Troch	0.447	-3.06 (30.0)	62%	-2.10	70%
Inter	0.699	-3.20 (29.0)	61%	-2.28	69%
TOTAL	0.594	-3.17 (28.0)	61%	-2.18	69%
Ward's	0.302	-4.49 (20.0)	38%	-2.18	56%

* Age and sex matched
T = peak bone mass
Z = age matched

Fig. 15.59

Case 16

A 56-year-old man with a ligamentous lesion in the shoulder joint and radiographic signs of osteoporosis.

Studies

Radiographs: lumbar spine, lateral view; pelvis, AP view. DXA: lumbar spine, PA (L1–L4); left proximal femur (femoral neck).

Findings

Spine. There is a reduction of the trabecular structures of the lumbar spine, with a column-like architecture as well as a slight spondylosis (Fig. 15.60).

Pelvis. The pelvic view radiograph reveals normal cortical bone and a reduced trabecular structure at the femoral neck (Singh grade III–IV) (Fig. 15.61).

Dual-Energy X-Ray Absorptiometry. Lumbar spine: the BMD is 0.695 g/cm², equivalent to a T score of –3.6 and a Z score of –3.0. (Fig. 15.62).

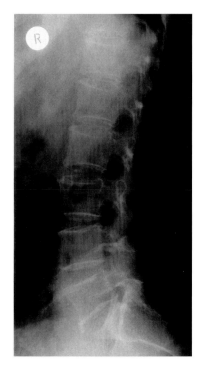

Fig. 15.60

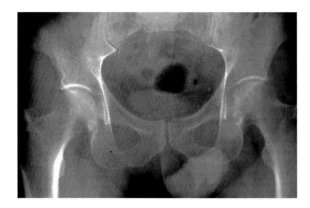

Fig. 15.61

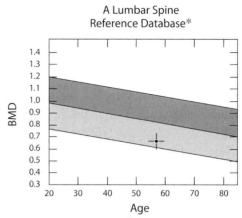

BMD (Neck[L]) = 0.653 g/cm²

Region	BMD	T (20.0)		Z	
Neck	0.653	-2.97	67%	-1.54	79%
Troch	0.544	-2.30	68%	-1.70	74%
Inter	0.923	-2.13	74%	-1.38	82%
TOTAL	0.775	-2.28	72%	-1.48	80%
Ward's	0.433	-3.33	52%	-1.39	72%

* Age and sex matched
T = peak bone mass
Z = age matched

Fig. 15.63

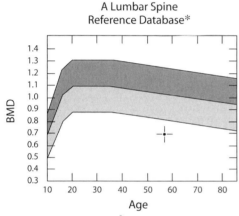

BMD (L1–L4) = 0.695 g/cm²

Region	BMD	T (30.0)		Z	
L1	0.704	-2.77	70%	-2.28	74%
L2	0.671	-3.85	61%	-3.31	65%
L3	0.732	-3.38	66%	-2.84	70%
L4	0.675	-4.28	59%	-3.72	62%
L1–L4	0.695	-3.60	64%	-3.07	67%

* Age and sex matched
T = peak bone mass
Z = age matched

Fig. 15.62

The BMD at the femoral neck is 0.653 g/cm², equivalent to a T score of –2.97 and a Z score of –1.54 (Fig. 15.63).

Diagnosis

Measurements at both sites show a BMD in the osteoporotic range according to the WHO criteria. The age-adjusted values are below the normal range for the lumbar spine and in the low normal range for the femoral neck.

Case 17

A 55-year-old man with suspected osteoporosis.

Studies

Radiographs: lumbar spine, lateral view; pelvis, AP view. DXA: lumbar spine, PA (L1–L4); left proximal femur.

Findings

Spine. The trabecular bone of the lumbar vertebral bodies is slightly reduced and has a column-like appearance. In addition, a moderate spondylotic reaction of the vertebral bodies of the lumbar spine is seen (Fig. 15.64).

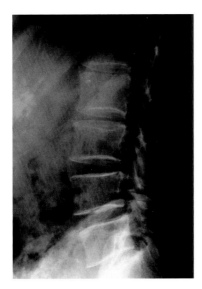

Fig. 15.64

Pelvis. The cortical border of the pelvis is normal, there is evidence of slight degenerative reactions of the right hip joint. The trabecular structure of the proximal femur is moderately reduced (Singh grade III) (Fig. 15.65).

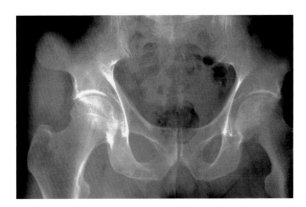

Fig. 15.65

Dual-Energy X-Ray Absorptiometry. Lumbar spine: the BMD is 0.871 g/cm², equivalent to a T score of –2.0 and a Z score of –1.51 (Fig. 15.66).

Left femoral neck: the BMD is 0.762 g/cm², equivalent to a T score of –1.97 and a Z score of –0.6 (Fig. 15.67).

Diagnosis

The conventional radiograph of the lumbar spine and pelvis are compatible with the presence of osteo-

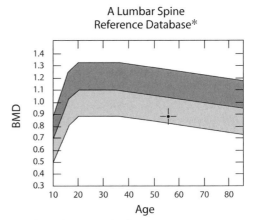

A Lumbar Spine
Reference Database*

BMD (L1–L4) = 0.871 g/cm²

Region	BMD	T (30.0)		Z	
L1	0.797	-1.92	79%	-1.46	83%
L2	0.875	-1.99	80%	-1.48	84%
L3	0.929	-1.58	84%	-1.08	89%
L4	0.868	-2.52	76%	-2.00	80%
L1–L4	0.871	-2.00	80%	-1.51	84%

* Age and sex matched
T = peak bone mass
Z = age matched

Fig. 15.66

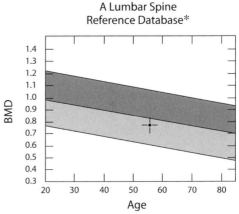

A Lumbar Spine
Reference Database*

BMD (Neck[L]) = 0.762 g/cm²

Region	BMD	T (20.0)		Z	
Neck	0.762	-1.97	78%	-0.60	92%
Troch	0.624	-1.57	78%	-0.99	85%
Inter	0.914	-2.19	74%	-1.46	81%
TOTAL	0.822	-1.92	77%	-1.14	85%
Ward's	0.441	-3.25	53%	-1.38	73%

* Age and sex matched
T = peak bone mass
Z = age matched

Fig. 15.67

porosis. The DXA measurements at both sites are consistent with the diagnosis of osteopenia; the age-adjusted values are in the normal range.

Case 18

A 39 year old male patient with a history of heart transplantation due to myocarditis, patient has been on steroids and immunosuppressants for 3 years.

Exam

Lumbar spine radiograph: AP view, DXA: lumbar spine, PA (L1–L4), DXA left proximal femur.

Findings

Spine. The ap view shows a pacemaker in a right paravertebral location at the height of L1, L2. (Fig. 15.68)

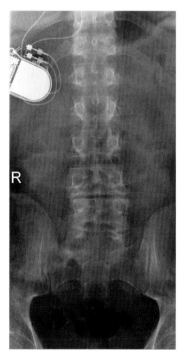

Fig. 15.68

Dual-Energy X-Ray Absorptiometry. L2 has to be excluded from the DXA analysis, as the software includes the area of the pacemaker into the L2 measurement (Fig. 15.69). Also L1 has to be excluded due to an unusual high T-score of 1.7 (Fig. 15.70). Average BMD at L3/L4 is 0.83 g/cm^2 corresponding to an T-score of –2.7 (Fig. 15.70). The DXA measurement of the left proximal femur (Fig. 15.71) gives a BMD-value of 0.67 g/cm^2 and a T-score of –1.9.

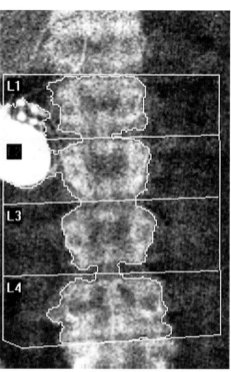

k = 1.139, d0 = 39.8

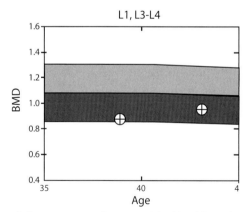

Reference curve and scores matched to white male

Fig. 15.69

Region	Area (cm²)	BMC (g)	BMD (g/cm²)	T-score	PR (Peak Reference)	Z-score	AM (Age matched)
L1	18.26	21.86	1.197	1.7	119	1.8	120
L2	19.89	39.47	1.985	8.1	181	8.2	184
L3	14.73	10.49	0.712	-3.6	65	-3.4	65
L4	18.53	17.11	0.923	-2.0	81	-1.9	82
TOTAL	71.40	88.93	1.245	1.4	114	1.6	116

Total BMD CV 1.0%, ACF = 0.998, BCF = 0.965

Region	Area (cm²)	BMC (g)	BMD (g/cm²)	T-score	PR (Peak Reference)	Z-score	AM (Age matched)
L3	14.73	10.49	0.712	-3.6	65	-3.4	65
L4	18.53	17.11	0.923	-2.0	81	-1.9	82
TOTAL	33.26	27.60	0.830	-2.7	74	-2.5	75

Total BMD CV 1.0%, ACF = 0.998, BCF = 0.965
Fracture risk: high; Classification: Osteoporosis

Fig. 15.70

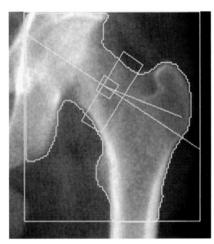

k = 1.444, d0 = 45.3

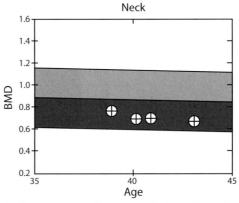

Reference curve and scores matched to white male

Region	Area (cm²)	BMC (g)	BMD (g/cm²)	T-score	PR (Peak Reference)	Z-score	AM (Age matched)
Neck	5.76	3.86	0.670	-1.9	72	-1.3	79
Troch	10.25	6.32	0.617	-1.3	79	-1.0	83
Inter	26.69	29.16	1.093	-0.6	91	-0.5	93
TOTAL	42.70	39.34	0.921	-0.7	89	-0.5	92
Ward's	1.14	0.61	0.535	-1.8	68	-0.8	82

Scan date	Age	BMD	T-score	BMD change vs baseline	BMD change vs previous
03.07.2006	43	0.670	-1.9	-12.2%	-3.9%
22.04.2004	40	0.697	-1.7	-8.6%	0.5%
30.07.2003	40	0.693	-1.7	-9.1%	-9.1%
24.04.2002	38	0.762	-1.2		

Fig. 15.71

Diagnosis

Osteopenic BMD values at the left hip and the diagnosis of osteoporosis at the lumbar spine.

Final diagnosis is osteoporosis with elevated fracture risk. The PM-generator near L1/L2 leads to falsely elevated BMD-values, thus L1 and L2 have to be excluded from analysis. The values of L3 and L4 are sufficient to establish the correct diagnosis in this case.

Case 19

A 48 year old male patient with a history of multiple vertebral fractures and vertebroplasty of L2 has been referred for assesement of bone mineral status.

Exam

DXA lumbar spine PA and lateral view (L1–L4), Lumbar spine radiograph: AP view, lateral view, DXA left proximal femur.

Findings

Dual-Energy X-Ray Absorptiometry. lumbar spine pa (L1–L4), bone cement is visible in projection of L2 (Fig. 15.72) The figures for the bone mineral densities are elevated for L2 and L2 has to be excluded. The DXA measurement of the lumbar spine gives a BMD-value of 0.832 g/cm^2 and a T-score of –2.3 (Fig. 15.73).

Lumbar spine radiographs show bone cement filling in wedge-shaped lumbar vertebral body L2 after prior vertebroplasty and fractured vertebral bodies L1–L4 (Figs. 15.74, 15.75).

The DXA measurement of the left proximal femur (Figs. 15.76, 15.77) gives a BMD-value of 0.832 g/cm^2 and a T-score of –1.0.

Diagnosis

Manifest osteoporosis at the lumbar spine, the calculated BMD L1, 3, 4 gives falsely elevated BMD-values due to vertebral fractures. Diagnosis should not be made from BMD-values at the lumbar spine. Osteopenia at the left hip.

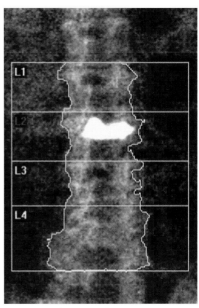

k = 1.444, d0 = 45.3

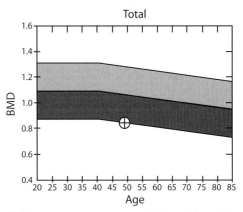

Reference curve and scores matched to white male

Fig. 15.72

Region	Area (cm²)	BMC (g)	BMD (g/cm²)	T-score	PR (Peak Reference)	Z-score	AM (Age matched)
L1	13.07	10.97	0.840	-1.5	83	-1.2	86
L3	12.70	11.07	0.871	-2.1	79	-1.8	82
L4	23.61	19.07	0.808	-3.1	71	-2.7	73
TOTAL	49.38	41.11	0.832	-2.3	76	-2.0	79

Fig. 15.73

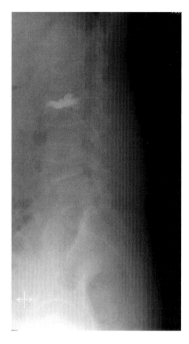

Fig. 15.74

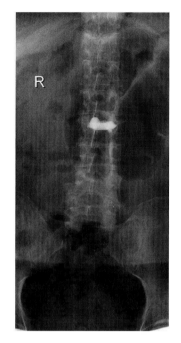

Fig. 15.75

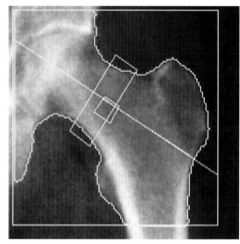

k = 1.446, d0 = 45.7

Fig. 15.76

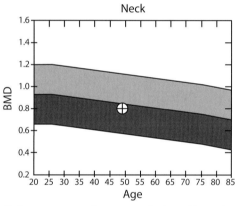

Neck

Reference curve and scores matched to white male

Region	Area (cm²)	BMC (g)	BMD (g/cm²)	T-score	PR (Peak Reference)	Z-score	AM (Age matched)
Neck	5.54	4.43	0.799	-1.0	86	-0.2	96
Troch	17.23	12.39	0.719	-0.5	93	-0.2	97
Inter	22.31	26.15	1.172	-0.1	98	0.1	101
TOTAL	45.08	42.96	0.953	-0.5	92	-0.2	97
Ward's	1.15	0.74	0.644	-1.0	82	0.2	105

Fig. 15.77

Case 20

A 78 year old male patient with a history of heart transplantation for ischemic cardiomyopathy 15 years ago, longterm treatment with steroids and immunosuppressents.

Exam

DXA lumbar spine PA (L1–L4), Lumbar spine radiograph: AP view, lateral view, DXA left proximal femur.

Findings

Lumbar spine radiographs show scoliosis of the lumbar spine and severe osteochondrosis of the segment L2/3, in addition calcification of the abdominal aorta is present (Figs. 15.78, 15.79).

DXA lumbar spine pa (L1–L4), pronounced density is visible in the segment L2/3 due to the osteochondrosis and have to be excluded for measurement of BMD (Fig. 15.80) The average figures for the bone mineral densities of L1 and L4 give a BMD of 0.949 g/cm^2 and a T-score of –1.2 (Fig. 15.81).

The DXA measurement of the left proximal femur (Figs. 15.82, 15.83) gives a BMD-value of 0.598 g/cm^2 and a T-score of –2.4.

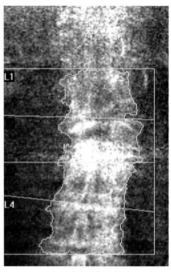

k = 1.446, d0 = 40.6

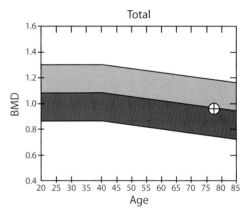

Reference curve and scores matched to white male

Fig. 15.80

Diagnosis

Osteopenic values at the lumbar spine and femoral neck. However BMD values of the lumbar spine despite exclusion of L2/3 are falsely elevated due to additional atherosclerosis of the abdominal aorta and should not be used for serial measurements.

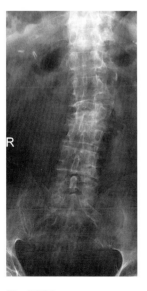

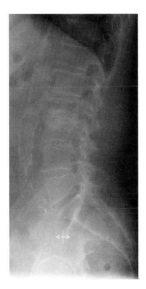

Fig. 15.78   **Fig. 15.79**

Region	Area (cm²)	BMC (g)	BMD (g/cm²)	T-score	PR (Peak Reference)	Z-score	AM (Age matched)
L1	16.77	13.48	0.804	-1.9	80	-0.8	90
L4	20.07	21.49	1.070	-0.7	93	0.5	105
TOTAL	36.85	34.97	0.949	-1.2	88	-0.1	98

Total BMD CV 1.0%, ACF = 0.998, BCF = 0.965

Fig. 15.81

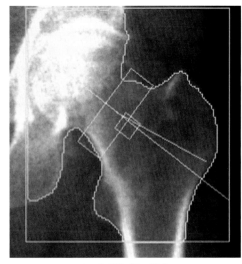

k = 1.444, d0 = 45.3

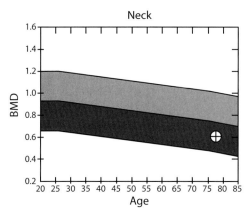

Reference curve and scores matched to white male

Fig. 15.82

Region	Area (cm²)	BMC (g)	BMD (g/cm²)	T-score	PR (Peak Reference)	Z-score	AM (Age matched)
Neck	6.25	3.74	0.598	-2.4	64	-1.0	81
Troch	14.25	6.07	0.426	-2.8	55	-2.1	61
Inter	25.46	20.32	0.798	-2.2	67	-1.3	77
TOTAL	45.96	30.13	0.656	-2.5	63	-1.6	74
Ward's	1.12	0.39	0.345	-3.1	44	-0.9	73

Total BMD CV 1.0%, ACF = 0.998, BCF = 0.965

Fig. 15.83

Case 21

A 80 year old female patient with a history of antiresorptive treatment for several years.

Exam

Lumbar spine radiograph: AP view, lateral view, DXA lumbar spine PA (L1–L4), DXA left proximal femur.

Findings

Lumbar spine radiographs show multisegmental osteochondrosis of the lumbar spine, in addition vertebral fractures (25%) of TH12 and L1 are diagnosed (Figs. 15.84, 15.85).

DXA lumbar spine pa (L1–L4), pronounced density is visible in the region of the upper endplate of L1. Serial measurement of BMD at the lumbar spine supports a 19.4% gain of BMD, however this can largely be explained by progressive degenerative changes at the lumbar spine (Fig. 15.86).

The DXA measurement of the left proximal femur (Figs. 15.88, 15.89) gives a BMD-value of 0.546 g/cm^2 and a T-score of –2.7 with a gain of 13.6% since 1999.

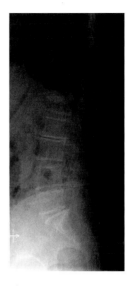

Fig. 15.85

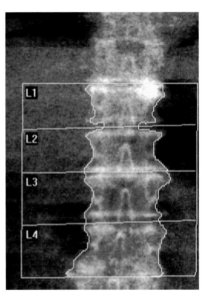

k = 1.440, d0 = 44.4

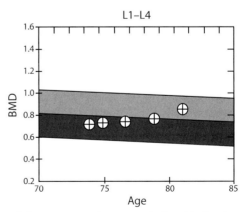

Reference curve and scores matched to white female

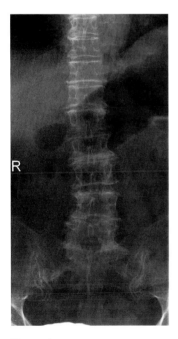

Fig. 15.84

Fig. 15.86

Results Summary

Region	Area (cm²)	BMC (g)	BMD (g/cm²)	T-score	PR (Peak Reference)	Z-score	AM (Age matched)
L1	11.53	9.86	0.856	-0.6	92	1.8	129
L2	12.14	9.74	0.802	-2.1	78	0.6	109
L3	15.01	12.18	0.811	-2.5	75	0.3	105
L4	17.99	16.42	0.913	-1.8	82	1.1	115
TOTAL	56.67	48.19	0.850	-1.8	81	0.9	114

Total BMD CV 1.0%, ACF = 0.998, BCF = 0.965

Results History

Scan date	Age	BMD	T-score	BMD change vs baseline	BMD change vs previous
04.07.2006	81	0.850	-1.8	19.4%	11.6%
15.04.2004	78	0.762	-2.6	7.0%	3.7%
18.01.2002	76	0.735	-2.8	3.2%	0.6%
12.04.2000	74	0.730	-2.9	2.5%	2.5%
09.04.1999	73	0.712	-3.0		

Fracture risk: increased; WHO Classifcation: Osteopenia

Fig. 15.87

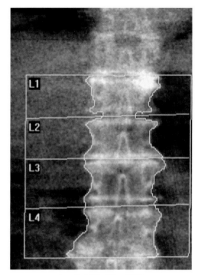

k = 1.440, d0 = 48.3

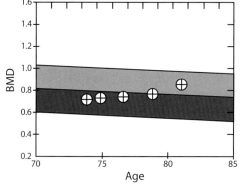

Reference curve and scores matched to white female

Fig. 15.88

Results Summary

Region	Area (cm²)	BMC (g)	BMD (g/cm²)	T-score	PR (Peak Reference)	Z-score	AM (Age matched)
Neck	5.67	3.09	0.546	-2.7	64	-0.4	93
Troch	11.27	6.27	0.556	-1.5	79	0.4	107
Inter	23.77	16.90	0.711	-2.5	65	-0.6	88
TOTAL	40.71	26.26	0.645	-2.4	68	-0.3	94
Ward's	1.12	0.37	0.332	-3.4	45	-0.4	88

Total BMD CV 1.0%, ACF = 0.998, BCF = 0.965

Results History

Scan date	Age	BMD	T-score	BMD change vs baseline	BMD change vs previous
04.07.2006	81	0.546	-2.7	13.6%	5.8%
15.04.2004	78	0.516	-3.0	7.4%	-2.5%
18.01.2002	76	0.529	-2.9	10.1%	9.1%
12.04.2000	74	0.485	-3.3	0.9%	0.9%
09.04.1999	73	0.481	-3.3		

Fig. 15.89

Diagnosis

Manifest osteoporosis with low BMD values at the lumbar spine and fractures at L1 and Th12. Serial measurements should not be performed at the lumbar spine in this patient due to progressive osteochondrosis. Diagnosis and change of BMD should be monitored at the femoral neck, as there are no degenerative changes expected. 13.6% gain of BMD is due to effective antiresorptive treatment.

References

Grampp S, Steiner E, Imhof H (1997) Radiological diagnosis of osteoporosis. Eur Radiol 7:11–19

Saville PD (1967) A quantitative approach to simple radiographic diagnosis of osteoporosis: its application to the osteoporosis of rheumatoid arthritis. Arthritis Rheum 10:416–422

Singh M, Nagrath AR, Maini PS (1970) Changes in trabecular pattern of the upper end of the femur as an index of osteoporosis. J Bone Joint Surg [Am] 52(3):457–467

Subject Index

List of Contributors

JUDITH E. ADAMS, MBBS, FRCR, FRCP
Professor, Department of Clinical Radiology
Imaging Science and Biomedical Engineering
Stopford Medical School
University of Manchester
Oxford Road
Manchester M13 9PT
UK

REINHARD BARKMANN, PhD
Medizinische Physik
Klinik für Diagnostische Radiologie
Universitätsklinikum Schleswig-Holstein
Campus Kiel
Michaelisstrasse 9
24105 Kiel
Germany

PETER M. BERNECKER, MD
Geriatric Center Baumgarten
Huetteldorferstrasse 188
1010 Vienna
Austria

DANIELE DIACINTI, MD
Department of Clinical Sciences
University "La Sapienza"
Roma
Italy

KLAUS ENGELKE, PhD
Henkestr. 91
91052 Erlangen
Germany
and
Synarc, Hamburg, Germany

HARRY K. GENANT, MD
Osteporosis and Arthritis Research Group
University of California, San Francisco
505 Parnassus Avenue
San Francisco CA 94143–0628
USA
and
Synarc, San Francisco, USA

STEPHAN GRAMPP, MD
Univ. Dozent
Dr. Grampp and Dr. Henk OEG
Röntgenordination
Lenaustrasse 23
2000 Stockerau
Austria

REINHARD GRUBER, PhD
Associate Professor, Department of Oral Surgery
Vienna University Clinic of Dentistry
Medical University of Vienna
Waehringer Strasse 25a
1090 Vienna
Austria

GIUSEPPE GUGLIELMI, MD
Professor of Radiology
University of Foggia
Viale Luigi Pinto
71100 Foggia
Italy

GEROLD HOLZER, MD
Department of Orthopedics
Medical University of Vienna
Vienna General Hospital
Waehringer Guertel 18–20
1090 Vienna
Austria

HERWIG IMHOF, MD
Universitätsklinik für Radiodiagnostik
Währinger Guertel 18–20
1090 Vienna
Austria

MICHAEL JERGAS, MD
Privat-Dozent
Department of Radiology and Nuclear Medicine
St. Elisabeth-Krankenhaus
Werthmannstrasse 1
50935 Cologne
Germany

Christian Krestan, MD
Universitätsklinik für Radiodiagnostik
Waehringer Guertel 18–20
1090 Vienna
Austria

Thomas M. Link, MD
Department of Radiology
University of California San Francisco
Department of Radiology
400 Parnassus Avenue, A 367
Box 0628
San Francisco, CA 94143
USA

Meinrad Peterlik, MD, PhD
Professor and Head of the Department of Pathophysiology
Medical University of Vienna
Waehringer Guertel 18–20
1090 Vienna
Austria

Peter Pietschmann, MD
Associate Professor of Pathophysiology and
Internal Medicine
Department of Pathophysiology
Medical University of Vienna
Waehringer Guertel 18–20
1090 Vienna
Austria
and
Ludwig Boltzmann Institute of Aging Research
Langobardenstrasse 122, 1220 Vienna, Austria

Sven Prevrhal, PhD
Musculoskeletal Quantitative Imaging Research Group
University of California, San Francisco
185 Berry Street, Suite 350
San Francisco, CA 94107
USA

Heinrich Resch, MD
Professor of Medicine
University of Vienna (Rheumatology, Osteology)
Head, Department of Internal Medicine II
St. Vincent Hospital Vienna
and
Ludwig Boltzmann-Institut für Altersforschung
Stumpergasse 13
1060 Vienna
Austria

Cornelis van Kuijk, MD, PhD
Department of Radiology
UMC Radbound
Geert Grooteplein-Zuid 10
6525 HB Nijmegen
The Netherlands

Rick R. van Rijn, MD, PhD
Department of Radiology
Academiv Medical Center
University of Amsterdam
Meibergdreef 9
1105 AZ Amsterdam
The Netherlands

MEDICAL RADIOLOGY Diagnostic Imaging and Radiation Oncology

Titles in the series already published

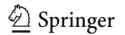

MEDICAL RADIOLOGY Diagnostic Imaging and Radiation Oncology

Titles in the series already published

RADIATION ONCOLOGY

Lung Cancer
Edited by C. W. Scarantino

Innovations in Radiation Oncology
Edited by H. R. Withers and
L. J. Peters

**Radiation Therapy
of Head and Neck Cancer**
Edited by G. E. Laramore

**Gastrointestinal Cancer –
Radiation Therapy**
Edited by R. R. Dobelbower, Jr.

**Radiation Exposure
and Occupational Risks**
Edited by E. Scherer, C. Streffer,
and K.-R. Trott

Radiation Therapy of Benign Diseases
Stanley E. Order and Sarah S. Donaldson

**Interventional Radiation
*Therapy Techniques – Brachytherapy***
Edited by R. Sauer

Radiopathology of Organs and Tissues
Edited by E. Scherer, C. Streffer,
and K.-R. Trott

**Concomitant Continuous Infusion
*Chemotherapy and Radiation***
Edited by M. Rotman
and C. J. Rosenthal

**Intraoperative Radiotherapy –
Clinical Experiences and Results**
Edited by F. A. Calvo, M. Santos,
and L. W. Brady

**Radiotherapy of Intraocular
and Orbital Tumors**
Edited by W. E. Alberti and
R. H. Sagerman

**Interstitial and Intracavitary
Thermoradiotherapy**
Edited by M. H. Seegenschmiedt
and R. Sauer

**Non-Disseminated Breast Cancer
*Controversial Issues in Management***
Edited by G. H. Fletcher and S. H. Levitt

**Current Topics in
Clinical Radiobiology of Tumors**
Edited by H.-P. Beck-Bornholdt

**Practical Approaches to
Cancer Invasion and Metastases
*A Compendium of Radiation
Oncologists' Responses to 40 Histories***
Edited by A. R. Kagan with the
Assistance of R. J. Steckel

Radiation Therapy in Pediatric Oncology
Edited by J. R. Cassady

Radiation Therapy Physics
Edited by A. R. Smith

Late Sequelae in Oncology
Edited by J. Dunst and R. Sauer

Mediastinal Tumors. Update 1995
Edited by D. E. Wood and
C. R. Thomas, Jr.

**Thermoradiotherapy
and Thermochemotherapy**
Volume 1:
Biology, Physiology, and Physics
Volume 2:
Clinical Applications
Edited by M. H. Seegenschmiedt,
P. Fessenden, and C. C. Vernon

**Carcinoma of the Prostate
*Innovations in Management***
Edited by Z. Petrovich, L. Baert,
and L. W. Brady

Radiation Oncology of Gynecological Cancers
Edited by H. W. Vahrson

**Carcinoma of the Bladder
*Innovations in Management***
Edited by Z. Petrovich, L. Baert,
and L. W. Brady

**Blood Perfusion and
Microenvironment of Human Tumors
*Implications for
Clinical Radiooncology***
Edited by M. Molls and P. Vaupel

**Radiation Therapy of Benign Diseases
A Clinical Guide
2nd Revised Edition**
S. E. Order and S. S. Donaldson

**Carcinoma of the Kidney and Testis,
and Rare Urologic Malignancies
*Innovations in Management***
Edited by Z. Petrovich, L. Baert,
and L. W. Brady

**Progress and Perspectives in the
Treatment of Lung Cancer**
Edited by P. Van Houtte,
J. Klastersky, and P. Rocmans

**Combined Modality Therapy of
Central Nervous System Tumors**
Edited by Z. Petrovich, L. W. Brady,
M. L. Apuzzo, and M. Bamberg

**Age-Related Macular Degeneration
*Current Treatment Concepts***
Edited by W. E. Alberti, G. Richard,
and R. H. Sagerman

**Radiotherapy of Intraocular and
Orbital Tumors
2nd Revised Edition**
Edited by R. H. Sagerman, and
W. E. Alberti

**Modification of Radiation Response
*Cytokines, Growth Factors,
and Other Biolgical Targets***
Edited by C. Nieder, L. Milas,
and K. K. Ang

Radiation Oncology for Cure and Palliation
R. G. Parker, N. A. Janjan,
and M. T. Selch

**Clinical Target Volumes in Conformal and
Intensity Modulated Radiation Therapy
*A Clinical Guide to Cancer Treatment***
Edited by V. Grégoire, P. Scalliet,
and K. K. Ang

**Advances in Radiation Oncology
in Lung Cancer**
Edited by B. Jeremić

New Technologies in Radiation Oncology
Edited by W. Schlegel, T. Bortfeld,
and A.-L. Grosu

**Multimodal Concepts for Integration of
Cytotoxic Drugs and Radiation Therapy**
Edited by J. M. Brown, M. P. Mehta,
and C. Nieder

**Technical Basis of Radiation Therapy
Practical Clinical Applications
4th Revised Edition**
Edited by S. H. Levitt, J. A. Purdy,
C. A. Perez, and S. Vijayakumar

**CURED I · LENT
Late Effects of Cancer Treatment
on Normal Tissues**
Edited by P. Rubin, L. S. Constine,
L. B. Marks, and P. Okunieff

**Radiotherapy for Non-Malignant Disorders
*Contemporary Concepts and Clinical Results***
Edited by M. H. Seegenschmiedt,
H.-B. Makoski, K.-R. Trott, and
L. W. Brady

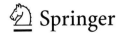 Springer